The warnings are clear: Cancer is on the rise, and much of the increase may have to do with how we eat, what vitamins we lack, and how little we exercise. But information about what to do has been scarce until now. Reports of cancer prevention and treatment miracles abound, yet many doctors are skeptical and don't know enough about natural remedies. In light of recent research on vitamin C, antioxidants, fiber, and so on, we're left wondering what to take, and how much, and what we are really supposed to eat every day. We need to know what's medically acceptable and what can cause harm.

How to Prevent and Treat Cancer with Natural Medicine answers these questions and more. Four of America's most prominent doctors of natural medicine advise you on what to eat, what combination of supplements to take, what to avoid before surgery, what helps heal the body during recovery, and what boosts the effectiveness of conventional medicine. It's all laid out in an easy-to-follow guide that gives you a daily protocol tailored to individual health needs, whether you have a family history of cancer and feel you're at risk, have a diagnosis of cancer and want to give your body the tools it needs to fight, or are in treatment and want to lessen the side effects. A unique risk assessment quiz will tell you how vigilant you need to be, and special recommendations for breast, prostate, lung, and colon cancer help you adapt the program to your specific needs. Besides creating a physical environment hostile to cancer, you can learn about the science that supports the significant roles that emotions and attitudes play in prevention and treatment.

This program was developed by doctors of natural medicine who work side by side with oncologists to give their patients the benefit of both conventional and natural medicine in fighting this deadly disease. All recommendations are backed by peer-reviewed medical studies. If you have cancer or are interested in preventing it, you cannot be without this book.

Turn the page for reviews of
How to Prevent and Treat Cancer with Natural Medicine . . .

PRAISE FOR

How to Prevent and Treat Cancer with Natural Medicine

"Packed with suggestions that cover the gamut of what makes a healthy life, from what you should eat, do and think to what you should not eat, do and think . . . the book provides sensible, easy-to-incorporate ways to reduce risk. The tools are right at hand."

—*The Denver Post*

"The authors . . . make hard-to-grasp information very accessible."

—*Natural Health*

"More than thirty-five books on alternative or complementary treatments for cancer have been published in the last ten years, not including those on specific cancers, but this title stands out. Besides being exceptionally well written and researched, it is also very reader-friendly."

—*Library Journal*

How to Prevent and Treat Cancer with Natural Medicine

Dr. Michael Murray

Dr. Tim Birdsall

Dr. Joseph E. Pizzorno

Dr. Paul Reilly

RIVERHEAD BOOKS

New York

Riverhead Books
Published by The Berkley Publishing Group
A division of Penguin Group (USA) Inc.
375 Hudson Street
New York, NY 10014

First Riverhead hardcover edition: September 2002
First Riverhead trade paperback edition: November 2003
Riverhead trade paperback ISBN: 1-57322-343-3

The Library of Congress has catalogued the Riverhead hardcover edition as follows:

How to prevent and treat cancer with natural medicine /
Michael Murray . . . [et al.].
p. cm.
Includes bibliographical references and index.
ISBN 1-57322-222-4
1. Cancer—Alternative treatment.   I. Murray, Michael T.
RC271.A62 H69   2002   2002021300
616.99'406—dc21

Printed in the United States of America

10   9   8   7   6   5   4   3   2   1

To our patients who have battled cancer
and taught us so much about life

Acknowledgments

First of all, it is important for us to acknowledge all the researchers, physicians, and scientists who over the years have sought to better understand the role of diet and natural medicines in the prevention and treatment of cancer. Without their work, this book would certainly not exist. Next, it is important to acknowledge the role that our agent, Bonnie Solow, played in linking us up with Amy Hertz and Riverhead Books. The original manuscript was prepared with the expert help of Ron Schaumburg, but the book's final form was significantly improved under Amy's leadership. We are grateful for her perseverance in making our book as reader-friendly and practical as possible.

Michael T. Murray, N.D.—Most of all, I would like to acknowledge my wife, Gina. Her love, support, and patience are the major blessings in my life, along with our two wonderful children, Alexa and Zachary.

Timothy Birdsall, N.D.—I would like to dedicate this book to my patients, those brave and wonderful individuals who have lived with the diagnosis of cancer. You have shown me how to see the beauty in each new day, to face life head-on, to celebrate every victory and to mourn each loss. In short, every day, you teach me how to live. Thank you. Also, without the understanding and loving support of my family, this book would not have been possible—thanks, guys! I also want to acknowledge the colleagues with whom I am privileged to work at Cancer Treatment Centers of America. Thank you for sharing your knowledge, enthusiasm, and vision of a different way to treat cancer.

Joseph E. Pizzorno, Jr., N.D.—In addition to dedicating this book to my patients with cancer who steadfastly searched for a better way to reestablish their health and taught me about the caring and indomitable power of the human spirit, I also dedicate this work to my dear wife, Lara, and my wonderful children, Raven and Galen. You mean the world to me.

Paul Reilly, N.D.—To those patients who have survived their cancer, for teaching me the awesome power of our bodies to heal. To those who are still fighting their cancer, for teaching me the power of determination. To those who have lost their battle with cancer, for teaching me the value of living each day with grace. To my wife Susan, who gives me a reason to be grateful every day.

Contents

Introduction

Rethinking the Way
We Look at Cancer

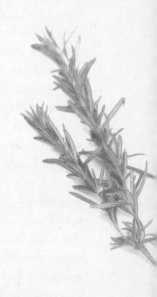

No other disease strikes as much fear deep within our souls as cancer. The reason? Most of us have witnessed firsthand the ravaging effect that cancer, as well as chemotherapy and radiation, has had on a loved one. Cancer statistics in the United States present us with some sobering facts. Each year:

1. Over 1,250,000 new cases of invasive cancers will be diagnosed.
2. An additional 1,500,000 new cases of non-invasive cancers will be diagnosed.
3. More than 500,000 people will die from cancer.
4. Cancer causes 1 in 5 of all deaths.

5. Cancer will affect 1 out of 3 people alive today.
6. Fifty percent of those diagnosed with cancer will die of the disease.
7. The economic toll of cancer will be greater than $110 billion.

Cancer is a dreaded disease for good reason. The biggest, perhaps, is that most of us have watched helplessly as this disease has robbed the body, mind, and spirit of someone close to us who at one time had so much life. Despite dedicating significant resources to the battle against cancer, conventional medicine alone has failed. Granted, there have been some tremendous advances, but for the most part we are losing the war on cancer. One of the key reasons is that conventional medicine has long ignored the greatest healer of all—nature.

How to Prevent and Treat Cancer with Natural Medicine is a valuable resource that provides not only the latest information on dietary and supplementation strategies to prevent cancer but also the critical guidance you need in preventing or treating cancer. Whether you want to prevent, treat, or deal with the side effects of conventional cancer care, we offer a comprehensive program of dietary measures and the proper use of vitamins, minerals, herbs, and other natural measures. You need this book because if you don't follow the guidelines we present, your cancer risk will be at least three times greater than if you do follow our recommendations. And if you have a family history of cancer it is even that much more important to follow the guidance we present because your cancer risk is higher. Simply stated, we provide a clear path to changing the environment within your body so that it will not support the growth of cancer. We provide a simple test to find out your relative risk for cancer, and if you have cancer we can help you provide the support you need to help you fight the disease or deal with the side effects as well as enhance the effectiveness of conventional cancer treatments like surgery, radiation, and chemotherapy.

How to Prevent and Treat Cancer with Natural Medicine provides a practical, focused program that will carefully detail how natural medicines can:

- Significantly reduce your risk for cancer
- Effectively change the internal environment to prevent cancer formation
- Improve the detoxification of harmful cancer-causing chemicals before they have the chance to do their damage

- Help keep chemotherapy or radiation therapy from causing cancer in the future
- Bolster the cancer patient's immune system
- Eliminate or dramatically reduce the common side effect of malnutrition and tissue wasting caused by chemotherapy
- Help to selectively starve the tumor cells
- Slow down cancer growth with natural compounds that are selectively toxic to tumor cells
- Lower the risk for recurrent tumors
- Significantly increase the chances for partial or complete remission—a cure

It is important to point out that the program given is not based on theory. It is based on real-life experience working with cancer patients. We have treated thousands of cancer patients successfully with the program detailed in *How to Prevent and Treat Cancer with Natural Medicine*. This experience has helped us learn firsthand what works and what does not.

If you have cancer, we want you to talk to your doctor about using the recommendations made in this book. Conventional oncologists will probably embrace the recommendations given in the book, because they will recognize that our recommendations are scientifically valid and supportive of many aspects of conventional cancer therapy. We believe that integrative therapy is the answer in the battle against cancer. To align your doctor with our program, we have provided extensive references from the medical literature.

Some Words of Caution

Although this book discusses numerous natural medicines and approaches, it is not intended as a substitute for appropriate medical care. Please keep the following in mind as you read:

- Do not self-diagnose. Proper medical care is critical to good health. If you have concerns about any subject discussed in this book, please consult a physician, preferably a naturopathic doctor (N.D.), holistic medical doctor (M.D.), or doctor of osteopathy (D.O.), chiropractor, or other natural health care specialist.

- Make your physician aware of all the nutritional supplements or herbal products you are currently taking to avoid any negative interactions with any of them.
- If you are currently taking a prescription medication, you absolutely must work with your doctor before discontinuing any drug or altering any drug regimen.
- Cancer is a multifactorial disease that requires a multifactorial solution: medical, nutritional, and lifestyle changes, as well as mental, emotional, social, and spiritual issues. Do not rely solely on a single area of focus. You can't just take pills and not change your diet, or do the diet and the pills but ignore the emotional or spiritual issues. Any truly effective approach for cancer must be truly integrated.

How to Use This Book

We have tried to make this book as reader-friendly as possible. As you will see, there is a massive amount of useful, practical information here. The book is organized into three major parts: Prevention, Treatment, and Support. We encourage you to read all three sections, but we realize that many may simply read what they feel is the most pertinent to them. In particular, individuals with cancer are likely to go straight to the sections on treatment and support. We have tried to make each section separate to itself with little need to flip back and forth from one chapter to another. Key points are reiterated concisely, and we always provide a page number for more information. We have also compiled useful information in the Appendixes and the Resources section; and physicians interested in our sources will find the chapter references quite useful. We have also included an open letter for cancer patients to take to their physicians (see Appendix F, page 343).

Our Hope

It is our sincere hope that you—or someone you care about—will use the information provided in the following pages to achieve greater health and happiness.

Live in good health with passion and joy!

Michael T. Murray, N.D.
Tim Birdsall, N.D.
Joseph E. Pizzorno, N.D.
Paul Reilly, N.D.

Part One

Preventing Cancer with

Natural Medicine

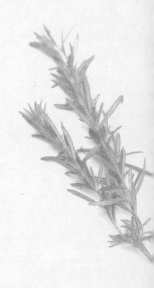

Chapter One

An Ounce of Prevention

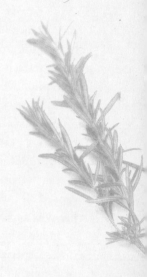

We've all heard it said: "An ounce of prevention is worth a pound of cure." When it comes to cancer, that old saying carries a ton of truth.

Can cancer really be prevented? Thankfully, in many cases, the answer is an emphatic "Yes!" This is true even if cancer runs in your family. As we'll explain in the first part of this book, by reducing or eliminating as many risk factors as possible and by practicing healthy habits that strengthen your body's defenses, you'll greatly reduce your chances of developing the disease.

Your campaign to prevent cancer requires a lifetime commitment, beginning here, now, today. Fortunately, many prevention strategies—a good diet, the right kind of exercise, a positive attitude—are not just good for you, they actually add to your quality of life. You'll not only live longer, you'll live better.

Self-Assessment of Cancer Risk

One key strategy in the prevention of cancer is to identify the presence of risk factors. The term *risk factor* refers to anything that might increase your chance of developing the disease. The higher the number of risk factors, the greater the likelihood that cancer will develop. On the other hand, reducing the number of risk factors increases the chances that prevention will succeed.

Cancer risk factors fall into two main categories: inherited and environmental. There's not a lot we can do to eliminate genetic risk factors, because they're passed on from generation to generation and are present at birth. But inherited genetic defects are responsible for only about 15 percent of all cancers. This statistic means that approximately 85 percent of all cancers result from environmental risk factors, such as diet, lifestyle, and exposure to harmful substances.

In assessing the likelihood that an individual will develop a certain disease, specialists in epidemiology (observational and statistical studies of people and diseases) use a concept known as relative risk. Relative risk (abbreviated RR) is a number that shows how much more likely it is that individuals who possess a certain trait will develop a condition compared with individuals who do not have that trait. For example, someone whose RR is 1.5 is 50 percent more likely to develop a condition than someone whose RR is 1. A relative risk of 2 means you are twice (100 percent) as likely, and so on.

Here's one dramatic statistic that should make the point. Compared with nonsmokers, cigarette smokers are said to have a relative cancer risk of 10. In other words, they are 10 times—*a thousand percent*—more likely to get lung cancer than someone who never smoked.

We have constructed for this book a self-assessment of cancer risk based on many variables. By completing this survey, you'll generate a score that indicates your relative risk of cancer. By reading the information in the Rationale column, you'll get a quick summary of the scientific data explaining why these variables are important.

A few words of caution: Relative risk is a statistic that's used to compare large numbers of people. So we cannot with any certainty predict your specific (absolute) risk as an individual. Some nonsmokers get lung cancer, while others, who are smokers, never develop the disease. If you are a nonsmoker, we have no idea if you will be the one person in ten who doesn't smoke but who still gets lung cancer. If you are a smoker, we cannot accurately predict if you will be the smoker who evades the disease.

Our solution to this difficult task of determining cancer risk was to insert as many variables as we possibly could into a single self-assessment questionnaire. For example, we know from our research that smokers who eat a diet rich in cabbage family vegetables—broccoli, cauliflower, cabbage, watercress, bok choy, kale, and so on—have a lower relative risk of developing lung cancer. So the smoker who does not eat cabbage family vegetables would still have a relative risk for developing lung cancer of 10, while the smoker who eats these foods would have a lower RR. By adding up two scores, one for factors that increase risk and another for factors that decrease risk, and then multiplying them together, you'll get a general sense of where you stand on the cancer-risk continuum compared with other people in this country.

Another caveat: This survey is for guidance only. We developed it based on our years of collective experience in the fields of nutrition and cancer management. It has not been scientifically validated in large clinical trials. Still, the information it provides may be useful as a guide to understanding your relative risk of developing cancer and may help inspire you to take certain steps to reduce that risk through natural strategies, diet, and nutritional support, as described in the following chapters.

Instructions

For each of the following, please enter a 1 if the cancer risk factor does *not* apply to you. Otherwise, enter the appropriate risk number as shown. (Note: Insert only one number for each factor 1 through 14.)

Section 1: Factors That Increase Risk

	FACTOR	RISK	SCORE	RATIONALE
1	Smoking Active (currently smoking) Ever active (formerly smoked, but have not smoked in at least 1 year) High exposure to passive smoke (especially as a child)	10.0 2.0 4.5		More than 30% of all cancer deaths are attributable to smoking. Quitting smoking dramatically reduces risk. For breast cancer, people who smoked at some time in their lives have a RR of 2.0 compared with people who never smoked or who were never exposed to high levels of passive smoke; for individuals exposed to passive smoke before age 12, the odds ratios for breast cancer is 4.5.[1]
2	Immediate family member with cancer: grandparent(s), parent(s), or sibling(s)	2.5		Family members have a 2- to 3-fold increased risk of developing the same type of cancer.
3	Electromagnetic radiation exposure (telephone installers, line workers, etc.)	2.0		Relative risk of 1.98 for pre-menopausal women in occupations with high electromagnetic field exposure in one study; 2.17 in all women who worked as telephone installers, repairers, and line workers in another study; 1.65 for system analysts/programmers; and 1.40 for telegraph and radio operators.[2]
4	Not eating fish	2.0		During 30 years of follow-up, men who ate no fish had a 2- to 3-fold higher frequency of prostate cancer than did those who ate moderate or high amounts.[3]
5	Red meat consumption 1 time per week or less >4 times per week If you usually eat meat well-done or smoked	 1.5 2.0 3.0		Researchers at the National Cancer Institute have found that those who ate their beef medium-well or well-done had more than 3 times the risk of stomach cancer than those who ate their beef rare or medium-rare. They also found that people who ate beef 4 or more times a week had more than twice the risk of stomach cancer than those consuming beef less frequently. Total meat intake of ≥1 time/week versus no meat intake

	FACTOR	RISK	SCORE	RATIONALE
				carries with it a relative risk for colon cancer of 1.90.[4] Well-done meats (burgers, beefsteak, bacon) increased risk of developing breast cancer by a factor of 4.6.[5]
6	Low consumption of fruits and vegetables (<1.5 servings/day)	1.65		Individuals who consumed less than 1.5 servings of fruits and vegetables per day had a relative risk for developing colorectal cancer of 1.65.[6]
7	Obesity/total calories	1.5		Obesity was associated with a statistically significant 50 to 60% increased risk of pancreatic cancer.[7] People who rank in the highest third of body mass index have a 1.9-fold higher risk of dying after breast cancer than those in the lowest third.[8]
8	Above-average consumption of sugar (American average is about 5 ounces/day)	1.6		High levels of sucrose intake were associated with 1.59 relative risk of colon cancer among younger men for highest fifth compared with those in lowest fifth.[9] High refined sugar consumption had a relative risk for colorectal cancer of 1.4.[10] Foods that produce sharper elevations in blood sugar levels were associated with a relative colorectal cancer risk of 1.8.[11]
9	Depression	1.4		Depression is associated with an increased cancer risk.[12]
10	Diesel emissions (heavy-equipment operators, tractor drivers	1.4		Thirty years of working on a job with diesel motor emission exposure combined showed an odds ratio of 1.43.[13]
11	Dairy (>1 serving/day)	1.4		Women who consumed the highest amount of lactose (1 or more servings of dairy per day) had a 44% greater risk for all types of invasive ovarian cancer compared with those who ate the lowest amount (≤3 servings monthly).[14] Men who consumed 2.5 servings a day of dairy products had a 50% increased risk of prostate cancer.[15]

Section 1: Factors That Increase Risk (continued)

	FACTOR	RISK	SCORE	RATIONALE
12	Refined-flour intake	1.3		Colon cancer: 1.32 for an increase of 1 serving per day of refined-flour product (e.g., white bread, pasta).[16]
13	Using omega-6 polyunsaturated oils (corn, saf-flower, sunflower, and soy oil), especially for cooking	1.4		Women who consumed the most polyunsaturated fats were 20% more likely to develop breast cancer.[17] Heating cooking oil to high tempera-tures was associated with a 1.64-fold increased risk of lung cancer.[18]
14	Alcohol Men >21 drinks/ week Women >10 drinks/week	1.2 1.2		Men who consumed 21 to 41 drinks per week or more than 41 drinks per week had relative risks of 1.23 and 1.57, respectively. Those who drank beer had a relative risk of 1.09 and 1.36, respectively. For spirits, the risk was 1.21 and 1.46, respectively.[19] Excessive alcohol poses a relative risk of 1.28 for colon cancer.[20] Consump-tion of more than 20 g/day of alcohol (approximately 10 drinks per week) led to a relative risk of breast cancer of 1.23.[21] One to 3 drinks per week, on average, did not increase the risk of breast cancer in this study.
	Total Score for Section 1:	_____		

Section 2: Factors That Decrease Risk

	FACTOR	RISK	SCORE	RATIONALE
1	Taking a multi-vitamin with folate >14 years 5–14 years	 0.25 0.8		Women who took multivitamin supplements containing folic acid for more than 15 years were 75% less likely todevelop colon cancer than women who did not use supplements. Women who took a multivitamin that contained folic acid between 5 and 14 years were about 20% less likely to develop cancer.[22]
2	Fluid consumption (>2.5 l/day)	0.5		Consuming more than 2.5 liters of fluid per day resulted in a 49% lower incidence of bladder cancer than consuming less than 1.3 l/day.[23]

	FACTOR	RISK	SCORE	RATIONALE
3	Selenium supplement (200 mcg/day)	0.50		Selenium supplementation is associated with reductions in incidence of all cancers, especially lung, colorectal, and prostate cancer, and is associated with a 50% decreased risk of mortality from cancer.[24]
4	Fish consumption ≥3 times/week	0.50		During 30 years of follow-up, men who ate no fish had a 2- to 3-fold higher frequency of prostate cancer than did those who ate moderate or high amounts.[25] Similar results have been seen in other cancers.
5	Cabbage family vegetables, including cabbages, kale, broccoli, Brussels sprouts, bok choy, and cauliflower (>5 servings/week)	0.50		Protective effect against lung, stomach, colon, and rectal cancers have been noted with cabbage family vegetables.[26, 27]
6	Legume or soy milk consumption of >5 servings/week	0.50		Soy milk (more than once a day) was associated with a 70% reduction in risk of prostate cancer,[28] while a relative risk of 0.53 was seen for all cancers with a legume intake of >2 times/week versus <1 time/week.[29]
7	Zinc supplement	0.55		Zinc supplementation reduced relative risk of prostate cancer to 0.55.[30]
8	Regular exercise of ≥5 hours/week	0.45		Risk for many cancers (e.g., colon and breast cancer) is reduced by 40 to 50% among the most active individuals, compared with the least active.[31]
9	Vegetable consumption of >4 servings/day or >28 servings/week	0.70		Colon cancer risk with frequent raw and cooked vegetable consumption was 0.85 and 0.69, respectively.[6] In a study comparing ≥28 servings of vegetables/week with <14 servings per week, the relative risk for prostate cancer was 0.65.[32]
10	Vitamin E supplement (400 IU/day)	0.70		Consumption of vitamin E showed a reduction in the rate of prostate cancer by 32%.[33] After 12 years of follow-up, bladder cancer risk was reduced by 30%.[34]

Section 2: Factors That Decrease Risk (continued)

	FACTOR	RISK	SCORE	RATIONALE
11	Green tea consumption of ≥3 cups per day or the use of green tea extract (300 mg/day)	0.70		A decreased recurrence of breast cancer was observed with consumption of ≥3 cups of green tea.[35] Green tea drinking decreased risk to 0.52 for stomach cancer.[36] Consumption of 10 cups per day decreased incidence of all cancers to 0.55.[37] However, this level produces caffeine side effects.
12	Garlic consumption of >20 g (5 cloves/week)	0.60		Garlic consumption reduces colorectal cancer risk to 0.69 and stomach cancer risk to 0.53.[38]
13	Olive oil consumption of >1 tablespoon/day	0.75		Women who consumed olive oil had a 25% lower risk of breast cancer.[17]
14	Wine consumption (1–13 glasses/week)	0.80		Drinkers of 1–13 glasses of wine per week had a relative risk of 0.78 compared with nondrinkers of wine.[39]
15	Whole grains	0.85		Colon cancer risk was reduced to 0.85 with consumption of whole grains versus refined flour products.[6]
16	Fruit, ≥2 servings/day	0.85		Citrus consumption reduced colon cancer relative risk to 0.86, other fruits to 0.85.[6]
	Total Score for Section 2:	_____		

Determining Your Cancer Risk

To determine your relative risk, add your score in Section 1 and place it on the line indicated. Remember that if a factor does not apply to you, then enter a "1" in the "Score" column. After adding all of the scores, divide that number by 14. Indicate the result here:

Total score (Section 1) = _____ divided by 14 = _____

Now repeat that process for Section 2, only this time divide the result by 16.

Total score (Section 2) = _____ divided by 16 = _____

Now take those two results and multiply them together.

Section 1 result _____ x **Section 2 result** _____ = **RR** _____

The result is an approximate guideline that indicates your risk of developing cancer. Remember, a relative risk of 2 means you are twice as likely to develop cancer as someone with a RR of 1. If your RR is 0.75, you are 25 percent *less* likely to develop cancer.

Identifying Risk Factors

Following is a description of the main cancer risk factors. When you finish the chapter, take the self-assessment survey (starting on page 4) to help you evaluate your risk of developing certain cancers. The higher the rating, the more aggressive your primary prevention strategies will need to be.

AGE | It's a fact of life: The older you are, the more likely you are to develop cancer. As we age, our cells become less proficient at repairing damage to our DNA. As a result, there are more cells present in the body that possess mutations and that are prone to develop cancer. In the year 2000, more than 60 percent of new cancer cases and more than 70 percent of all cancer-related deaths occurred in people over age 65.

GENES | Studies on identical twins (who share the exact same DNA) confirm that most cancers do not arise from genetic defects. Instead, diet and lifestyle usually play a significant role. Surprisingly, that's true even for cancers that tend to run in families. Still, researchers have identified about thirty genetic defects that increase risk for certain cancers. Some of these cancers are rare; they also tend to be types that develop more often in childhood.

FAMILY HISTORY | Some (but not most) cancers seem to run in families. For example, if a woman has two first-degree relatives (mother, aunt, or sister) who developed breast cancer, her risk for breast cancer is two to five times greater than a woman without such a family history. The same sort of relationship exists concerning prostate cancer in men. Even with a family history, in most cases lifestyle and dietary factors have been found to have a greater impact than genetics on cancer risk.

RACE | Overall, black Americans are more likely to develop cancer than persons of other racial and ethnic groups (Table 1-1). Each year,

Should You Have Genetic Testing?

Perhaps the best-known example of cancer with a genetic basis is an inherited mutation in two genes whose function is to suppress the development of breast cancer. Overall, these genes (known as BRCA1 and BRCA2; the letters stand for "breast cancer") are responsible for about 10 percent of all cases of the disease. A little more than half of women who inherit mutations in these genes will develop breast cancer by age 70. These women also have a greater risk of ovarian cancer.

If you have a strong family history of cancer, it's worthwhile to talk to your doctor about blood tests that can identify genetic mutations. It's important to understand and weigh the benefits and risks of genetic testing before these tests are done. Testing is expensive and is not covered by some health plans. There is concern that people with abnormal genetic test results will not be able to get life insurance, or coverage may be available only at a much higher cost.

We do not recommend genetic testing as a cancer screening method. This advice is especially true with respect to identifying the mutated BRCA genes, since only about 1 woman out of 850 carries these mutations. From the public health perspective, not enough women at risk would be identified to justify the enormous cost of widespread testing. In addition, even if you have the BRCA1 or BRCA2 mutation, you still have only about a 50/50 chance of developing breast cancer before age 70.

If you elect to undergo genetic testing and a mutated gene is found, you will need to be more aggressive in your prevention plan and schedule more frequent exams to monitor for early signs of cancer. (For specific recommendations for some of the more common forms of cancer, see Chapter 4.)

Table 1-1. Overall Incidence of Cancer Among Ethnic/Racial Groups[40]

GROUP	RATE (PER 100,000)
Blacks	445
Whites	402
Asian/Pacific Islanders	280
Hispanics	273
Native Americans	153

about 445 out of 100,000 blacks develop the disease. The incidence of certain types of cancers also varies by race. Compared with other groups, black men are more likely to have cancers of the prostate, colon and rectum, and lung. In fact, black men have at least a 50 percent higher rate of prostate cancer than any other group. In contrast, female breast cancer rates are highest among white women (114 per 100,000) and lowest among Native American women (33.4 per 100,000).

Some of the differences in cancer rates among racial and ethnic groups may be due to factors associated with social class rather than race or ethnicity. Such factors include education, access to health care, occupation, income, and exposure to harmful substances in the environment. Diet is also critical to look at when evaluating data on race and cancer.

MEDICAL HISTORY | Sometimes, having one disease can increase your risk for developing another. Diseases known to increase risk of certain cancers include alcoholism, chronic hepatitis, diabetes, history of genital warts, HIV infection, inflammatory bowel disease (Crohn's disease and ulcerative colitis), and peptic ulcers. The presence of any of these conditions requires a more concerted effort to reduce cancer risk. The use of certain medications such as long-term corticosteroids, immunosuppressive drugs, or chemotherapy agents can also increase the risk of cancer.

HORMONES | Certain cancers, most notably prostate and breast cancer, are affected by hormonal factors. In prostate cancer, the primary hormonal factor is testosterone, while in breast cancer the hormone of concern is estrogen. For more information, see Chapter 4, Special Steps for Preventing Lung, Breast, Prostate, and Colon Cancer.

ENVIRONMENT | Exposure to tobacco smoke is a leading cause of cancer, especially lung cancer. A long and growing list of other environmental factors linked to certain cancers includes pesticides, herbicides, heavy metals, asbestos, solvents, and possibly exposure to power lines. The risk depends on the concentration, intensity, and duration of exposure. Substantial increases in risk have been demonstrated in occupational settings where workers have been exposed to high concentrations of certain chemicals, metals, and other substances. In Chapter 2, we'll discuss natural ways to support the body's detoxification system to help it remove harmful, cancer-causing chemicals.

CERTAIN MEDICAL TREATMENTS | Sometimes medical treatment increases the risk of certain cancers. For example, radiation therapy and many chemotherapy drugs carry with them an increased risk for producing new cancers later on. Estrogen and oral contraceptives have been linked to an increased risk of breast cancer. The term *iatrogenic* refers to the diseases that arise inadvertently as a result of medical or surgical treatment.

LIFESTYLE | The importance of a healthy lifestyle in cancer prevention cannot be overstated. The key components are avoiding tobacco use and exposure to cigarette smoke, exercising regularly, and avoiding alcohol or drinking only moderate amounts.

Smoking history: The evidence is overwhelming that smoking is the most preventable cause of cancer and premature death in the United States. Smoking is responsible for nearly 90 percent of all lung cancers. Lung cancer mortality rates are more than 20 times higher for current male smokers and 12 times higher for current female smokers compared with people who have never smoked. Smoking is also associated with an increased risk for virtually every other cancer and accounts for at least 30 percent of all cancer deaths. Smoking is also a major cause of heart disease (the leading cause of death in the United States), strokes, chronic bronchitis, and emphysema.

Passive smoking—exposure to "secondhand" smoke—is an important risk for cancer (particularly lung and breast cancers), and is an even greater risk for causing heart disease. People who don't smoke but who inhale smoke from the environment may be even more susceptible to free radical damage to their heart and arteries than smokers are, because their bodies just aren't used to dealing with such a heavy toxic load. One study found that a woman who has never smoked has an estimated 24 percent greater risk of getting lung cancer if she lives with a smoker.[41] The U.S. Environmental Protection Agency estimates that passive smoking causes 3,000 lung cancer deaths each year.

Exercise level: A number of studies have found a link between low physical activity levels and an increased cancer risk. On the other hand, increased physical activity, whether from structured exercise or physical labor, has been found to cut the overall cancer risk nearly in half. The greater the activity level, the lower the risk. The association is strongest for colon and breast cancers. The preventive effects of exercise are seen even in people who have other risk factors, such as poor diet, excess body weight, and smoking.[42,43]

Alcohol consumption: There is a clear association between alcohol consumption and many forms of cancer. The higher the dose (amount of alcohol), the greater the risk. While moderate consumption (that is, less than one or two glasses of wine; one beer; or 1 ounce of alcohol per day) poses little risk, drinking alcohol beyond this amount greatly increases the chance of getting cancer of the throat, liver, colon, or breast. Alcohol is metabolized into highly reactive compounds like acetaldehyde that act as free radicals and damage DNA repair mechanisms, further raising the risk.

PSYCHOLOGICAL HEALTH | Stress, personality, attitude, and emotional state are thought to predict the development of many diseases, including cancer. Although somewhat controversial, personality stereotypes have emerged that reflect an increased risk for certain diseases. For example, the so-called Type A personality of being easily angered, competitive, and hard-driving is associated with an increased risk for heart disease. The prototypical cancer personality is Type C, associated with the denial and suppression of emotions—in particular, anger. Other features of this pattern are "pathological niceness," avoidance of conflicts, exaggerated social desirability, harmonizing behavior, overcompliance, and overpatience, as well as high rationality and a tendency toward feelings of helplessness. The Type C personality displays on the outside a façade of pleasantness, but this outward expression quickly dissolves during times of stress. Typically the Type C personality deals with stress through excessive denial, avoidance, suppression and repression of emotions.[44] This internalization is thought to contribute to the development of cancer by amplifying the negative effects that stress produces on the immune system.

What research continues to tell us is that how a person handles stress is more crucial than the stressor itself and that the response to stress is highly individualized. Two people might have the same stressful experience, but they may react to it in entirely different ways, and as a result, some may develop cancer and others may not.[45]

It is our belief that helping a person develop an effective method to deal with stress is more important than identifying a particular cancer personality. Put simply, dealing with stress in a positive manner through exercise, relaxation techniques, and counseling appears to offer protection against cancer and boost immune function regardless of the personality type. In contrast, inappropriate ways of dealing with stress—such as suppression of emotion, denial, drinking alcohol, using drugs, or overeating—will likewise have a negative effect.

In Chapter 5 we discuss in much more detail the importance of attitude and emotions in cancer prevention, while in Chapter 9 we discuss the healing power of faith, hope, and prayer in cancer therapy and provide specific relaxation exercises that fight cancer and boost immune function.

DIET | Poor diet is a major cause of cancer in the United States. There are two main reasons. One is that a poor diet fails to supply the body with the nutrients it needs to maintain healthy cells and tissues. A poor diet means the immune system is less able to defend against foreign invaders that can trigger the onset of cancer.

The other reason poor diet is a concern is that it promotes obesity (extreme overweight). A recent report by RAND Corporation researchers found that obesity contributes as much or more to the development of chronic degenerative disease—including cancer—as smoking does.[46] Obesity severely disturbs the body's ability to regulate the complex interactions among diet, metabolism, physical activity, hormones, and growth factors. Women who are obese after menopause have a 50 percent higher relative risk of breast cancer. Obese men have a 40 percent higher relative risk of colon cancer. Gallbladder and endometrial cancer risks are 5 times higher among obese individuals, and obesity appears to raise the risk of cancers of the kidney, pancreas, rectum, esophagus, and liver.

Table 1-2. Diet and Cancer

DIETARY FACTORS THAT INCREASE CANCER RISK	DIETARY FACTORS THAT DECREASE CANCER RISK
Meats	Fish
Dairy	Whole grains
Total fat	Legumes
Saturated fats	Cabbage
Refined sugar	Vegetables
Total calories	Nuts
Alcohol	Fruits

In Chapter 2, we identify seven key dietary recommendations for cancer prevention. The goal of these recommendations is to reduce the intake of dietary factors that increase cancer risk while increasing the intake of substances that protect against cancer. Table 1-2 presents a quick overview of these factors.

How Cancer Develops

To understand why natural prevention strategies are so effective, it helps to know some basic facts about the cells in your body and cancer. Your body contains trillions of cells. Within each cell is a central core known as the nucleus. Inside the nucleus lies the key to life itself: the long, twisted molecule of deoxyribonucleic acid—better known as DNA. Put simply, DNA contains the instructions (the genes) that the cell needs to make its vital proteins as well as replicate itself. Abnormal changes in a cell's DNA are called mutations. Usually cells with mutations simply die. But sometimes they continue to divide at a rapid, uncontrolled rate to form clumps of cells that grow into the mass of tissue we call a malignant tumor.

There are two types of tumors: benign and malignant.

- Benign tumors are not cancer because the cells are normal (non-mutated) and do not pose a threat to life. They can usually be surgically removed or treated with drugs. Cells from benign tumors do not spread to other parts of the body. Once treated, such tumors usually do not come back.

- Malignant tumors are cancerous. Their mutated cells divide without control or order, and they can invade and damage nearby tissues and organs. Also, cancer cells can break away from a malignant tumor and enter the bloodstream or the lymphatic system, forming new tumors in other organs.

Free Radicals Damage DNA

Cancer-causing injury to cells and their DNA molecules usually comes from toxic atoms known as free radicals. Free radicals assault us from all directions. Some of these come from our environment, in pollutants such as chemicals or cigarette smoke, or from our diet in the form of fats damaged by frying or the presence of nitrates in smoked or cured meats. Even sunlight produces free radical damage. But free radicals also result from the cell's own metabolic activity.

Simply defined, a free radical is a highly reactive atom that can destroy body tissues. All atoms contain small particles called electrons. Normally, electrons come in pairs. But sometimes one of the electrons can get stripped away. By carrying an unpaired electron, the atom—now a free radical—becomes unstable. It sets off on a frantic search to find another electron to complete its set, grabbing on to any electron it can find. But by stealing electrons, free radicals destroy those other molecules. Because the oxygen atom is most often involved as the donor of the electron, this damaging process is known as oxidation, and it is similar to the process that causes apples to turn brown or cars to get rusty.

Like tiny ornery BBs, free radicals shoot through the cell's membranes, tearing gaping holes and putting the cell at risk. A free radical can also knock apart segments of DNA, leading to mutations and the development of cancer.

Because free radicals damage the cell's delicate structures, including DNA, the cumulative damage they cause leads to cellular aging. This, in turn, contributes to a number of diseases, including the two biggest killers of Americans: heart disease and cancer. Most carcinogens (cancer-causing compounds) are dangerous because they cause severe free-radical or oxidative damage to cell structures.

Fortunately, Nature counteracts free radicals and the oxidation they cause by neutralizing them with other molecules known as antioxidants. These work by quenching the unpaired electron by donating one of its own electrons, effectively "calming down" the free radical. By mopping up free radicals, antioxidants are powerful weapons in the fight against cancer and other degenerative diseases. Because they protect cell integrity, antioxidants slow down the aging process, enhance immune function, reduce inflammation, and fight allergies.

The Immune System

The immune system is one of your body's most important defenses against cancer. Cells of the immune system circulate throughout the body, alert for the presence of invading organisms and abnormal cells. When the immune system detects an attack by bacteria or viruses, or notices the presence of proteins that did not originate within the body, it sounds an alert. In response, blood cells, proteins, and other compounds signal one another to attack the intruder, destroy it, and eliminate its remains from the body. The presence of cancer can be a sign that the immune system is not functioning well or that it has been outfoxed by the disease. One of the key principles in the natural prevention and treatment of cancer is to enhance immune function.

So if you want to reduce your risk of cancer, it's important to:

- Reduce free-radical formation in the body
- Limit exposure to dietary and environmental sources of free radicals
- Increase your intake of antioxidant nutrients and other substances that support immune function

We will tell you exactly how to do this in subsequent chapters.

How Cancer Progresses

Of course, preventing cancer from ever starting in the first place is the best way to avoid the disease. But there are no guarantees; cancer is so insidious that it can develop in people despite their best efforts to eat right, stay in shape, and lead a healthy lifestyle. If cancer does arise, the focus shifts. Now the goal is to keep it from getting worse.

Let's take a look now at how cancer runs its course. Understanding this aspect of the disease will help you see why diet and additional nutritional support are so important once a diagnosis of cancer has been made.

Segments of your cell's DNA, known as proto-oncogenes, are responsible for cell growth and activity. They control how often a cell divides. They also regulate the way a cell develops and carries out its specialized functions, a process called differentiation. Mutations in these genes can turn them into oncogenes (*onco-* means "tumor"). These abnormal genes stay "switched on" all the time, ordering the cell to keep dividing at an accelerated rate. The cell continues to produce abnormal copies of itself; these cells, too, continue to proliferate, causing a tumor to grow.

Like all living things, cells eventually die. Their life span—the number of times they can reproduce—is programmed into their genetic code. The medical word for programmed cell death is *apoptosis*. Although it's necessary that old cells die, their "daughter" cells live on, reproducing as often as needed before they, too, die. But damage to a gene known as p53 can disrupt the apoptosis program. When that happens, the cells become "immortal," reproducing faulty copies in an endless cycle. Mutations in the p53 gene are thought to be involved in more than 50 percent of human cancers, including cancers of the lung, colon, and breast.

Your cells don't take this abuse lying down. Cells contain other genes, called tumor-suppressor genes, whose job is to be alert for such damage. When a dangerous mutation arises, these tumor-suppressor genes go into action, repairing the damage to DNA. But like other genes, tumor-suppressor genes are also susceptible to damage and may lose their ability to function.

Like normal cells, cancerous cells need nutrients to survive. They get those nutrients from the same source as your other cells: the blood supply. Tumor cells secrete proteins that cause the growth of new blood vessels. This process is known as angiogenesis. The growth of the tumor is critically dependent on developing these new blood vessels to deliver the nutrients it needs to grow.

Over time, the tumor grows, eventually taking over the part of the body where it originated. Sometimes the tumor damages the organ's cells so much that the organ can no longer perform its normal functions. In other cases the tumor simply grows so big that it presses on the organ and on neighboring tissues. Cancer pain often results from such pressure on nearby nerves.

Normal tissue cells are well connected to their neighbors. But that's not true of cancer cells. They're loosely connected and are likely to break off. These detached cells can enter the bloodstream or the lymphatic system and travel to other parts of the body. The lymphatic system is another circulatory system in your body, responsible for carrying fluid and filtering out many of the waste products. Eventually these migrating cells can lodge in other organs, where they create new tumors. The spread of cancer to a new site is called metastasis.

Typically, cancer spreads first to the liver, lungs, bones, or brain. But even when it has spread to another location, the cancer retains the characteristics of the original tumor. For example, breast cancer that spreads to the liver is known as metastatic breast cancer, not as liver cancer. That's an important distinction to make when it comes time to decide on the appropriate treatment strategy.

Cancer is classified by its appearance under a microscope, as well as by the part of the body in which it began. Different types of cancer vary in their rates of growth, patterns of spread, and responses to treatment.

- Carcinomas are malignant tumors that begin in the lining layer (epithelial cells) of organs. Approximately 80 percent of all cancers are carcinomas.
- Sarcomas are malignant tumors growing from connective tissues, such as cartilage, fat, muscle, or bone.
- Leukemias are cancers involving the blood and blood-forming organs (bone marrow, lymphatic system, and spleen), and lymphomas are cancers involving the lymphatic system. Leukemias do not usually form a tumor. Instead, these cancer cells circulate in the blood and through other tissues where they can accumulate.

The Importance of a Regular Checkup

As expressed clearly above, one key strategy in the prevention of cancer is to identify the presence of risk factors and take the appropriate actions to eliminate or reduce them. Another important step is periodic

Table 1-3. American Cancer Society Recommendations for the Early Detection of Cancer

SITE	RECOMMENDATION
Cancer-related checkup	A cancer-related checkup is recommended every 3 years for people ages 20–40 and every year for people ages 40 and older. This exam should include health counseling and, depending on a person's age and sex, might include examinations for cancers of the thyroid, oral cavity, skin, lymph nodes, testes, or ovaries, as well as for some nonmalignant diseases.
Breast	Women ages 40 and older should have an annual mammogram and an annual clinical breast examination (CBE) by a health care professional. They also should perform monthly breast self-examination. The CBE should be conducted close to the scheduled mammogram. Women ages 20–39 should have a CBE by a health care professional every 3 years and should perform monthly breast self-examination.
Colon and rectum	Beginning at age 50, men and women should follow one of the examination schedules below: • A fecal occult blood test every year and a flexible sigmoidoscopy every 5 years • A colonoscopy every 10 years • A double-contrast barium enema every 5 to 10 years A digital rectal exam should be done at the same time as a sigmoidoscopy, colonoscopy, or double-contrast barium enema. People who have a family history of colon cancer should talk with a doctor about a different testing schedule.
Prostate	The ACS recommends that both the prostate-specific antigen (PSA) blood test and the digital rectal examination be offered annually, beginning at age 50, to men who have a life expectancy of at least 10 years and to younger men who are at high risk. Men in high-risk groups, such as those with a strong familial predisposition (2 or more affected first-degree relatives) or blacks, may begin at a younger age (35 years).
Uterus	Cervix: All women who are or have been sexually active or who are 18 and older should have an annual Pap test and pelvic examination. After 3 or more consecutive satisfactory examinations with normal findings, the Pap test may be performed less frequently. Discuss the matter with your physician. Endometrium: Women with a family history of cancer of the uterus should have a sample of endometrial tissue examined when menopause begins.

Source: Modified from information from the American Cancer Society, Inc.

screening. Screening means getting a regular checkup to look for cancer. Screening is especially important for people who have certain risk factors, such as a family history of certain cancers or exposure to environmental toxins.

The major benefit of regular screening examinations by a health care professional is that it can lead to early detection of cancer (Table 1-3). Screening-accessible cancers—especially cancers of the breast, colon, rectum, cervix, prostate, testicles, oral cavity, and skin—account for about half of all new cancer cases. The earlier a cancer is discovered, the more likely it is that treatment will be successful. Self-examinations for cancers of the breast and skin may also result in detection of tumors at earlier stages. We can't stress enough the importance of having a complete regular physical exam. Your life may depend on it!

Chapter Two

Seven Tips for Creating an Environment That Is Hostile to Cancer

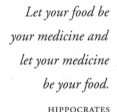

> *Let your food be*
> *your medicine and*
> *let your medicine*
> *be your food.*
>
> HIPPOCRATES

Without question, a good diet is essential for good health. Mounting scientific evidence makes it clear that poor dietary habits cause or contribute to many diseases, including cancer. By the same token, a nourishing diet can minimize the risk of cancer and may actually prevent many forms of the disease. What's more, certain foods offer benefit to people with cancer, either because they help treat the condition or because they boost the effectiveness of other therapies. And finally, just as critical as the food you eat is how your body breaks down, absorbs, and eliminates what is ingested. All these issues will be discussed in this chapter as we strive to help you create an environment within your body that is hostile to the development of cancer.

Seven Key Principles of the Cancer-Prevention Diet

By following seven important guidelines, you'll give your body its best chance of avoiding not just cancer but a range of other chronic diseases as well.

1. Eat a "rainbow" assortment of fruits and vegetables.
2. Reduce exposure to pesticides.
3. Reduce the intake of meat and other animal foods.
4. Eat the right type of fats by increasing the intake of omega-3 fatty acids.
5. Avoid high-calorie, low-nutrient foods such as junk foods, candy, and soft drinks.
6. Keep salt intake low, potassium intake high.
7. Choose foods that help your body detoxify and eliminate waste.

1. Eat a "rainbow" assortment of fruits and vegetables

A diet rich in fruits and vegetables is your best bet for preventing cancer. That fact has been established time and again in scientific studies on large numbers of people.[1-3] The evidence in support of this recommendation is so strong that it has been endorsed by U.S. government health agencies and by virtually every major medical organization, including the American Cancer Society. By "rainbow," we simply mean that by selecting foods of different colors—red, orange, yellow, green, blue, and purple—you'll be giving your body the full spectrum of cancer-fighting compounds as well as the nutrients it needs for optimal function and protection against disease.

Why are fruits and vegetables so important in fighting cancer?

The simplest answer—and the one that is most deeply rooted in history—has to do with the way humans evolved. We are omnivorous, which means we can digest foods from both plant and animal sources. In prehistoric times, our survival as a species depended on our ability to get food both by hunting other animals and by gathering fruits and vegetables.[4]

Still, anthropologists tell us that our bodies are built primarily to process foods from plant sources. They base that conclusion on the shape and arrangement of our teeth, the way our jaws move, and the long length of our digestive tract (our intestines are more than 20 feet long, while most carnivores have intestines only a few feet in length). The human body is designed to function efficiently by getting most of its energy and nutrition from plant sources.[5]

In fact, some experts have said—and we believe—that cancer is a result of a "maladaptation" over time to a reduced level of intake of fruits and vegetables. In fact, we agree with the statement, "Vegetables and fruit contain the anticarcinogenic cocktail to which we are adapted. We abandon it at our peril."[6] For the earliest humans, eating animal foods was possible—perhaps even a luxury—but was not absolutely crucial for survival. But over the millennia, the balance in the human diet shifted to include more foods from animal sources and fewer fruits and vegetables. The digestive system does the best it can with what we provide it, but without the important vitamins and minerals available in plant foods, the chances of cell damage increase. And that raises the risk of cancer.

A vast number of substances found in fruits and vegetables are known to protect against cancer. Some experts refer to these as chemopreventers to emphasize their potent anticancer effects. Such substances include antioxidant nutrients, such as vitamin C and folic acid, and a group of other compounds known as phytochemicals (Table 2-1).

Phytochemicals include pigments such as carotenes, chlorophyll, and flavonoids; dietary fiber; enzymes; vitamin-like compounds; and other minor dietary constituents. Although phytochemicals work in harmony with antioxidants like vitamin C, vitamin E, and selenium, phytochemicals exert considerably greater protection against cancer than these simple nutrients.

A CLOSER LOOK AT PLANT PIGMENTS | Among the most important groups of phytochemicals are the pigments. As you might have guessed, pigments give foods their color. Color contributes to food's eye appeal. Equally important for survival, color helps us recognize when a food has spoiled. But pigments do more than just make food look pretty or rotten. They are powerful chemicals that contribute to your body's cancer-fighting activity.

Table 2-1. Examples of Anticancer Phytochemicals

PHYTOCHEMICAL	ACTIONS	SOURCES
Carotenes	• Antioxidants • Enhance immune functions	Dark-colored vegetables such as carrots, squash, spinach, kale, tomatoes, yams, sweet potatoes; fruits such as cantaloupe, apricots, citrus fruits
Coumarin	• Antitumor properties • Enhance immune functions • Stimulate antioxidant mechanisms	Carrots, celery, fennel, beets, citrus fruits
Dithiolthiones, Glucosinolates, and Thiocyanates	• Block cancer-causing compounds from damaging cells • Enhance detoxification	Cabbage family vegetables— broccoli, Brussels sprouts, kale, etc.
Flavonoids	• Antioxidants • Direct antitumor effects • Immune-enhancing properties	Fruits, particularly richly colored fruits such as berries, cherries, citrus fruits; also tomatoes, peppers, greens
Isoflavonoids	• Block estrogen receptors	Soy and other legumes
Lignans	• Antioxidants • Modulate hormone receptors	Flaxseed and flaxseed oil; whole grains, nuts, seeds.
Limonoids	• Enhance detoxification • Block carcinogens	Citrus fruits, celery
Polyphenols	• Antioxidants • Block carcinogen formation • Modulate hormone receptors	Green tea, chocolate, red wine
Sterols	• Block production of carcinogens • Modulate hormone receptors	Soy, nuts, seeds

The carotenes are the best-known pigments and the ones found most widely in foods. These are the red and yellow pigments found in vegetables such as carrots, peppers, yams, and tomatoes, and in fruits such as apricots, watermelons, and cherries. Carotenes are also found in green leafy vegetables, such as spinach, and in legumes, grains, and seeds. Over 600 carotenes exist in nature, including perhaps 50 that the body can transform into vitamin A. Beta-carotene is the most active of the carotenes (because more of it is converted to vitamin A), but several other carotenes, such as lutein and lycopene, may exert greater anticancer effects.[7,8]

The leading sources of carotenes are the dark-green leafy vegetables: kale, collards, and spinach. The deeper the green color, the greater the concentration of carotenes.

Another important group of plant pigments are the flavonoids. These are sometimes called nature's biological response modifiers because of their anti-inflammatory, antiallergic, antiviral, and anticancer properties. Good dietary sources of flavonoids include citrus fruits, berries, onions, parsley, legumes, green tea, and red wine.

HOW TO EAT A RAINBOW ASSORTMENT | Everyone knows it's important to eat fruits and vegetables. In 1992, the National Cancer Institute launched a campaign called "Five a Day for Better Health" to get people to eat more of these essential foods.

But Americans still aren't getting the message. Sad to say, if French fries, potato chips, and the lettuce and tomatoes from hamburgers are taken out of the equation, *less than half* of all Americans actually consume even a single serving of a fruit or vegetable in the course of a day! Only about 10 percent of people actually achieve the five-a-day recommendation, and virtually no one is eating enough of the fruits and vegetables that are the most important in fighting cancer.[9]

We cannot stress it enough: *The key dietary recommendation for you to reduce your risk of cancer is to consume liberal amounts of cancer-fighting fruits and vegetables.* In fact, we go well beyond the five-a-day recommendation. We recommend ten servings a day. That sounds like a lot, but the serving size is actually quite small. Serving size equals 1 cup raw leafy vegetables (such as lettuce or spinach); ½ cup raw nonleafy or cooked vegetables; ½ cup cooked green beans or peas; 1 medium fruit or ½ cup small or cut-up fruit, or 100 percent juice; and ¼ cup dried fruit.

In Appendix A, Daily Plan for Preventing Cancer, we will provide additional guidance to help you achieve this goal. Right now, we want to encourage you to choose at least one food per day from the five key color groups—red, dark green, yellow and light green, orange, and purple from Table 2-2.

Table 2-2. The Rainbow Assortment

RED	DARK GREEN	YELLOW AND LIGHT GREEN	ORANGE	PURPLE
Apples (red)	Artichoke	Apples (green or yellow)	Apricots	Beets
Bell peppers (red)	Asparagus	Avocado	Bell peppers (orange)	Blackberries
Cherries	Bell peppers (green)	Bananas	Butternut squash	Blueberries
Cranberries	Broccoli	Bell peppers (yellow)	Cantaloupe	Cabbage (purple)
Grapefruit	Brussels sprouts	Bok choy	Carrots	Cherries
Grapes (red)	Chard	Cabbage	Mangoes	Currants
Plums (red)	Collard greens	Cauliflower	Oranges	Eggplant
Radishes	Cucumber	Celery	Papaya	Grapes (purple)
Raspberries	Grapes (green)	Fennel	Pumpkin	Onions (red)
Strawberries	Green beans	Kiwi fruit	Sweet potatoes	Pears (red)
Tomatoes	Honeydew melons	Lemons	Yams	Plums (purple)
Watermelon	Kale	Lettuce (light-green types)		Radishes
	Leeks	Limes		
	Lettuce (dark-green types)	Onions		
	Mustard greens	Pears (green or yellow)		
	Peas	Pineapple		
	Spinach	Squash (yellow)		
	Turnip greens	Zucchini (yellow)		

WHICH IS BETTER—RAW OR COOKED? | On one level, the answer to this question is: It doesn't matter! What's important is to make sure you're eating enough fruits and vegetables, in whatever form.

As a rule, we recommend eating fruits and most vegetables in their raw state. But we must note that some of the carotenes (like lycopene and lutein) are better absorbed from cooked foods. In addition, it may not be wise to consume more than four servings per week of raw cabbage family vegetables (including broccoli, cauliflower, and kale),

Grapefruit—Not Such a Great Fruit?

Citrus fruits are an important part of a cancer-fighting diet because they provide vitamin C, other essential nutrients, and important phytochemicals. But grapefruit contains high levels of a flavonoid (plant compound) called naringin that can be a problem if people are taking certain drugs. Naringin reduces the activity of CYP3A enzymes, part of the P450 enzyme family. These enzymes are the ones your body uses to break down certain drugs, such as calcium channel blockers (used in the treatment of high blood pressure), sedatives (for example, midazolam), and cyclosporin (an immune suppressant given to people who have received organ transplants). If the drugs are not metabolized, they remain in the body in higher concentrations, increasing the risk of unwanted toxic effects.

If you are taking a prescription medication, ask your doctor if you should avoid eating grapefruit or drinking grapefruit juice. Some drugs, such as Neoral (oral cyclosporin), already carry a warning. For citrus lovers, there are plenty of other choices. Oranges, tangerines, and tangelos do not contain significant amounts of naringin but have lots of other important nutrients and flavonoids.

because these foods in their raw state contain compounds that can interfere with thyroid hormone production. When you cook vegetables, we recommend lightly steaming them or stir-frying them in olive oil.

If you can't eat fresh produce, then frozen is the next-best thing. We do not advocate eating canned fruit or vegetables, as many of the naturally occurring cancer-fighting phytochemicals are destroyed in the canning process.

It is important to eat at least two of the servings of fruits or vegetables in their raw, fresh state. Many of the compounds with anticancer properties are found in much higher concentrations in raw foods than in their cooked counterparts. For example, ellagic acid, found in fresh apples and raspberries, exhibits significant anticancer activity.[10–12] A potent antioxidant, it protects against damage to the chromosomes. It also blocks the cancer-causing actions of many pollutants, such as polycyclic aromatic hydrocarbons (PAH) found in cigarette smoke and toxic chemicals such as benzopyrene. Ellagic acid is not destroyed by freezing or freeze-drying, but it is destroyed by heat.[13] While fresh whole apples and fresh apple juice contain approximately 100 to 130 mg per 100 g (roughly 3½ ounces) of ellagic acid, the amount found in cooked or commercial apple products is at or near zero.

DETOXIFICATION: SPOTLIGHT ON GLUTATHIONE | Many fresh fruits and vegetables contain glutathione, an important antioxidant found in all tissues in the body. Glutathione is an important anticancer agent that helps detoxify and eliminate toxins such as heavy metals, pesticides, and solvents.[14] The average glutathione content for various food classes per 100 g is fresh fruit, 4.5 mg; fresh vegetables, 6.5 mg; red meat, fish, and poultry, 10 mg; walnuts, 15 mg; and breads, cereals, legumes, and nuts other than walnuts, less than 1 mg per 100 g. Fresh fruits and vegetables provide excellent levels of glutathione, but—not surprisingly—cooked foods contain far less (Table 2-3).[15] It's also worth noting that your body absorbs glutathione from foods, but it absorbs very little when glutathione is taken as a supplement.

Glutathione's combination of detoxification and free-radical protection makes it one of the most important cancer and aging fighters in our cells. The greater your exposure to toxins, the faster your body uses up its supply of glutathione. Without the protection of glutathione, your cells die at a faster rate, making you age quicker and putting you at risk for toxin-induced diseases including cancer. People who smoke,

Table 2-3. Glutathione Content of Uncooked vs. Cooked Foods

FOOD	UNCOOKED	COOKED
Apples	21.0	0.0
Carrots	74.6	0.0
Grapefruit	70.6	0.0
Peaches	65.1	16.6
Spinach	166.0	27.1
Tomatoes	169.0	0.0

who are chronically exposed to toxins, or who suffer from inflammatory conditions such as rheumatoid arthritis or chronic conditions such as diabetes, AIDS, or cancer typically have lower levels of glutathione. It's a vicious circle: Health problems deplete your supply of glutathione, and reduced levels of glutathione increase your risk of health problems.

Don't depend on supplements containing glutathione to boost levels of glutathione in the body. While dietary forms of glutathione appear to be efficiently absorbed into the blood, the same may not be true for glutathione supplements in humans. When healthy subjects were given a single dose of up to 3000 mg of glutathione, researchers found, there was no increase in blood glutathione levels.[16]

To boost glutathione levels in your cells, we recommend supplementing your diet with at least 500 mg of vitamin C each day[17] and focusing on the best dietary sources of glutathione, such as fresh fruits, asparagus, avocados, walnuts, and cabbage family foods such as cabbage, broccoli, and Brussels sprouts. You can also step up your body's production of glutathione by eating foods that contain a compound called limonene, such as citrus, dill weed, and caraway seeds.

Additional recommendations for boosting glutathione in the support of conventional treatment of some cancers are given in Chapter 13.

2. Reduce exposure to pesticides

In the United States, more than 1.2 billion pounds of pesticides and herbicides are sprayed or added to food crops each year. That's roughly 5 pounds of pesticides for each man, woman, and child. There is a growing concern that in addition to these pesticides directly causing a significant number of cancers, exposure to these chemicals damages your body's detoxification mechanisms, thereby increasing your risk of getting cancer and other diseases.[18]

We all are exposed to pesticides and other toxins in the air that we breathe, the environment, and the food that we eat. To illustrate just how problematic pesticides can be, let's take a quick look at the health problems of the farmer. The lifestyle of farmers is generally healthy: Compared with city dwellers, they have access to lots of fresh food; they breathe clean air, work hard, and have a lower rate of cigarette smoking and alcohol use. Yet studies show that farmers have a higher risk of de-

Easy Tips to Reach Your Ten-a-Day Goal

- Buy many kinds of fruits and vegetables when you shop, so you have plenty of choices.
- Stock up on frozen vegetables for easy cooking, so that you always have a vegetable dish with every dinner.
- Use the fruits and vegetables that go bad easily (peaches, asparagus) first. Save hardier varieties (apples, acorn squash) or frozen goods for later in the week.
- Keep fruits and vegetables where you can see them. The more often you see them, the more likely you are to eat them.
- Keep a bowl of cut-up vegetables on the top shelf of the refrigerator.
- Keep a fruit bowl on your kitchen counter, table, or desk at work.
- Pack a piece of fruit or some cut-up vegetables in your briefcase or backpack; carry moist towelettes for easy cleanup.
- Add fruits and vegetables to lunch by having them in soup or salad, or cut-up raw.
- At dinner, serve vegetables steamed, sautéed in olive oil, or microwaved.
- Choose fresh fruit for dessert. For a special dessert, try a fruit parfait with low-fat yogurt or sherbet topped with lots of berries.
- Add extra varieties of vegetables when you prepare soups, sauces, and casseroles (for example, add grated carrots and zucchini to spaghetti sauce).
- Take advantage of salad bars, which offer ready-to-eat raw vegetables and fruits and prepared salads made with fruits and vegetables.
- Use vegetable-based sauces such as marinara sauce and juices such as low-sodium V-8 or tomato juice.

veloping lymphomas, leukemias, and cancers of the stomach, prostate, brain, and skin.[19]

There is significant evidence linking pesticide use to the risk of non-Hodgkin's lymphoma (NHL).[20] This blood cancer currently accounts for about 3 percent of all cancer diagnosed in the United States and affects about 55,000 Americans each year. In the last thirty years the incidence of NHL has increased more rapidly than that of any other cancer except for prostate, skin, and lung cancers. Large studies of farmers in Canada, Australia, Europe, New Zealand, and the United States have demonstrated that the greater the exposure to pesticides, the greater the risk for non-Hodgkin's lymphoma.

But in dealing with cancer risk, it can be difficult to establish a clear link between cause and effect. In addition to pesticide exposure, other suspected risk factors for NHL include use of hair dyes, exposure to toxic chemicals, history of prior blood transfusion, smoking, and several dietary factors, such as a higher intake of meat, animal fats (including butter), soft drinks (especially colas), and milk, and lower intakes of cabbage family vegetables, citrus fruits, dark-green vegetables, vitamin C, and beta-carotene.[21–25]

Perhaps the most problematic pesticides are those that belong to the halogenated hydrocarbon family, such as DDE, PCB, PCP, dieldrin, and chlordane. These chemicals persist almost indefinitely in the environment. For example, a similar pesticide, DDT, has been banned for nearly thirty years, yet it can still be found in the soil and in root vegetables such as carrots and potatoes. Our bodies also have a tough time detoxifying and eliminating these compounds, so they end up being stored in our fat cells. What's more, inside the body these chemicals can act like the hormone estrogen. They are thus suspected as a major cause of the growing epidemic of estrogen-related health problems, including breast cancer.[26–28] Some evidence also suggests that these chemicals increase the risk of lymphomas, leukemia, and pancreatic cancer as well as play a role in low sperm counts and reduced fertility in men.

The bottom line is that while pesticides may increase risk, they are not necessarily the only factor involved. Overall diet, genetic history, and other factors may come into play (see the cancer risk self-assessment in Chapter 1). We believe that by following the dietary recommendations given in this chapter, you'll go a long way in overcoming harmful effects of these compounds. A lot of this protection is the result of im-proved detoxification of these potentially dangerous compounds (dis-cussed more fully below).

Here are our recommendations for avoiding pesticides in your diet.

- Do not overconsume foods that concentrate pesticides, such as animal fat, meat, eggs, cheese, and milk.
- Buy organic produce, which is grown without the aid of synthetic pesticides and fertilizers. Although less than 3 percent of the total produce in the United States is grown without pesticides, organic produce is widely available.
- Develop a good relationship with your local grocery store produce manager. Explain your desire to reduce the exposure to pesticides and waxes. Ask what measures the store takes to assure that pesti-cide residues are within approved limits. Ask where the store gets its produce; make sure the store is aware that foreign produce is much more likely to contain excessive levels of pesticides as well as pesticides that have been banned in the United States.
- Try to buy local produce, in season.
- Peel off the skin or remove the outer layer of leaves of some pro-duce; that may be all you need to do reduce pesticide levels. The downside of this is that many of the nutritional benefits are con-centrated in the skin and outer layers. An alternative measure is to remove surface pesticide residues, waxes, fungicides, and fertilizers by soaking the item in a mild solution of additive-free soap such as Ivory or pure castile soap. All-natural, biodegradable cleansers are also available at most health food stores. To use, spray the food with the cleanser, gently scrub, and rinse.

The possible presence of pesticides in fruits and vegetables should not deter you from eating a diet high in these foods. The concentrations in fruits and vegetables are much lower than the levels found in animal fats, meat, cheese, whole milk, and eggs. Furthermore, the various antioxi-dant components in fruits and vegetables are necessary to help the body deal with the pesticides.

3. Reduce the intake of meat and other animal foods

Study after study confirms one basic truth: The higher your intake of meat and other animal foods, the higher your risk of cancer—especially for the major cancers, such as colon, breast, prostate, and lung cancers.[29]

There are many reasons for this association. Meat lacks the antioxidant and phytochemicals that protect us from cancer. At the same time, it contains lots of saturated fat and other potentially carcinogenic (cancer-causing) compounds—including pesticide residues, heterocyclic amines, and polycyclic aromatic hydrocarbons, which form when meat is grilled, fried, or broiled. The more well done the meat, the higher the level of amines.

Some proponents of a diet high in meat claim that we should eat the way our caveman ancestors did. That argument doesn't really hold up. The meat of wild animals that early humans consumed was much different from the industrially produced, shrink-wrapped meat we find in supermarkets today. The demand for tender meat has led to the breeding of cattle whose meat contains 25 to 30 percent fat or more. In contrast, meat from free-living animals and wild game has a fat content of less than 4 percent.

It's not just the amount of fat. The composition is also different. Domestic beef contains primarily saturated fats and virtually no beneficial omega-3 fatty acids (discussed on page 40), while the fat of wild animals contains more than 5 times the polyunsaturated fat per gram and has substantial amounts (about 4 percent) of omega-3 fatty acids.

Range-fed animals also contain 10 times as much conjugated linoleic acid (CLA) as grain-fed animals. CLA is a slightly altered form of the essential fatty acid linoleic acid. It occurs naturally in meat and dairy products. CLA was discovered in 1978 when researchers at the University of Wisconsin were looking for cancer-causing compounds that result from cooking. Instead, they found CLA, which appears to be an anticancer compound. Preliminary animal and test tube studies show that CLA might reduce the risk of cancers at several sites, including the breast, prostate, colorectal, lung, skin, and stomach. Whether CLA will produce a similar protective effect in humans is yet to be determined.[30]

HIGHLIGHT: NITRATE- AND NITRITE-CONTAINING FOODS | Cured or smoked meats such as ham, hot dogs, bacon, and jerky contain sodium nitrate and/or sodium nitrites—compounds that keep the food from spoiling but that dramatically increase the risk for cancer. These chemicals react with amino acids in foods in the stomach to form highly carcinogenic compounds known as nitrosamines.

Research in adults makes a convincing argument to avoid these foods. Even more compelling is the evidence linking consumption of nitrates to a significantly increased risk of the major childhood cancers (leukemias, lymphomas, and brain cancers):[31,32]

- Children who eat 12 hot dogs per month have nearly 10 times the risk of developing leukemia compared with children who do not eat hot dogs.
- Children who eat hot dogs once a week double their chances of brain tumors; eating them twice a week triples the risk.
- Pregnant women who eat two servings per day of any cured meat have more than double the risk of bearing children who have brain cancer.
- Kids who eat the most ham, bacon, and cured sausage have 3 times the risk of lymphoma.
- Kids who eat ground meat once a week have twice the risk of acute lymphocytic leukemia compared with those who eat none; eating two or more hamburgers weekly tripled the risk.

Fortunately, vegetarian alternatives to these standard components of the American diet are now widely available, and many of them actually taste quite good. Consumers can find soy hot dogs, soy sausage, soy bacon, and even soy pastrami at their local health food store as well as in many mainstream grocery stores.

If you choose to eat red meat:

- Limit your intake to no more than 3 to 4 ounces daily—about the size of a deck of playing cards. And choose the leanest cuts available (it is important to point out that the USDA allows the meat and dairy industries to label fat content by weight rather than by percent of calories).
- Avoid consuming well-done, charbroiled, and fat-laden meats.
- Don't eat cured meats (bacon, hot dogs, etc.), especially if you are pregnant or a child under age 12.

Table 2-4. Healthier Food Choices

REDUCE INTAKE OF:	SUBSTITUTE WITH:
Red meat	Fish and white meat of poultry
Hamburgers and hot dogs	Soy-based or vegetarian alternatives
Eggs	Egg Beaters and similar reduced-cholesterol products Tofu
High-fat dairy products	Low-fat or nonfat products
Butter, lard, other saturated fats	Olive oil
Ice cream, pies, cake, cookies, etc.	Fruits
Fried foods, fatty snacks	Vegetables, fresh salads
Salt and salty foods	Low-sodium foods, light salt
Coffee, soft drinks	Herbal teas, green tea, fresh fruit and vegetable juices
Margarine, shortening, and other sources of trans fatty acids or partially hydrogenated oil	Cook with olive oil or canola oil, use vegetable spreads that contain no trans fatty acids (available at most health food stores)

- Consider buying free-range meats or wild game such as grass-fed beef or buffalo, venison, and ostrich.

4. Eat the right type of fats by increasing the intake of omega-3 fatty acids

There is no room for debate: A diet high in fat, particularly saturated fat and cholesterol, has been linked to numerous cancers. Both the American Cancer Society and the National Cancer Institute recommend a diet that supplies less than 30 percent of calories as fat. However, just as important as the amount of fat is the *type* of fat you consume. The goal is to *decrease* your total fat intake (especially intake of saturated fats) while *increasing* your intake of omega-3 fatty acids and monounsaturated fatty acids.

Some of these terms can be confusing. To help you understand, here's a quick chemical lesson.

Fat molecules are made of atoms of carbon, hydrogen, and oxygen. Each of the separate atoms attaches to the others only in certain predetermined ways. The backbone of a fat is a chain of carbon atoms (C):

$$| \quad | \quad | \quad |$$
$$-C-C-C-C-$$
$$| \quad | \quad | \quad |$$

Hydrogen (H) and oxygen (O) atoms can then attach to the carbons. A saturated fat is a fat molecule in which all the available binding sites are occupied with another atom. In other words, the carbons are saturated with all the atoms they can hold:

$$H \quad H \quad H \quad H$$
$$| \quad | \quad | \quad |$$
$$H-C-C-C-C-O$$
$$| \quad | \quad | \quad |$$
$$H \quad H \quad H \quad H$$

An unsaturated fat has one or more bonding sites left unoccupied, so the two neighboring carbon atoms will take up the slack by forming a double bond:

$$H \qquad \qquad H$$
$$| \qquad \qquad |$$
$$H-C-C=C-C-O$$
$$| \quad | \quad | \quad |$$
$$H \quad H \quad H \quad H$$

A fat molecule with one double bond is called a monounsaturated fat. Molecules with more than one double bond are called polyunsaturated fats. *Mono-* means "one"; *poly-* means "many." When an unsaturated fat contains the first double bond at the third carbon, it is referred to as an omega-3 fatty acid. If the first double bond is at the sixth carbon, it is an omega-6 fatty acid, and if it occurs at the ninth carbon, it is an omega-9 fatty acid.

The human body absolutely requires two essential fatty acids—linoleic acid (an omega-6 fat) and alpha-linolenic acid (an omega-3 fat). But most Americans eat way too much of the omega-6 oils found in meats and most vegetable oils, and suffer a relative deficiency of the omega-3 fats found in fish and flaxseed oil—a situation that is associated with an increase risk for cancer and about sixty other conditions, including heart disease, stroke, high blood pressure, skin diseases, and diabetes. Particularly important to good health are the longer-chain omega-3 fatty acids, such as eicosapentaenoic acid (EPA) and docosahexaenoic acid (DHA) found in fish, especially cold-water fish such as salmon, mackerel, herring, and halibut. Although the body can convert alpha-linolenic acid from flaxseed and other vegetable sources, it is much more efficient to get them from the diet.

Essential fatty acids are transformed into regulatory compounds known as prostaglandins. These compounds carry out many important tasks in the body. They regulate inflammation, pain, and swelling; they play a role in maintaining blood pressure; and they regulate heart, digestive, and kidney function. Prostaglandins also are involved in blood clotting. They participate in the response to allergies, help control transmission of signals along the nerves, and are used in the production of steroids and other hormones. Prostaglandins derived from the omega-6 fatty acids tend to stimulate cancer cell growth, while those from the omega-3 fatty acids inhibit cancer. Having higher dietary levels of omega-3 and reduced levels of the omega-6 acids can protect against not only cancer but also heart disease and Alzheimer's disease. All told, fish oils have been shown to benefit about sixty different health conditions, including rheumatoid arthritis and other autoimmune diseases, psoriasis, eczema, asthma, attention deficit disorder, and depression.

What else makes saturated fats and margarine "bad" and omega-3 fatty acids "good"? The answer has to do with the function of fats in cellular membranes. Membranes are made mostly of fatty acids. What determines the type of fatty acid present in the cell membrane is the type of fat you consume. A diet composed mostly of saturated fat, animal fatty acids, cholesterol, and margarine acids results in membranes that are much less fluid in nature than the membranes in a person who consumes optimum levels of both essential fatty acids.

An alteration in cell membrane function is the main cause of cell injury and death. Without healthy membranes, cells lose their ability to hold water, vital nutrients, and electrolytes. They also lose their ability to communicate with other cells and to be controlled by regulating hormones. They simply do not function properly. Cell membrane dysfunction is a critical factor in the development of cancer. Particularly harmful to cell membrane function are margarine and other foods containing trans fatty acids and partially hydrogenated oils. These "unnatural" forms of fatty acids interfere with the body's ability to utilize important essential fatty acids and have been linked to several human cancers. We strongly urge you to avoid them.

Along with the healthier food choices given in Table 2.4 above, here is a key recommendation for making sure you get higher levels of the beneficial omega-3 fats: Increase your intake of fish. Fish consumption offers significant protection against many forms of cancer.[33-35] Particularly beneficial are cold-water fish such as salmon, mackerel, herring, and halibut, because of their high levels of omega-3 fats. If you don't eat at least two servings of cold-water fish per week, we recommend taking fish oil capsules. Take enough capsules to provide 120 to 360 mg of EPA and 80 to 240 mg of DHA per day.

For women we also recommend taking one tablespoon of organic flaxseed oil daily. Flaxseed oil is unique because it contains both essential fatty acids: linoleic (omega-6) and alpha-linolenic (omega-3). The level of alpha-linolenic acid is a whopping 58 percent by weight. Flaxseed oil can be used as a salad dressing, or as a bread dip (instead of butter), or mixed with yogurt or cottage cheese. We do not recommend flaxseed oil use in men at this time, because researchers report conflicting information concerning the possible role of alpha-linolenic acid in prostate cancer (discussed more fully in Chapter 4).

HIGHLIGHT: FISH CONSUMPTION, CANCER—AND A CAUTION | Fish consumption offers significant protection against many forms of cancer, especially the major cancers like lung, colon, breast, and prostate.[33-35] While we are encouraging you to eat more fish, we need to give you some guidelines. Nearly all fish contain trace amounts of methyl mercury. Usually, this is of little concern, because the level is so low. The fish most likely to have the lowest level of methyl mercury are salmon (usually nondetectable levels), cod, mackerel, cold-water tuna, farm-raised catfish, and herring. But certain seafoods—particularly swordfish, shark, and some other large predatory fish—may contain high levels of methyl mercury. Fish absorb methyl mercury from water and aquatic plants. Larger predatory fish also absorb mercury from their prey. Methyl mercury binds tightly to the proteins in fish tissue, including muscle; cooking does not reduce the mercury content significantly.

We suggest limiting fish intake to no more than about two pounds (one kilogram) per week. That translates to six 7-ounce servings per week maximum. Limit your intake of swordfish, shark, and warm-water tuna to no more than once a week (or once a month if you are a woman of childbearing age who might get pregnant).

5. Avoid high-calorie, low-nutrient foods such as junk foods, candy, and soft drinks

High-sugar diets are associated with increased risk of breast, colorectal, biliary, and pancreatic cancers. Refined sugars are quickly absorbed into the bloodstream, causing a rapid rise in blood sugar. In response, the body boosts secretion of insulin by the pancreas. And too much insulin, as it turns out, can promote the growth of certain kinds of cancer cells, including breast, stomach, colon, endometrial, ovarian, lung, and prostate cancer.[36] High insulin levels may be the best predictor of whether a woman's breast cancer returns after treatment, since high insulin levels increase the risk of recurrence and death at least eightfold.

We'll make this simple: Don't eat "junk foods."

According to the third National Health and Nutrition Examination Survey, which studied eating habits among 15,000 American adults, one-third of the average diet in this country is made up of unhealthy foods, including potato chips, crackers, salted snack foods, candy, gum, fried fast food, and soft drinks. These items offer little in terms of protein, vitamins, or minerals. What they do have, though, is lots of "empty calories" in the form of sugar and fat. They fill you up so you don't have room for the good stuff—the foods that give your body a fighting chance to prevent cancer.

Here are guidelines for making healthier eating choices:

- Read labels carefully. If sugar, fat, or salt is one of the first three ingredients listed, it is probably not a good option.
- Be aware that words appearing on the label such as sucrose, glucose, maltose, lactose, fructose, corn syrup, or white grape juice concentrate mean that sugar has been added.

- Look not just at the percentage of calories from fat but also at the number of grams of fat. For every 5 grams of fat in a serving, you are eating the equivalent of one teaspoon of fat.
- If a snack doesn't provide at least 2 grams of fiber, it's not a good choice.

6. Keep salt intake low, potassium intake high

The electrolytes—potassium, sodium, chloride, and magnesium—are mineral salts that can conduct electricity when dissolved in water. For optimal health, it's important for you to consume these nutrients in the proper balance. Too much sodium in the diet from salt, sodium chloride, can disrupt this balance. Many people know that a high-sodium, low-potassium diet can cause high blood pressure, but not as many are aware that such a diet also increases the risk of cancer, including esophageal and colon cancers.[37]

In our society, only 5 percent of sodium intake comes from the natural ingredients in food. Prepared foods contribute 45 percent of our sodium intake, 45 percent is added in cooking, and another 5 percent is added as a condiment.

Tips for reducing your sodium intake:

- Take the salt shaker off the table.
- Omit added salt from recipes and food preparation.
- If you absolutely must have the taste of salt, try the salt substitutes such as NoSalt and Nu-Salt. These products are made with potassium chloride and taste very similar to sodium chloride.
- Learn to enjoy the flavors of unsalted foods.
- Try flavoring foods with herbs, spices, and lemon juice instead of salt.
- Read food labels carefully to determine the amount of sodium. Learn to recognize ingredients that contain sodium. Salt, soy sauce, salt brine, or any ingredient with sodium (such as monosodium glutamate) or baking soda (sodium bicarbonate) as part of its name contains sodium.
- In reading labels and menus, look for words that signal high-sodium content, such as smoked, barbecued, pickled, broth, soy

sauce, teriyaki, Creole sauce, marinated, cocktail sauce, tomato base, Parmesan, and mustard sauce.
- Don't eat canned vegetables or soups; these are often extremely high in sodium.
- Choose low-salt (reduced-sodium) products when available.

Many of us have already learned to watch our salt intake. We'd like to encourage you to increase your potassium intake as well.

Most Americans have a potassium-to-sodium (K:Na) ratio of less than 1:2. In other words, they ingest twice as much sodium as potassium. But experts believe that the optimal dietary potassium-to-sodium ratio is greater than 5:1—*ten times higher* than the average intake. Even this may not be optimal. A natural diet rich in fruits and vegetables can easily produce much higher K:Na ratios, because most fruits and vegetables have a K:Na ratio of at least 50:1. For example, here are the average K:Na ratios for several common fresh fruits and vegetables:

Apples	90:1
Bananas	440:1
Carrots	75:1
Oranges	260:1
Potatoes	110:1

If you are following the dietary recommendations here and in Appendix A, Daily Plan for Preventing Cancer, there is no question that you are reaching your daily potassium goals.

HIGHLIGHT: POTASSIUM SUPPLEMENTS | The FDA restricts the amount of potassium available in dietary supplements to a mere 99 mg per dose because of problems associated with high-dosage potassium salts. However, so-called salt substitutes (such as NoSalt and Nu-Salt) are in fact potassium chloride that provides 530 mg of potassium per one-sixth teaspoon. Therefore, to boost potassium levels, it is much easier to use one of the salt substitutes than a potassium supplement.

Potassium chloride preparations are also available by prescription in a vast array of formulations (timed-release tablets, liquids, powders, and effervescent tablets) and flavors. Potassium salts are commonly prescribed by physicians at doses of 1.5 to 3 g per day. However, potassium salts can cause nausea, vomiting, diarrhea, and ulcers when given in pill form in high doses. These effects are not seen when potassium levels are increased through the diet only. This difference highlights the advantages of using foods or food-based potassium supplements to meet the human body's high potassium requirements.

Most people can handle any excess of potassium without experiencing adverse effects. The exception is people with kidney disease, who are unable to metabolize potassium in the normal way. Such individuals are likely to experience heart disturbances and other signs of potassium toxicity. If you have a kidney disorder, you probably need to restrict potassium intake and should follow the dietary recommendations of your physician.

7. Choose foods that help your body detoxify and eliminate waste

Incomplete protein digestion or poor intestinal absorption of protein breakdown products can result in the formation of compounds that can dramatically stimulate cell growth and increase the risk of cancer. Specifically, gut bacteria convert the amino acids arginine and ornithine into compounds known as polyamines, which include the nasty-sounding compounds putrescine and cadaverine, respectively. As their names imply, these compounds are also associated with decaying flesh—a process known as putrefaction. Clearly, we do not want this process occurring within our living body.

The role of polyamines in cancer development and growth has been established best in colon cancer, although there is also research that suggests they play a role in virtually all forms of cancer, including breast, prostate, and brain cancers.[38–40] When cancer cells grown in the laboratory are exposed to polyamines, their already excessive growth rate increases exponentially. And when the formation of polyamines is inhibited, so is the growth of the tumor.

There are a number of natural compounds that can inhibit the formation of polyamines in the gut, such as Bifidobacteria,[41] vitamin A,[42] selenium,[43] volatile oils from peppermint and other plants,[44] and the alkaloids of goldenseal *(Hydrastis canadensis)*.[45] But the best way to prevent the excessive formation of polyamines is to ensure optimal digestive function and elimination.

The following questionnaire can be used to determine whether you may be suffering from incomplete protein digestion. Circle the number that best describes the intensity of your symptoms on the following scale:

0 = I do not experience this symptom
1 = Mild
2 = Moderate
3 = Severe

1. Abdominal cramps	0	1	2	3
2. Indigestion or belching 1 to 3 hours after eating	0	1	2	3
3. Fatigue after eating	0	1	2	3
4. Lower bowel gas	0	1	2	3
5. Alternating constipation and diarrhea	0	1	2	3
6. Diarrhea	0	1	2	3
7. Large, greasy (shiny) stools	0	1	2	3
8. Poorly formed stools	0	1	2	3
9. Three or more large bowel movements daily	0	1	2	3
10. Foul-smelling stools or flatulence	0	1	2	3
11. Dry, flaky skin and/or dry brittle hair	0	1	2	3
12. Pain in left side under rib cage	0	1	2	3
13. Acne	0	1	2	3
14. Food allergies	0	1	2	3

Interpreting Your Score

If you scored higher than 9, we recommend supplementation with protein-digesting (proteolytic) enzymes. These enzymes are discussed fully on page 166. To enhance digestive function, take the enzymes just before meals at the low end of the dosage recommendation (higher doses may be needed by people who have cancer).

PROMOTING ELIMINATION | There are four primary ways the body gets rid of toxins: through the feces, the urine, the skin, and respiration.

To assist the body's elimination of toxic chemicals, it's important to eat a high-fiber diet and drink plenty of bottled, filtered, or purified water.

Fiber is important because it traps the toxins excreted in the bile. Each day the liver manufactures approximately one quart of bile, which serves as a carrier that helps eliminate toxic substances from the body. Sent to the intestines, the bile and its toxic load are absorbed by fiber and excreted. However, a diet low in fiber means that these toxins are not bound and are more likely to be reabsorbed. Even worse, bacteria in the intestine often modify these toxins so that they become even more damaging and cancer-causing. In addition to eliminating unwanted toxins, the bile emulsifies fats and fat-soluble vitamins in the intestine, improving the body's ability to absorb them.

Dietary fiber, particularly the soluble fiber found in legumes (beans), fruit, and vegetables, is effective in lowering cholesterol levels. Many studies have found that high intake of fiber, especially soluble fiber, is associated with a significant reduction in the level of serum total cholesterol. An intake of 20 g or more typically lowers total cholesterol levels by 10 to 20 percent. Our recommendation is to consume at least 35 g of fiber a day from a variety of food sources, especially vegetables. To help you achieve this goal, we have provided a list of foods and their fiber content (see Appendix G, page 344). If you are eating your five servings of fruits and vegetables each day or you are following one of our meal plans, you are probably coming close to meeting these goals, but we urge you to keep a diet diary to calculate your daily fiber intake. Focus on sources of soluble fiber, since that's the most beneficial kind. Breads, cereals, and pastas that contain bran (wheat, rice, oat, or corn bran) supply fiber, but they also supply high amounts of starch and sugar. Again, try to focus on vegetables and legumes as your source of dietary fiber.

Some warning is necessary if you are not used to eating a high-fiber diet. You can have too much of a good thing. Increasing your fiber intake can increase the amount of intestinal gas (flatulence). Don't worry, this side effect will not be a problem after your body has had a chance to adjust. We suggest that you increase the amount of dietary fiber gradually. Start with small amounts and build up to the recommended level over the course of a few weeks. You'll know you're overdoing it if you experience excessive gas or other abdominal symptoms. Cut back until the symptoms resolve, and then proceed more slowly until you reach a level you can tolerate.

PROMOTING DETOXIFICATION | As you've learned, the main dietary strategies for preventing cancer are to eat foods containing necessary nutritional substances and to avoid ingesting potentially harmful substances. There's another vital link in the process, one that's no less important: helping your body neutralize and eliminate toxic substances through detoxification processes involving your own enzymes.

Enzymes are busy little proteins made by your cells. Their role is to promote chemical changes. Typically, enzymes act like chemical scissors, snipping apart larger molecules into smaller chunks. They also act like a needle and thread, stitching the molecules together in different forms. Various enzymes serve different functions, some helping to break down food, allowing nutrients to be digested and absorbed by cells, and others changing harmful compounds into inactive ones; still others repair damage to DNA; and so on.

A family of about 100 enzymes, known as the P450 family, that reside in the liver is responsible for much of the detoxification process. Differences in people's P450 enzyme levels or activities explain, at least partly, why some people can smoke without developing lung cancer and why certain individuals are more susceptible to the harmful effects of toxic chemicals.[46] Scientists refer to such differences as biochemical individuality.

Further evidence supporting the critical role of the P450 system in preventing cancer is an imbalance in the manner in which it handles toxins.[46] Detoxification of harmful compounds is usually a two-step process—Phase I and Phase II detoxification. During Phase I, many toxins are transformed into an intermediate compound that is actually even more damaging than the original toxin. It is important to have an active Phase II system so that the intermediate compound can be quickly neutralized. Scientific studies are clearly showing that people who have a very active Phase I system but a slow or inactive Phase II system have a substantially increased risk for lung, colon, breast, and prostate cancers.

The first step in supporting detoxification is to supply the body with the necessary building blocks for the manufacture of detoxification enzymes. Nutrients such as proteins, vitamins, and minerals are essential ingredients for making enzymes and their partners, the coenzymes (molecules that help the enzymes do their job). A healthy diet, plus a high-potency multiple vitamin and mineral formula, help ensure that your body will have an adequate supply of hardworking enzymes.

The second step in supporting detoxification is to promote balance between Phase I and Phase II reactions. The dietary and supplement measures recommended in this chapter and the next go a very long way to provide balance between the two phases. We want to add a couple more here: Regularly consume certain spices and herbs in your food. Specifically, make sure that you frequently eat foods that contain turmeric, red pepper (cayenne or chili pepper), black pepper, dill, caraway, garlic, onion, basil, and oregano. When you regularly consume these spices, toxic intermediate products spend less time in the body and have less of a chance to damage cells. One component that's particularly helpful in this regard is curcumin, the stuff that gives turmeric its yellow color. (Turmeric is a key ingredient in curry.) In animal studies, curcumin has been found to inhibit carcinogens such as benzopyrene (the carcinogen found in charcoal-broiled meat) and to neutralize toxic compounds from cigarette smoke.[47] It appears that the curcumin exerts its effects both by making carcinogens less active and by speeding up their detoxification. Curcumin has also been shown to exert many other beneficial actions against cancer and is discussed more fully in Chapter 4.

We suggest that people who smoke, or who are exposed to secondhand smoke, eat a lot of curries. The curcumin in the turmeric can help limit the cancer-causing activity. In one human study, 16 chronic smokers were given 1.5 g of turmeric daily, while 6 nonsmokers served as a control group. At the end of the 30-day trial, the smokers who received turmeric had a significant drop in the level of cancer-causing compounds as measured in urine. Their levels were almost the same as those of the nonsmokers.[48]

THE IMPORTANCE OF WATER | Drink water! Low fluid consumption in general and low water consumption in particular increase the risk for cancers of the breast, colon, and urinary tract.[49] Drinking enough water is another basic axiom for good health that you've probably heard a thousand times. But it's true: You need to drink at least six to eight glasses of bottled, filtered, or purified water (48 to 64 ounces) each day. That means having a glass of water every two waking hours. Don't wait until you're thirsty; instead, schedule regular water breaks throughout the day.

Water is essential for life. The average amount of water in your body is about 10 gallons. We need to drink at least 48 ounces of water per day to replace the water that is lost through urination, sweat, and breathing. If we don't, we are likely to become dehydrated.

Even mild dehydration results in impaired physiological and performance responses. Many nutrients dissolve in water, so they can be absorbed more easily in your digestive tract. Similarly, many metabolic processes need to take place in water. Water is a component of blood and thus is important for transporting chemicals and nutrients to cells and tissues. Each of your cells is constantly bathed in a watery fluid. Water also carries waste materials from cells to the kidneys so that they can be filtered out and eliminated. Water absorbs and transports heat. For example, heat produced by muscle cells during exercise is carried by water in the blood to the surface, helping your body maintain the right temperature balance. The skin cells also release water as perspiration, which helps keep you cool.

Several factors are thought to increase the likelihood of chronic mild dehydration: a faulty thirst "alarm" in the brain; dissatisfaction with the taste of water; regular exercise that increases the amount of water lost through sweat; living in a hot, dry climate; and consumption of the natural diuretics caffeine and alcohol. Diuretics are substances that draw water out of your cells and increase the rate of urination. Surprisingly, if you drink two cups of water and two cups of coffee, cola, or beer, you may end up with a net water intake of zero! Be aware of your "water budget." If you drink coffee or other dehydrating beverages, compensate by drinking an additional glass of water.

Chapter Three

Taking the Right Natural Products to Prevent Cancer

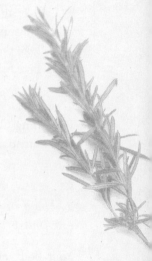

In this age of processed foods and fast-paced, stressful lifestyles, it can be very hard—if not actually impossible—for you to nourish your body completely through diet alone. That's especially true if you want to give yourself the best chance to prevent cancer and other chronic diseases. If you're like most people, you may need a little help in the form of nutritional supplements.

The recommendations we offer here are *supplementary* measures. Vitamin and mineral supplements by themselves cannot provide all the benefits you seek. In fact, taking certain supplements without the support of a diet rich in phytochemicals may actually pose some serious risks. Supplements are of greatest value when used as part of a health-promoting diet and lifestyle.

Key Dietary Supplements for Preventing Cancer

We offer five key dietary supplement recommendations to significantly reduce the risk of cancer:

1. Use a high-potency multiple vitamin and mineral, especially one that provides sufficient levels of antioxidant nutrients.
2. Take an appropriate herbal extract rich in flavonoids.
3. Consume green drinks regularly (see page 63).
4. Take probiotics.
5. Take fish oil supplements.

These dietary supplements are an important part of the Daily Plan for Preventing Cancer given in Appendix A. Here's a closer look at these recommendations.

1. Use a high-potency multiple vitamin and mineral, especially one that provides sufficient levels of antioxidant nutrients

Your body needs essential vitamins and minerals—each in the right amount—for your tissues to do their jobs. Every one of your billions of cells must have these ingredients to maintain the strength and integrity of their delicate membranes and other vital structures.

One of the most crucial functions of your cells is to produce hundreds of different enzymes—molecules that trigger and control chemical reactions. Among other tasks, enzymes are in charge of repairing damage to cells. For example, DNA is fragile and can become "chipped" when it reproduces or if it gets bombarded by a toxic molecule. Such damage can cause cells to mutate. One possible result: cells that grow out of control—cancer.

Normally enzymes rush to the scene and restore DNA to its original form. But if your cell's enzyme-manufacturing system isn't up to par— for example, because your body lacks one or more of the key nutrients—you are far more vulnerable to cell malfunction. Cancer is one possible result. Other consequences include accelerated aging and chronic diseases other than cancer.

Most enzymes in the body have both a vitamin portion and a mineral portion. That's why we recommend taking a high-quality product—one that provides adequate levels of all (or most) of these essential vitamins and minerals. See page 286 in Appendix A for the proper dosage.

Read labels carefully to find multiple vitamin/mineral formulas that contain doses in the right ranges. Be aware that you will not find a formula that provides all these nutrients at these levels in one single pill—it would simply be too big. Usually, you'll need to take at least three to six tablets per day to meet these levels. While many one-a-day supplements provide good levels of vitamins, they tend to be insufficient in the amount of some of the minerals they provide. Your body needs the minerals as much as the vitamins—remember: the two work hand in hand.

THE IMPORTANCE OF ANTIOXIDANT NUTRIENTS | The antioxidant nutrients are the carotenes, vitamins C and E, selenium, and zinc. There is no question that antioxidant nutrients in the diet protect against cancer. What is not yet clear is how aggressive you need to be in taking supplemental amounts of antioxidants. Many scientific studies are under way that should help answer this question, but the results won't be available for several years. From our reading of the available literature, and from our experience with thousands of patients over the past decades, we believe that making sure you get optimal levels of antioxidant nutrients is a key step in the battle against cancer. The levels that we recommend are listed in the recommendations for a high-quality multiple in Appendix A on page 286.

There are three main points to keep in mind when discussing antioxidants:

- The antioxidant system of the body relies on a complex interplay of many different dietary antioxidants.
- Taking any single antioxidant nutrient is not enough. Total protection requires a strategic, comprehensive supplement program.
- Although dietary supplements are important, they cannot replace the importance of consuming a diet rich in antioxidants.

Clinical trials utilizing antioxidant vitamins have produced inconsistent results.[1,2] While the scientific research is quite clear that diets high in antioxidants are protective against many cancers, the evidence is not as solid with antioxidant supplements. Several explanations have been offered, including the focus on a single antioxidant rather than a more complete formulation; inadequate dosages; and failure to address confounding dietary and lifestyle habits (antioxidant supplements are likely to offer less benefit to people who do not consume adequate levels of phytochemicals or who engage in harmful habits such as smoking or drinking excessively).

THE PROBLEM OF SINGLE-NUTRIENT ASSESSMENT | A shortcoming of many dietary studies is that researchers often focus on the effects of just one factor. In a way, this is like judging an entire symphony by listening to a single trombone. Such research has its value, but it's not complete and often raises more questions than it answers. It seems that many researchers become too focused on the tree instead of looking at the forest, because they fail to understand the importance of the way individual antioxidants interact within the entire antioxidant system of the human body to produce their anticancer benefits.

Another issue is that not all antioxidants are created equal. When it comes to mopping up free radicals, each may have a somewhat different (and usually very narrow) range of activity. Most, in fact, only do one or two things, but they do those things very well. For example, beta-carotene is an effective quencher of a free radical known as singlet oxygen, but it is virtually powerless against the dozens of other types of free radicals. As a result, it has a very narrow range of benefit and is very susceptible to being damaged itself without additional support.

Most antioxidants require some sort of "partner" antioxidant that allows them to work more efficiently. And scientists have discovered that beta-carotene itself can become damaged if it's used alone (that is, without its partner antioxidants vitamin C, vitamin E, and selenium). Damaged beta-carotene is extremely toxic to the liver, the lining of the arteries, and the lungs. This fact may explain some of the disappointing results from recent beta-carotene studies. These studies showed that synthetic beta-carotene supplements, *given alone,* actually increase the risk of cancer in smokers.[3,4] In contrast, when beta-carotene is given along with vitamin E and selenium, it may reduce cancer deaths (by a significant 13 percent in one study).[3]

Similarly, selenium functions primarily as a component of the antioxidant enzyme glutathione peroxidase. This enzyme works closely with vitamin E to prevent free-radical damage to cell membranes. We believe that some of the studies looking only at vitamin E's ability to reduce cancer and heart disease were faulty because they failed to factor in the critical partnership between selenium and vitamin E.

MULTINUTRIENT SUPPLEMENTATION IS THE BEST APPROACH | Mounting scientific evidence confirms that a combination of antioxidants will provide greater protection than any single nutritional antioxidant. To illustrate this fact, let's take a look at a double-blind trial using a combination of vitamins and minerals with the goal of reducing recurrence of bladder cancer.[5] Although the combination still provided less than the ideal supplement program that we recommend, impressive results were achieved. The 65 patients who had undergone surgical removal of the bladder cancer were randomized to receive either a multivitamin/zinc supplement with RDA concentrations of all components or the RDA multivitamin/zinc supplement plus 40,000 IU vitamin A acetate, 100 mg vitamin B_6, 2000 mg vitamin C, 400 IU vitamin E, and 90 mg zinc per day. During five years of supplementation, tumor recurrence was seen in 80 percent of the RDA vitamin-supplemented group, but in only 40 percent of those receiving the megadose vitamin therapy. The probability of this occurring by chance was extremely small ($P = 0.0011$).

This study provides two very important points. First, the RDA is simply less than ideal in preventing cancer. Second, supplementation of antioxidants and supportive nutrients as a group is more effective than any single antioxidant.

VITAMIN C | Vitamin C is the first and most effective line of antioxidant defense. It's a water-soluble vitamin. That means it dissolves in water, so it does its work in the body's aqueous (watery) environments, both outside and inside cells. Its primary antioxidant partners are vitamin E, selenium, and beta-carotene. These antioxidants are fat-soluble; they dissolve in fat and thus work in other types of cells than vitamin C. Vitamin C is also responsible for regenerating damaged (oxidized) vitamin E in the body.

Vitamin C has several actions that may offer protection against cancer. It protects cellular structures, including DNA, from damage. Vitamin C also helps the body deal with environmental pollution and toxic chemicals, enhances immune function, and inhibits the formation of cancer-causing compounds such as nitrosamines.

A high vitamin C intake has been shown to reduce the risk for virtually all forms of cancer including leukemia, non-Hodgkin's lymphoma, and cancers of the bladder, breast, cervix, colorectum, esophagus, lung, pancreas, prostate, salivary glands, and stomach. Most of this evidence is based on a high vitamin C intake from foods that are also rich in carotenes and other nutrients that protect against cancer, but a few of the studies also looked at the benefits of supplementation by itself.

The use of vitamin C supplementation in the treatment of cancer is discussed in Chapter 7. Popularized by two-time Nobel Prize winner Linus Pauling, vitamin C as a cancer treatment has shown both positive and no effect in clinical trials.[6–12]

VITAMIN E | Vitamin E, also known as alpha-tocopherol, is the most important fat-soluble antioxidant in the human body. Without vitamin E to defend them, your cells—especially their delicate membranes— would suffer severe damage.

As is the case with other dietary antioxidants, population studies (studies conducted on large groups who have certain traits in common) have shown that a high vitamin E intake appears to offer significant protection against cancer.[13,14] More than a dozen such studies have shown that low levels of vitamin E (especially when selenium levels are also low) are associated with an increased risk of certain types of cancer, particularly colon, prostate, breast, and lung cancers.[15] In contrast, higher levels of vitamin E appear to exert considerable immune-enhancing and antitumor effects. Intervention studies (in which patients receive measured doses of vitamin E for treatment or prevention) are now under way to judge vitamin E's effectiveness in preventing breast and prostate cancer.

One of the key anticancer effects of vitamin E may be its positive impact on the immune system. As we age, immune function tends to decline, in part because of the buildup of free-radical damage to the membranes of white blood cells, particularly the type known as T cells. Age-related impairment of T cell function appears to be a factor in many diseases of the elderly, including cancer, arthritis, autoimmune diseases, and infections. Much of the age-related decline in immune function may be related to nutritional factors, including low vitamin E levels.[16] In recent years, several studies have shown that antioxidants (including vitamin E at daily doses between 400 to 800 IU) are crucial for preserving T cell function and thus for keeping the immune system humming.[17,18]

Be sure that the vitamin E that you take is a natural form. Such forms are designated *d-*, as in d-alpha-tocopherol, while synthetic forms are *dl-*, as in dl-alpha-tocopherol. (The letters *d* and *l* indicate mirror images of the vitamin E molecule.) The human body recognizes and responds only to the *d-* form, and several studies indicate that natural forms of vitamin E exert far greater anticancer effects.[19,20] The *dl-* form may actually prevent the *d-* form from entering cell membranes. But you don't need to be a biochemist to take our advice: Use the natural form.

SELENIUM | Selenium, a trace mineral, is a vital ingredient of the antioxidant enzyme glutathione peroxidase. This enzyme works closely with vitamin E and vitamin C to prevent free-radical damage to cell membranes. Selenium supports all components of the immune system. It stimulates white blood cells and thymus function. Selenium deficiency lowers resistance to infection because it impairs the ability of white blood cells and the thymus to fight off invading bacteria and viruses. Low levels of selenium have been linked to a higher risk for virtually all cancers.[21] In contrast, selenium supplementation offers significant protection against several cancers, especially cancers of the lung, colon, prostate, stomach, esophagus, and liver, and it is associated with a 50 percent decreased risk of mortality from cancer.[21,22]

You don't have to have a selenium deficiency to benefit from this important nutrient. One study found that people who had normal selenium concentrations but who took selenium supplements showed a 118 percent increase in the ability of lymphocytes to kill tumor cells. There was also an 82 percent increase in the activity of natural killer cells, so called because of their ability to destroy cancer cells and microorganisms. These benefits were apparently due to the fact that selenium stimulates cells to produce a powerful immune compound called interleukin-2.[23]

Selenium is available in various forms. Inorganic salts such as sodium selenite are less effectively absorbed and are not as biologically active as organic forms. For those reasons, we recommend use of a selenium supplement in the form of either selenomethionine or high-selenium-content yeast.

The human body requires just a small amount of selenium (100 to 200 mcg per day is enough). Don't overdo it; doses of 900 mcg per day taken over a long time can be toxic. Signs and symptoms of selenium toxicity include depression, nervousness, emotional instability, nausea and vomiting, a garlic odor of the breath and sweat, and, in extreme cases, loss of hair and fingernails.

CAROTENES | In the last chapter we told you about the benefit of a "rainbow diet." Pigments known as carotenes are the "warm" colors of that rainbow, responsible for giving foods their red, orange, and yellow hues. All organisms, whether plant or microbe, that survive through photosynthesis—converting sunlight into energy—contain carotenes. Carotenes are fat-soluble and are important for preserving the integrity of cell membranes. Without protection from carotenes, the organism would be destroyed by the oxidative damage that results during the process of photosynthesis.

In humans, carotenes act as antioxidants. Our bodies also convert certain carotenes into vitamin A. These forms of carotene are known as provitamins. Of the over 600 known carotenes, about 30 to 50 are believed to have some degree of vitamin A activity. The most well known are alpha-carotene and beta-carotene. Carotenes that lack vitamin A activity but that still act as powerful antioxidants are lutein, lycopene, and zeaxanthin (Table 3-1).[24,25]

A number of studies have concluded that the higher the intake of dietary carotenes, the lower the rate of lung, skin, uterine, cervix, and gastrointestinal tract cancers.[2,13,14] But can taking supplements (especially beta-carotene supplements) reduce the risk of cancer? Not, apparently, if the beta-carotene is in a synthetic form and if it is given without other supportive antioxidants. The negative effects from trials featuring synthetic all-trans-beta-carotene in smokers were discussed above.[3,4] These studies may have failed to show benefit because the patients were not also given adequate doses of supportive antioxidants, or their failure to show benefit may have been due to the fact that they used the synthetic form of beta-carotene.

Most multiple-vitamin products supply 5000 to 15,000 IU of beta-carotene. If you are consuming a rainbow assortment of carotene-rich foods each day, it is unlikely that you really need to take supplemental

Table 3-1. Carotenes, Vitamin A Activity, and Food Sources

CAROTENE	VITAMIN A ACTIVITY (%)	FOOD SOURCES
Beta-carotene	100	Green plants, carrots, sweet potatoes, squash, spinach, apricots, green peppers
Cryptoxanthin	50–60	Corn, green peppers, persimmons, papayas, lemons, oranges, prunes, apples, apricots, paprika, poultry
Alpha-carotene	50–54	Green plants, carrots, squash, corn, watermelons, green peppers, potatoes, apples, peaches
Gamma-carotene	42–50	Carrots, sweet potatoes, corn, tomatoes, watermelons, apricots
Beta-zeacarotene	20–40	Corn, tomatoes, yeast, cherries
Lycopene	0	Tomatoes, carrots, green peppers, apricots, pink grapefruit
Zeaxanthin	0	Spinach, paprika, corn, fruits
Lutein	0	Green plants, corn, potatoes, spinach, carrots, tomatoes, fruits
Canthaxanthin	0	Mushrooms, trout, crustaceans
Crocetin	0	Saffron
Capsanthin	0	Red peppers, paprika

carotenes for prevention. If you do elect to use additional amounts of carotenes, we recommend using natural mixed carotenes such as palm oil carotene products, mixed carotenes from an alga called *Dunaliella,* carrot oil, and the various "green drinks" on the market, such as dehydrated barley greens or wheat grass. Of these, palm oil appears to be the best, because its carotene complex closely mirrors that found in high-carotene foods. Palm oil carotenes are about 4 to 10 times better absorbed than synthetic all-trans-beta-carotene.

HIGHLIGHT: CAROTENES IN SKIN CANCER PREVENTION | A diet high in carotenes is very important in protecting against skin cancer—the most commonly occurring cancer in the United States. There are three types of skin cancer: basal cell carcinoma, squamous cell carcinoma (together referred to as nonmelanoma skin cancer), and melanoma. The outer layer of the skin is made up of squamous cells. Basal cells are found below the squamous cells. Melanoma develops from melanocytes—pigment-producing cells located in the deepest layer of the skin.

Keys to reducing the risk of skin cancer:

- Reduce exposure to ultraviolet (UV) radiation. Ultraviolet radiation is invisible high-energy rays that come from the sun and from artificial sources such as tanning booths and sunlamps. Wear protective clothing when exposed to sunlight, and adequate amounts of sufficiently protective sunscreen.
- Follow the dietary and supplement recommendations given in this book, emphasizing a high intake of carotene-rich foods—especially if you have a tendency to sunburn.

FOLIC ACID | Folic acid is a member of the B vitamin family that plays a vital role in many body processes including the formation of normal DNA. A deficiency of folic acid is thought to contribute to cancer by leading to DNA abnormalities, inappropriate activation of proto-oncogenes, and induction of the transformation of normal cells into cancerous ones.[26]

Folic acid functions along with vitamin B_{12} and B_6 and a form of the amino acid methionine known as SAM (S-adenosyl-methionine) in reducing body concentrations of a damaging compound known as homocysteine—an intermediate in the conversion of the amino acid methionine to cysteine. If a person is relatively deficient in folic acid, there will be an increase in homocysteine. This compound has been implicated in a variety of conditions, including atherosclerosis and osteoporosis. There is emerging evidence that elevated homocysteine levels or low folic acid status also plays a role in many cancers, particularly cervical, colon, lung, and breast cancers.[27–29] Long-term folic acid supplementation has been shown to reduce the risk of colon cancer by 75 percent[30] and may produce equally impressive results for other cancers.

VITAMIN D | Since vitamin D can be produced in our bodies by the action of sunlight on the skin, many experts consider it more of a hormone than a vitamin. Nonetheless, by current definitions vitamin D is both a vitamin and a hormone. Vitamin D is best known for its ability to stimulate the absorption of calcium, but it is also showing great promise in the prevention of cancer via additional mechanisms. There is emerging evidence that vitamin D levels are very important in fighting against the development of colon, breast, and prostate cancers.[31]

Colon, breast, and prostate cancer rates are generally higher in regions where winter sunlight is reduced because of a combination of high or moderately high latitude, high-sulfur-content air pollution (acid haze), higher-than-average stratospheric ozone thickness, and persistently thick winter cloud cover. Experimental studies have shown that vitamin D interacts with the hormonal system of the body in the control of cancer development and proliferation, and apoptosis in colon, breast, and prostate cells.[31-33]

The RDA for vitamin D is 200 to 400 IU daily. For adults not exposed to sunlight or living in the northern latitudes, a daily intake of 400 to 800 IU seems reasonable. Since vitamin D is fat-soluble and can build up in the body, it does have the potential to cause toxicity. Dosages greater than 800 IU per day are certainly not recommended. Toxicity is characterized by increased blood concentration of calcium (a potentially serious situation), excessive accumulation of calcium into internal organs, and kidney stones.

2. Take an appropriate herbal extract rich in flavonoids

A group of plant pigments known as flavonoids exert antioxidant activity that is generally more potent and effective against a broader range of oxidants than the traditional antioxidant nutrients vitamins C and E, beta-carotene, selenium, and zinc.[34] Besides lending color to fruits and flowers, flavonoids are responsible for many of the medicinal properties of foods, juices, herbs, and bee pollen. More than 8,000 flavonoid compounds have been characterized and classified according to their chemical structure. Flavonoids are sometimes called "nature's biological response modifiers" because of their anti-inflammatory, antiallergic, antiviral, and anticancer properties.[35-37]

Certain flavonoids have been studied extensively for their anticancer properties. Of these, quercetin and green tea extract are among our key recommendations for fighting existing cancer.

Flavonoids are sometimes considered "semi-essential" nutrients, but in our view they are as important to human nutrition as the so-called essential nutrients. Because they have a broader range of antioxidant activity as well as other important anticancer effects, we recommend taking flavonoid-rich extract or supplemental doses of specific flavonoids. Doing so will provide extra insurance that your body can mop up any type of free radical or oxidant that escapes the other protective systems.

Because certain flavonoids concentrate in specific tissues, it is possible to take flavonoids that target specific conditions. For example, one of the most beneficial group of tissue-specific plant flavonoids is the proanthocyanidins (also referred to as procyanidins). These molecules are found in high concentrations (up to 95 percent) in grape seed and pine bark extracts. We recommend grape seed extract for most people under the age of 50 for general antioxidant support, as it appears to be especially useful in protecting against heart disease. For those over 50, Ginkgo biloba extract is generally the best choice. If there is a strong family history of cancer, however, the best choice is clearly green tea extract (see page 63). In Appendix A you can identify which flavonoid or flavonoid-rich extract is most appropriate for you, and take it according to the recommended dosage. There is tremendous overlap among the mechanisms of action and the benefits of flavonoid-rich extracts, so the key point here is to take the one that is most specific to your personal needs.

In one of the more interesting human studies of flavonoids in cancer, Ginkgo biloba extract was shown to reduce the levels of substances known as clastogenic factors in Chernobyl accident workers.[38] Clastogenic factors are found in the blood of persons irradiated accidentally or therapeutically and are associated with increased tendency to form cancers. In the study, 30 workers with elevated clastogenic factors were treated with Ginkgo biloba extract at a daily dose of one 40 mg tablet three times daily for 2 months. The clastogenic activity of the plasma was reduced to normal levels within the time span of the study. A 1-year follow-up showed that the benefit of the treatment persisted for at least 7 months. One-third of the workers again had clastogenic factors after 1 year, demonstrating that the process that produced clastogenic factors continued. Although this observation that Ginkgo biloba extract did not have to be given continuously is encouraging, we believe that continued use offers the greatest benefit. Given the ever-increasing radiation load associated with modern living, it certainly seems important to protect against this cancer-causing potential by taking a flavonoid-rich extract like Ginkgo biloba extract or any of the other extracts listed on page 287.

3. Consume green drinks regularly

The term *green drinks* refers to green tea and a number of commercially available products containing dehydrated barley grass, wheat grass, or algae sources such as chlorella or spirulina. Such formulas are rehydrated by mixing with water or juice. Some of the more popular brands are Enriching Greens, Green Magma, Kyo-Green, Greens +, Barlean's Greens, and ProGreens. These products—packed full of phytochemicals, especially carotenes and chlorophyll—are more convenient than trying to sprout and grow your own source of greens. An added advantage is that they tend to taste better than, for example, straight wheat grass juice.

Green foods such as young barley grass, wheat grass, spirulina, and chlorella are exceptionally high in nutritional value. Using any of the popular brands listed above results in a more concentrated and convenient source of phytochemicals than eating two cups of a well-rounded salad. We recommend drinking one to two servings daily in addition to eating a diet rich in phytochemicals. Try to consume these drinks 20 minutes before or two hours following a meal.

The green foods are particularly rich in natural fat-soluble chlorophyll—the green pigment that converts sunlight to chemical energy in plants, algae, and some microorganisms. Like the other plant pigments, chlorophyll also possesses significant antioxidant and anticancer effects. It has been suggested that chlorophyll be added to certain beverages,

Warning

Green tea, other green drinks, and some other natural products (see page 274) can interfere with the blood thinner coumadin (Warfarin). This drug blocks blood clotting in part by interfering with the actions of vitamin K. Since green drinks are a good source of vitamin K, they may reduce the effectiveness of coumadin. However, coumadin can effectively be used even if you drink green tea, as long as the quantities you drink remain constant from day to day. The standard blood tests done when you are taking coumadin will show any effects from the extra vitamin K contained in green tea or other green drinks, and your doctor can simply adjust the coumadin dose to compensate.

foods, chewing tobacco, and tobacco snuff to reduce cancer risk. A better recommendation would be to include green drinks and fresh green vegetable juices regularly in the diet.

Both green tea and black tea are derived from the same plant, *Camellia sinensis*. Of the nearly 2.5 million tons of dried tea produced each year, only 20 percent is green tea. In other words, four times as much black tea is produced and consumed than green tea. But green tea is healthier for you, because it contains compounds called polyphenols that have high levels of therapeutic activity, including anticancer activity.

The difference between green and black teas results from the manufacturing process. To produce black tea, the leaves are allowed to oxidize. During oxidation, enzymes present in the tea convert polyphenols into substances with much less biological activity. In contrast, green tea is produced by lightly steaming the fresh-cut leaf. Steaming prevents the enzymes from converting polyphenols, so oxidation does not take place.

The major polyphenols in green tea are flavonoids, the most active of which is epigallocatechin gallate. In addition to serving as antioxidants, green tea polyphenols may increase the activity of antioxidant enzymes in the small intestine, liver, and lungs. A number of experiments conducted in test tube and animal cancer models have shown that green tea polyphenols inhibit cancer by blocking the formation of cancer-causing compounds such as nitrosamines, suppressing the activation of carcinogens, and detoxifying or trapping cancer-causing agents. The forms of cancer that appear to be best prevented by green tea are cancers of the gastrointestinal tract, including cancers of the stomach, small intestine, pancreas, and colon; lung cancer; estrogen-related cancers, including most breast cancers; and prostate cancer.[39,40] Although important in fighting all these cancers, it is especially important in preventing breast and prostate cancers.[41-43]

Green tea can be consumed as a beverage made from either loose green tea leaves or tea bags. Green tea extracts concentrated to contain 70 to 99 percent polyphenol content are available commercially in capsules or tablets.

Studies have suggested that cancer rates are lower in Japan in part because people there typically drink about three cups of green tea daily. At this rate they consume about 3 g of soluble components, which yields a daily dose of roughly 240 to 320 mg of polyphenols. To achieve the same degree of protection from pills containing green tea extract standardized for 80 percent total polyphenol content would mean taking a daily dose of 300 to 400 mg.

Some green teas contain caffeine. Drinking three cups provides about the same dose of caffeine as one cup of coffee. Drinking green tea or taking caffeine-containing extract may be overstimulating, leading to such symptoms as nervousness, anxiety, insomnia, and irritability. Fortunately, decaffeinated green teas and decaffeinated green tea extracts are now widely available. If you have a family or personal history of cancer, then we recommend using green tea extract as your "tissue-specific" flavonoid. If not, then we simply recommend the regular consumption of green tea.

4. Take probiotics

The term *probiotics* literally means "for life." Probiotics are friendly microflora (bacteria and other organisms) that are vital to our health. Normally at least 400 different species of these little critters colonize the human gastrointestinal tract. The most important healthful bacteria are *Lactobacillus acidophilus* and *Bifidobacterium bifidum*.

Probiotics play a vital role in determining how we absorb the nutrients from the food we eat. They are also involved in maintaining immune system function, regulating cholesterol metabolism, and processing toxin loads. They may hold the key to preventing many forms of cancer, both within the intestinal tract and in other tissues, such as breast, lung, and prostate cancers.

Several studies have suggested that the consumption of high levels of cultured milk products, such as yogurt and buttermilk, may reduce the risk of colon cancer.[44,45] That's because these products contain high levels of lactobacilli. The beneficial effects of lactobacilli extend well beyond the colon, however. Various probiotic species have demonstrated immune-enhancing and antitumor effects, but they also play a critical role in the detoxification of many cancer-causing substances including hormones, meat carcinogens, and environmental toxins.

One of the key ways in which the body gets rid of "bad" substances, such as excess estrogen and fat-soluble toxins, is by attaching them to a molecule called glucuronic acid and then excreting this complex in the bile. But the bond between the "bad" molecule and its escort can be broken by glucuronidase, an enzyme secreted by certain types of undesirable bacteria in the intestinal tract. Excess glucuronidase activity means more of the "bad" molecules are present in the body. This, in turn, is associated with an increased cancer risk, particularly the risk of estrogen-dependent breast cancer. Glucuronidase activity is higher in people who eat a diet high in fat and low in fiber. The level of glucuronidase activity may be one of the key underlying factors explaining why certain dietary factors cause breast cancer and why other dietary factors are preventive.

The activity of harmful bacterial enzymes can be reduced by making sure your digestive system maintains the proper balance of bacterial flora. One way to do so is by eating foods known to reduce glucuronidase activity, including onions and garlic, and foods that are high in glucuronic acid, such as apples, Brussels sprouts, broccoli, cabbage, and lettuce. Another strategy is to supplement the diet with the "friendly bacteria" *Lactobacillus acidophilus* and *Bifidobacterium bifidum.*

There is clinical evidence of a significant protective effect against cancer with probiotic supplementation. In a double-blind trial conducted in 138 patients surgically treated for bladder cancer, patients were divided into three groups: (A) those with multiple primary tumors, (B) those with recurrent single tumors, and (C) those with recurrent multiple tumors. In each of these groups, patients were randomly allocated to receive an oral lactobacillus preparation or placebo. The lactobacillus preparation was better than the placebo in preventing cancer recurrences in groups A and B. No significant effect was noted in group C, however.[46]

Lactobacillus preparations are available in powder, liquid, capsule, and tablet forms. Proper manufacturing, packaging, and storing of the product are necessary to ensure viability, the right amount of moisture, and freedom from contamination. We prefer products that have been "enteric-coated" to prevent the capsule from breaking down in the stomach, thereby increasing the delivery of the organisms to the small and large intestines. Examples of enteric-coated products are Protec (Natural Factors), JarroDophilus EPS (Jarrow), and PrimaDophilus (Nature's Way).

The dosage is based on the number of live organisms. The ingestion of 4 to 10 billion viable lactobacillus and bifidobacteria cells daily is a sufficient dosage for most people. Amounts exceeding this may induce mild gastrointestinal disturbances, while smaller amounts may not be able to colonize the gastrointestinal tract.

A new probiotic product called Innersync Plus may prove even more beneficial than other probiotics. Rather than supply only lactobacillus or bifidobacteria, Innersync Plus also provides the bacterium *Propionibacterium freudenrichii,* historically used in the production of Emmenthal Swiss cheese. This bacteria has been shown to dramatically increase the growth of the beneficial bacteria like lactobacillus or bifidobacteria in human studies while exerting some beneficial actions of its own, including enhanced immune function and protection against colon cancer.[47,48] The dosage for Innersync Plus is one to two capsules (i.e., 5 to 10 billion organisms) daily—equal to approximately 100 to 200 g (3.5 to 7 oz) of Emmenthal Swiss cheese, but without the fat and calories.

5. Take fish oil supplements

The benefits of the omega-3 oils from fish oils were described on page (40). Adding a fish oil supplement to your daily routine provides extra insurance that you are getting sufficient levels of these important oils. Take enough capsules to provide 120 to 360 mg of EPA and 80 to 240 mg of DHA daily. We prefer the fish oils to flaxseed oil, because although the body can convert alpha-linolenic acid from flaxseed oil into the more potent molecules of EPA and DHA, it is much more efficient to use fish oils. All told, about sixty different health conditions have been benefited by fish oil supplementation, including cancer, heart disease, rheumatoid arthritis and other autoimmune diseases, psoriasis, eczema, asthma, attention deficit disorder, and depression.[49]

When selecting a fish oil supplement, it is essential to use a brand that you trust. Quality control is an absolute must to ensure the product is free from heavy metals like lead and mercury, pesticides, damaged fats (lipid peroxides), and other contaminants. Three brands of fish oil products that we recommend are Natural Factors, Enzymatic Therapy, and Nordic Naturals. All three are widely available at your local health food store.

Chapter Four

Special Steps for Preventing Lung, Breast, Prostate, and Colon Cancer

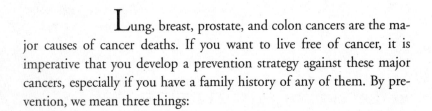

Lung, breast, prostate, and colon cancers are the major causes of cancer deaths. If you want to live free of cancer, it is imperative that you develop a prevention strategy against these major cancers, especially if you have a family history of any of them. By prevention, we mean three things:

- Stopping your body's cells from becoming damaged in the first place
- Keeping any microscopic cancer cells that do appear from progressing to life-threatening tumors
- Getting an accurate diagnosis early enough in the course of the disease to give yourself the best chance of a complete recovery

Lung Cancer

Lung cancer kills more Americans each year than any other form of cancer. In 2001, an estimated 150,000 people in this country died from the disease, representing more than one-fourth of all cancer-related deaths. Each year, 14 percent of new cancer cases involve lung cancer. This is tragic, because lung cancer is the most easily preventable form of the disease.

Risk Factors

The epidemic of lung cancer over the last 100 years is due largely to tobacco use. There is no longer any debate about the issue: Smoking causes lung cancer. For every 100 cases of lung cancer, 90 of them result from smoking. This is true whether you're talking about using cigarettes, cigars, or pipes. Even exposure to smoke in the air—so-called environmental tobacco smoke or secondhand smoke—causes cancer.

The best way to prevent the disease? Simple: Don't smoke. If you do smoke, do everything you can to stop.

But what about the 10 percent of lung cancers that develop in people who don't smoke? What causes them? The main culprits appear to be two carcinogenic (cancer-causing) substances, radon and asbestos.

Radon is a gas that results when molecules of uranium and radium decay. Invisible and odorless, radon can seep into houses. The Environmental Protection Agency estimates that about 1 out of 15 homes in the United States has an unsafe level of radon. Many schools and businesses may also be affected. Each year, approximately 15,000 cases of lung cancer result from radon exposure.

Asbestos is a naturally occurring mineral complex that was once considered a miracle product because of its unique qualities. Specifically, its fibers can be woven into lightweight, fire-resistant, and extremely strong materials. Asbestos was widely used for insulation in homes and office buildings until 1989, when it was banned by the Environmental Protection Agency because of its cancer-causing effects. Asbestos was also common in shipbuilding and brake repair. Asbestos fibers break easily into particles that can float in the air and stick to clothes. Inhaled particles lodge in the lungs, damaging cells and triggering the development of cancer. Workers who have been exposed to asbestos, including those involved in its mining and manufacture, have 3 to 4 times the risk of lung cancer. The risk is even higher among asbestos workers who also smoke.

Detecting Lung Cancer

In the early stages, lung cancer causes no symptoms, so the best method for detecting it is regular yearly exams by your physician. See a physician immediately if you have any of the following common signs and symptoms:

- A cough that doesn't go away and gets worse over time
- Constant chest pain
- Coughing up blood
- Shortness of breath, wheezing, or hoarseness
- Repeated problems with pneumonia or bronchitis
- Swelling of the neck and face
- Loss of appetite or weight loss
- Fatigue

Since a number of respiratory diseases cause similar symptoms, your doctor will take specific steps to determine what's causing the problem. You'll be asked questions about your medical history, smoking history, and possible exposure to environmental carcinogens. The doctor will also perform a physical exam and may order a chest x-ray and other tests. Even more sensitive than a chest x-ray in detecting lung cancer at an earlier stage is a spiral computed tomography (CT) scan. The earlier cancer is found, the greater the chances for a cure. If you are at high risk for lung cancer, talk to your doctor about whether a spiral CT scan is an appropriate option.[1]

If lung cancer is suspected, your doctor will order a lab test to study cells found in a sample of mucus from your lungs. If the results of this test (known as sputum cytology) are positive, you'll probably be asked to undergo a lung biopsy. A small sample of tissue will be removed for study under the microscope by a pathologist trained in analyzing tumors.

Smoking

Here's the good news: If you quit smoking now, it's possible for you to reduce your risk of lung cancer to the same level as that in people who never smoked. Studies have found that ten years after quitting, an ex-smoker's risk of dying from lung cancer is 30 to 50 percent less than the risk for those who continue to smoke. After fifteen years, an ex-smoker's risk is almost the same as that of a person who never smoked. Quitting smoking also reduces the risk for developing heart disease, emphysema, and cancers elsewhere in the body. You'll live longer, and you'll live better.

As physicians, we know that stopping smoking is not easy. We've seen many of our patients struggle to meet the challenge. There is no magic formula, but it can be done. You may need several tries before you hit on the right strategy for you. Some of the natural approaches to support your effort to quit may help you.

According to several published studies, for many people the best strategy for quitting smoking may be to just stop—to go "cold turkey." Nicotine-replacement therapy (using gum, a skin patch, or an inhaled form) is effective for about 13 percent of people who try it. Behavioral modification (rewards and punishments) works for about two people in every hundred. Acupuncture is only slightly better. Some people have been able to quit following hypnosis. Sad to say, in our experience, the most successful aid to smoking cessation is hearing a doctor say, "You have lung cancer."

It is especially important to reduce smoking among youths, because younger lung tissue appears to be more sensitive to the cancer-causing effects of tobacco smoke. We also know that preventing teens from smoking reduces their risk of becoming smokers later in life.

Diet

Environmental poisons cause lung cancer, and some people may be genetically vulnerable to these poisons. But your diet may be the key to whether you get cancer. If two people with the same protective genes are exposed to the same level of pollutants, the one who follows a cancer-protective diet has a lower risk than the one who eats junk food every day.

Here's an example. The rate of smoking among the Japanese is much higher than the rate in the United States, yet the Japanese have a lower incidence of lung cancer. Research suggests that it's because they have more of the dietary factors that protect against cancer: a higher intake of soy, green tea, and fish and a lower intake of dairy products and red meat.[2,3]

The guidelines in Chapters 2 and 3 will help you with an effective lung cancer–prevention diet and supplement program. But there are some areas that you should try to put even more focus on. For example, as mentioned previously, one way to protect the body against toxins from smoke and pollution is to increase the intake of curries. Curry dishes get much of their flavor from a spice, turmeric. Turmeric's distinctive yellow color comes from a pigment called curcumin. In the body, curcumin acts as an antioxidant and also aids in detoxification reactions. When you smoke or are exposed to secondhand smoke, cancer-causing compounds are taken in by the body, metabolized, and eliminated through the urine. Adding turmeric to the diet helps the body to neutralize these toxic compounds more efficiently. It's as much as 300 times more effective than vitamin E. Curcumin also possesses other significant anticancer effects, as we'll discuss in Chapter 8.

Supplemental Support

Curry dishes are a delicious way to get healthy doses of curcumin. It's also available as a natural supplement. The recommended dose is 200 to 400 mg daily. An alternative supplement for lung cancer protection is to take quercetin (200 to 400 mg daily). Flavonoids like quercetin and those found in green tea reduce the risk of lung cancer. A study published in the *Journal of the National Cancer Institute* looked at the diets of nearly 600 people living in Hawaii who had lung cancer and compared them with diets in a matched group without cancer.[4] The researchers discovered that people who ate the most apples, white grapefruit, and onions—foods especially rich in quercetin—were 40 to 50 percent less likely to develop lung cancer.

Fish Oils

Given the significant protection against lung cancer of the omega-3 fatty acids from fish consumption,[2,5] we recommend, in addition to eating at least two servings of cold-water fish per week, taking enough cap-

> ## Warning
>
> Smokers should not supplement their diet with *synthetic* beta-carotene unless they also take a multivitamin containing the other key antioxidant nutrients: vitamins C and E and selenium. Taking synthetic beta-carotene alone and continuing to smoke may increase your risk of lung cancer. The best strategy to get the protection of carotenes against lung cancer for smokers is to increase the intake of natural carotenes from food sources.

sules of a fish oil product to provide 120 to 360 mg of EPA and 80 to 240 mg of DHA daily for anyone at risk for lung cancer.

SELENIUM | A long-term cancer prevention trial studied more than 1,300 patients with skin cancer and found that selenium appeared to reduce the rate at which new skin tumors formed. The results were exciting, because they showed that simply adding a nutritional supplement to a normal diet could prevent cancer.

But what about other cancers? To find out, the researchers expanded their study, to that "gold standard" of scientific research: It was a randomized, double-blind study, which means neither patients nor doctors know who is receiving the intervention. This minimizes the chances of a significant placebo effect. Patients took a tablet containing either 200 mcg of selenium or a placebo daily for four-and-a-half years and were followed for an additional six-and-a-half years.[6]

The outcome was so positive that the researchers stopped the trial two years sooner than planned. The overall cancer rate was significantly lower in the selenium group than in the placebo group (77 cases versus 119). The selenium group had fewer lung cancers (17 versus 31), fewer colorectal cancers (8 versus 19), and fewer prostate cancers (13 versus 35).

The results also showed that the death rate from cancer was 50 percent less in the selenium-treated group than the control group (29 versus 57). Lung cancer deaths were lower in the selenium-treatment group than in the placebo group (12 versus 26). There was no significant difference between the two groups for other causes of death.

Clearly, selenium is a valuable part of the cancer-prevention strategy. As noted in Chapter 3, we recommend taking a vitamin and mineral supplement that gives you 100 to 200 mcg of selenium per day. In order to fully realize the benefit of any single antioxidant like selenium, it is important that it be taken with the other important antioxidant nutrients.

Breast Cancer

For many women, breast cancer is the disease they fear most. The frightening statistic is that about one in seven or eight women will develop breast cancer in their lifetime. Fortunately, there are many effective strategies that can help reduce your risk. One is to know the factors that can contribute to the disease. Of course, lifestyle and diet are among the biggest factors that determine your risk of breast cancer. Here is a quick guide to the important risk factors.

Risk Factors

Age: The risk of breast cancer increases as a woman gets older. Breast cancer is uncommon in women under age 35. Most breast cancers occur in women over the age of 50, and the risk is especially high for women over 60.

Race: Breast cancer occurs more often in white women than among blacks, Hispanics, or Asian women.

Family history: A woman's risk for developing breast cancer increases if her mother, sister, or daughter had breast cancer, especially at a young age.

Genetics: The presence of certain genes increases the risk of breast cancer, although this is mainly true if most or all of the women in your family have actually developed breast or ovarian cancer. Women of Ashkenazi (central and eastern European) Jewish ancestry tend to have a higher-than-average rate of breast cancer.

Estrogen: The female hormone estrogen stimulates breast cells. The longer a woman is exposed to estrogen in any form (made by the body, taken as a drug, or delivered by a patch), the more likely she is to develop breast cancer. For example, risk is higher among women who began menstruation at an early age (before age 12), experienced menopause late (after age 55), never had children, or took hormone replacement therapy for long periods of time.

Later childbearing: Women who have their first child after about age 30 have a greater chance of developing breast cancer than women who have a child at a younger age. The most protection comes from childbirth followed by breast-feeding enough to suppress the return of ovulation.

Breast density: Breast cancers nearly always develop in dense tissue (lobes and ducts), not in fatty tissue. That's why cancer is more likely to occur in women who have "dense" breasts than in those with "fatty" ones. Complicating the picture is that abnormal areas in dense breasts are harder to detect on a mammogram.

Environment: Among the factors that have been linked to breast cancer in varying degrees are exposure to xenoestrogens (synthetic compounds that mimic estrogen), secondhand smoke, pesticides, herbicides, power lines, electric blankets, radiation, and lack of exposure to sunlight.

Exercise: Taking into account other established risk factors for breast cancer, women who regularly exercise have up to a 60 percent reduction in the risk of breast cancer compared with women with low levels of activity.

Alcohol consumption: Women who drink one drink a day have a 10 percent greater risk; those who drink two drinks have a 20 percent increased risk, and so on.

Smoking: As with most other cancers, cigarette smoking increases the risk of developing breast cancer.

Diet: Important dietary factors include body weight (the more overweight you are, the greater the risk); increased intake of saturated fat; and decreased intakes of antioxidants, dietary fiber, omega-3 fatty acids (particularly alpha-linolenic acid), and dietary phytoestrogens (estrogen-like compounds found in foods such as legumes, nuts, and seeds).

Detecting Breast Cancer

Early detection of breast cancer improves the likelihood of preventing it from progressing to a life-threatening condition. The earlier it can be detected, the better. Monthly breast self-exams are important steps toward this goal. But mammography (a special type of breast x-ray) can detect breast cancer long before it can be felt. Most medical doctors, as well as the National Cancer Institute, recommend that women age 40 and older have mammograms every 1 to 2 years.

Recently, however, this practice of routine mammography has come under fire. An increasing number of studies suggest that for women under 50 who have not yet gone through menopause, screening mammograms may not be necessary.[7] According to many experts in the field, screening mammograms don't work very well for these women because:

- They have a high rate of false negatives (results that show no cancer when in fact cancer is present). The dense, healthy breast tissue of younger women can obscure tumors. Routine mammograms miss approximately 40 percent of the breast cancers that develop among women ages 40 to 49.
- Mammograms expose women to radiation that may cause breast cancer. With modern mammography equipment the risk is small (no more than 1 in 2,700). On the downside, the risk is cumulative, meaning that the chances increase with each subsequent mammogram.
- Screening mammography has not always been shown to increase the chances that premenopausal women will survive breast cancer, even though it's been detected.
- In women over the age of 50, it appears that mammography is best used to evaluate suspicious lumps rather than screen for cancer (that is, to look for cancers when there is no sign the woman might have the disease). Results from a major study, The Canadian National Breast Screening Study-2, involving nearly 40,000 women, showed that yearly mammograms in women 50 to 59 years old did not lower breast cancer mortality compared with yearly physical examination alone. The authors of the study concluded that for women older than 50, thorough annual physical breast examinations, plus teaching of breast self-examination, may be a valid alternative to yearly mammography.[8]

Prophylactic Mastectomy?

A highly publicized report in the *New England Journal of Medicine* in early 1999 on the value of prophylactic mastectomy in women with a family history of breast cancer raises many interesting questions.[9] The retrospective study consisted of all women with a family history of

> ## Important
>
> The debate about the value of regular mammograms has been heating up in recent years. Many women, understandably, are confused. Before deciding on your approach to breast care, be sure you speak with your primary caregiver, gynecologist, or other qualified health expert. Be sure to discuss your family history, lifestyle, and other issues to be sure you get advice that's right for you. In our clinical practice we have seen numerous women who discovered during an annual mammogram breast cancer too small to feel with a self breast-exam. If a woman is at extremely low risk for breast cancer, it may make sense to get mammograms every 2 to 3 years instead of annually to reduce the risk of radiation. If a woman has significant risk for breast cancer because of family history of breast or ovarian cancer, however, then annual mammograms probably still make sense at this time.

breast cancer who underwent bilateral (both breasts) prophylactic mastectomy at the Mayo Clinic between 1960 and 1993. The women were divided into two groups—high risk and moderate risk—on the basis of family history. A control study of the sisters of the high-risk women was used to predict the number of breast cancers expected in these two groups if they did not receive a prophylactic mastectomy. The researchers identified 639 women with a family history of breast cancer who had undergone prophylactic mastectomy of both breasts: 214 at high risk and 425 at moderate risk. The median length of follow-up was 14 years. The median age at prophylactic mastectomy was 42 years. According to the Gail model, 37.4 breast cancers were expected in the moderate-risk group, but only 4 breast cancers occurred. This difference correlated to an 89.5 percent reduction in risk. In high-risk women, breast cancer was diagnosed in 1.4 percent (3 of 214) of the high-risk women who elected to have a mastectomy. In contrast, 38.7 percent of their 403 sisters were diagnosed with breast cancer (115 cases were diagnosed before the respective sister's prophylactic mastectomy, 38 were diagnosed afterward, and the time of the diagnosis was unknown in 3 cases). What all of these results indicate is that a prophylactic mastectomy was associated with a reduction in the incidence of breast cancer of at least 90 percent in these high-risk women.

Given the growing number of women who will now have a family history of breast cancer, do these results indicate that prophylactic mastectomy should be the primary preventive measure for these women? It is hard to argue against the numbers, but prophylactic mastectomy seems to be a very aggressive preventive measure. Instead, the focus should be on diet and lifestyle. In fact, it is estimated that dietary interventions alone could reduce the risk for breast cancer by at least 80 percent, which is pretty close to the level produced with prophylactic mastectomy.

The Night Shift–Melatonin–
Breast Cancer Connection

Several studies have shown quite dramatically that women working the so-called graveyard shift have an increased risk of developing breast cancer.[10,11] In fact, in one study graveyard shift work was associated with a 60 percent increased breast cancer risk.[10] The risk seems to be related to how much time was spent on the job.

The explanation given for this link is that exposure to light at night appears to increase the risk of breast cancer by suppressing the normal nighttime production of melatonin—a hormone secreted by the pineal gland (a small pea-sized gland at the base of the brain). The exact function of melatonin is still poorly understood, but it is critically involved in regulating the natural biorhythm of hormone secretion referred to as the circadian rhythm. Melatonin exerts significant anticancer effects and is described in more detail in Chapter 13.

Release of melatonin is stimulated by darkness and suppressed by light. Nighttime exposure to bright light therefore suppresses melatonin manufacture and secretion. To offset the increased risk of breast cancer with night shift work, we recommend taking 3 mg of melatonin at bedtime for night shift workers (regardless of when that bedtime might be).

Breast Is Best

There's a special lifestyle factor that appears to offer some protection against breast cancer: breast-feeding. Several studies have shown that women who breast-feed their infants for at least three months have a lower incidence of breast cancer.[12] This may be because breast-feeding causes estrogen levels to fall, delaying ovulation so the new mother won't get pregnant again too soon. Since estrogen is a known risk factor, any reduction in total estrogen exposure over the course of a lifetime reduces the risk of breast cancer.

Of course, breast-feeding does the baby a lot of good too. Besides offering wholesome natural nutrition, babies who are breast-fed have fewer and less severe illnesses; they are less likely to have diarrhea, lower respiratory infections, ear infections, and bacterial meningitis. Some research indicates that breast-feeding may also protect against sudden infant death syndrome, allergic diseases, and chronic digestive diseases.

Diet

Diet is one of the critical factors in the prevention of breast cancer. The research on diet and breast cancer is a bit muddy, because investigators often look only to dietary factors in the United States. For example, let's take a look at the research on saturated fats and breast cancer. It is difficult to determine true risk when looking at women in the United States, because the lowest percentile for saturated fat intake in the United States often translates to the highest percentile in other countries. To gauge all dietary risk factors in breast cancer, it is extremely important to examine data from a global perspective. In an extensive multinational population study, investigators explored diets from around the world to determine the components that most affect breast cancer risk.[13] The information

Table 4-1. Dietary Factors in Breast Cancer

FACTORS THAT MAY INCREASE RISK	FACTORS THAT MAY LOWER RISK
Meats	Fish
Total fat	Whole grains
Saturated fats	Soy and other legumes
Dairy	Cabbage
Refined sugar	Vegetables
Total calories	Nuts
Alcohol	Fruits

collected provides much more valuable insight into dietary factors and breast cancer. Table 4-1 lists these factors in order of importance.[13]

One of the most interesting aspects of the population study was the tremendous protective effect of fish consumption. Fish—particularly cold-water fish such as salmon, mackerel, halibut, and herring—is a rich source of the omega-3 fatty acids. As described in Chapter 2 and elsewhere, this group of fats is very useful in fighting against cancer, especially breast cancer. In contrast, the omega-6 fatty acids found in most animal products—as well as in common vegetable oils such as corn, safflower, and soy—are associated with promoting breast cancer.

THE MOST IMPORTANT FOODS TO AVOID: MEATS GRILLED OR BROILED AT HIGH TEMPERATURES | It may not be simply that meat intake is associated with breast cancer. What may eventually be shown is that the manner in which the meat is prepared determines whether it is carcinogenic. When broiled or grilled at high temperatures, meat forms many potent carcinogens, including toxic lipid peroxides (especially those from alpha-linolenic acid) and heterocyclic amines. These compounds are extremely harmful to breast tissue.

Researchers from the University of South Carolina gave questionnaires to 273 women who were diagnosed with breast cancer between 1992 and 1994 as well as 657 women who were cancer-free. They found that women who routinely ate three meats—hamburger, beefsteak, and bacon—very well done had a 462 percent greater chance of developing breast cancer. Women who regularly consumed these meats individually had lower increases in risk for breast cancer. The risk for very well done versus rare or medium was 50 to 70 percent greater for hamburger and bacon, and 220 percent greater for beefsteak. These results, coupled with other evidence, suggest that avoiding well-done meats can dramatically reduce breast cancer risk.[14]

THE MOST IMPORTANT FOODS TO EAT: FISH, FLAXSEED, AND FLAXSEED OIL | The omega-3 fatty acids from fish have shown tremendous effects against breast cancer in experimental and population-based studies.[15,16] In contrast, the omega-6 fatty acids found in most animal products—as well as in common vegetable oils such as corn, safflower, and soy—are associated with promoting breast cancer in experimental studies.[17] The protective effect of fish intake against breast cancer was thought to be due primarily to its high omega-3 fatty-acid levels.

In addition to a diet that features fish, eating ground flaxseed and supplementing the diet with flaxseed oil appear to offer significant protection against breast cancer for a couple of different reasons. First of all, flaxseed oil contains nearly twice the level of omega-3 fatty acids as fish oils, although it is the smaller-chain alpha-linolenic acid rather than the longer-chain fats like EPA and DHA. Data derived from biopsies of adipose breast tissue at the time of diagnosis from women with breast cancer compared with benign breast disease indicated that the relative risk of breast cancer for women in the highest breast tissue level of alpha-linolenic acid level was 64 percent less compared with those in the lowest level.[18] In another study, the higher the level of alpha-linolenic acid in breast tissue, the less likely the cancer was to spread into the lymph nodes of the armpit or to be invasive.[19]

The second reason is that, besides containing high doses of alpha-linolenic acid, flaxseed and flaxseed oil are the most abundant sources of lignans. These components are fiber compounds that can bind to estrogen receptors and interfere with the cancer-promoting effects of estrogen on breast tissue. Lignans also increase the production of a compound known as sex hormone binding globulin (SHBG). This protein regulates estrogen levels by escorting excess estrogen from the body.

Population studies, as well as experimental studies in humans and animals, have demonstrated that lignans exert significant anticancer effects.[20–22] In one recent study, researchers followed 28 postmenopausal nuns for a year and tracked blood levels of two cancer-related estrogens: estrone sulfate and estradiol.[23] In addition to their normal diets, the nuns received daily supplements of 0, 5, or 10 g of ground flaxseed. Estrogen levels fell significantly in the women taking ground flaxseed, but they remained stable in the control group (those taking no flaxseed).

Ground flaxseed provides more nutritional benefits than does whole seed. That's because flaxseed is very hard, making it difficult to crack, even with careful chewing. But flaxseed is easy to grind in a coffee grinder, food processor, or blender. You can also buy FortiFlax from Barlean's at your local health food store. This product contains ground flaxseed in a special nitrogen-flushed container for maximum freshness. Grinding makes flaxseed easier for the body to digest. We recommend 1 to 2 tablespoons daily added to foods such as hot cereals, salads, or smoothies. We also recommend 1 tablespoon flaxseed oil daily. Flaxseed oil can be used as a salad dressing or for dipping bread, or it can be mixed with yogurt or cottage cheese.

Paul Gross, director of the breast cancer prevention program at the Princess Margaret Hospital and the Toronto Hospital, has reported that flaxseed in the diet may shrink breast cancers. His study involved 50 women who had recently been diagnosed with breast cancer. While waiting for their surgery, the women were divided into two groups. One group received a daily muffin containing 25 g (a little less than 2 table-spoons) of ground flaxseed. The others were prescribed ordinary muffins. After surgery, the investigators found that women who had received the flaxseed muffins had slower-growing tumors than the others.

Don't cook with flaxseed oil Flaxseed oil has high levels of polyunsaturated fats, which can be damaged by heat. Never cook with flaxseed oil—use olive or canola oil instead. Buy flaxseed oil in small, opaque bottles and keep it refrigerated at all times. Some manufacturers also add antioxidants, such as vitamin E or rosemary, to the oil to further protect it. Put a label indicating the date of purchase on the bottle. If the oil is not used within three months, throw it out and replace it with a fresh bottle. Also dispose of any flaxseed oil that has a bitter or rancid taste.

Soy: It's interesting to note that among Japanese women (living in Japan), the rate of breast cancer is about one-fifth the rate in the United States. When Japanese women move to the West, however, the rate increases, until by the third generation after immigration, the risk of breast cancer is about the same. Researchers explain this rise by noting that most "Westernized" Japanese begin eating the standard American diet (high-fat, low-fiber, not enough fruits and vegetables).

One reason might be that Japanese women eat much more soy than

Westerners do. Soy is gaining in popularity. Since the 1970s, there has been a marked increase in the consumption of traditional soy foods, such as tofu, tempeh, and miso, and in the development of so-called second-generation soy foods that simulate traditional meat and dairy products. Consumers can now find soy milk, soy hot dogs, soy sausage, soy cheese, and soy frozen desserts at their grocery stores. One of the big reasons for the increase in soy consumption is that there is now considerable evidence from laboratory and human studies that indicates a possible anticancer effect of soy, particularly in hormone-sensitive cancers such as breast and prostate cancers.[24,25]

As an anticancer nutrient, soy isoflavonoids:

- act as antioxidants
- reduce estrogen levels, particularly free estrogen (Lower levels of estrogen have been associated with a decreased risk of breast cancer.)
- prevent the formation of new blood vessels, thus preventing tumors from obtaining the blood supply necessary for continued growth
- prevent tumor cells from dividing and growing by inhibiting enzymes involved in cell replication

Population studies have consistently found that soy consumption may help reduce a woman's risk of developing breast cancer. Clinical and experimental studies further support the benefits of soy. Such studies show, for instance, that when healthy women add soy products to their diets, their levels of estrogen and other hormones fall. They also have lower levels compared with women who do not eat soy.

In recent years, growing evidence suggests that two isoflavones found in soy—daidzein and genistein—are the sources of soy's benefits. That's because these substances act as phytoestrogens, naturally occurring plant compounds that bind to estrogen receptor sites in human cells, including breast cells. By blocking these receptors, they reduce the effects of estrogen.

The amount of soy found to be protective against the development of breast cancer delivers 25 to 100 mg per day of isoflavones. We strongly recommend getting this amount from foods rather than from dietary supplements of purified isoflavones. Many soy foods now state the level

Table 4-2. Soy Foods and Isoflavone Content

PRODUCT	SERVING SIZE	APPROXIMATE ISOFLAVONE CONTENT
Cooked soybeans	1/2 cup	40 mg
Roasted soybeans (soy nuts)	1/2 cup	40 mg
Tempeh	4 ounces	40 mg
Tofu	4 ounces	40 mg
Soymilk	1 cup	40 mg
Soy protein	1/2 cup	35 mg

of isoflavones per serving. As you can see from Table 4-2, you do not need to eat huge amounts of soy foods to meet the recommended levels.

New evidence suggests that soy contains other substances besides isoflavones that provide even more benefit.[27] Researchers at the University of Chicago tested soy on lab animals with mammary gland tumors. One group of animals received pure soy protein (without isoflavones), another group got pure isoflavones, and a third group got a mix that had both. All three groups had fewer tumors than the untreated animals. Surprisingly, the treatment that worked best was soy *without* isoflavones. Clearly, something else is at work.

The greatest benefits of soy consumption may occur during adolescence.[28] Studies indicate that preadolescent intake of soy enhances the maturation (differentiation) of breast cells. These more mature cells are

Warning

Women who have estrogen-sensitive breast tumors should restrict soy intake and should avoid soy isoflavone supplements. Studies in test tubes and in animals show that the isoflavone genistein stimulates growth of estrogen-receptor positive tumors.[24–26] It inhibits the growth of breast cancer cells that lack estrogen receptors, however. Whether these results apply to humans is not yet clear, but until more information is available it makes sense that women who have estrogen-receptor positive breast cancer should restrict soy intake (no more than four servings per week) and should avoid soy isoflavone supplements.

less susceptible to carcinogens. The anticancer effects of soy intake after adolescence appear to be more valuable in preventing the onset of cancer in the premenopausal women through more favorable estrogen levels and metabolism.[29] The take-home message: Start eating soy as a child or, at the latest, before menopause.

CABBAGE FAMILY VEGETABLES | Cabbage family vegetables include cabbage, broccoli, cauliflower, and kale. These flavorful foods, also called cruciferous vegetables, contain anticancer phytochemicals known as glucosinolates. The most important of these is indole-3-carbinol (I3C), a compound formed when the vegetables are crushed or cooked. I3C and other glucosinolates are antioxidants and potent stimulators of natural detoxifying enzymes in the body. Studies have shown that increasing the intake of cabbage family vegetables or taking I3C as a dietary supplement significantly increases the conversion of estrogen from cancer-producing forms to nontoxic breakdown products.[30–32] Thus I3C is thought to be especially protective against breast and cervical cancers.

To help you understand how this works, here's a quick lesson in biochemistry. The body breaks down estrogen in several ways. Some estrogen is converted into a substance called 16-alpha-hydroxyestrone, a compound that promotes breast tumors. Another method of breakdown produces 2-hydroxyestrone, which does not stimulate breast cancer cells. Increasing the intake of cabbage family vegetables or taking supplements containing I3C shifts the ratio so that your body produces more of the "good" estrogen breakdown product and less of the "bad."

In high-risk women, we recommend either eating four to five servings of cabbage family foods per week or supplementing the diet with I3C at a dosage of 200 to 400 mg daily. No side effects or drug interactions have been reported with I3C supplementation. Broccoli sprouts have been reported to have the highest levels. In terms of glucosinolates, 1 pound of broccoli sprouts equals 40 pounds of fresh broccoli.

REDUCING GLUCURONIDASE | One of the key ways in which the body gets rid of estrogen is by attaching glucuronic acid to the estrogen in the liver and then excreting this complex in the bile. Bacteria in your body also produce an enzyme called glucuronidase, however, which breaks the bond between estrogen and glucuronic acid. When that happens, the level of estrogen rises. Not surprisingly, excess glucuronidase activity is associated with an increased risk of cancer, particularly estrogen-dependent breast cancer. The activity of this enzyme is higher in people whose diet is high in fat and low in fiber. High glucuronidase activity may be one of the key underlying factors explaining why certain dietary factors cause breast cancer and why other dietary factors are protective.

Glucuronidase activity can be reduced by eating lots of plant foods, especially onions and garlic and foods high in glucuronic acid, such as apples, Brussels sprouts, broccoli, cabbage, and lettuce. You can further reduce glucuronidase by supplementing the diet with the "friendly bacteria" *Lactobacillus acidophilus* and *Bifidobacterium bifidum*. (For more information, see the section on probiotics in Chapter 3.)

Another option for inhibiting glucuronidase activity is to use a supplement called calcium d-glucarate. Researchers at major cancer centers are studying this natural substance as a possible preventive measure in women at high risk for breast cancer.[33,34] In the animal studies, calcium d-glucarate reduced glucuronidase levels by over 50 percent, resulting in a drop in blood estrogen levels of over 20 percent and a 50 to 70 percent reduction in mammary cancer. The recommended daily dose for prevention is 200 to 400 mg; higher doses (400 to 1200 mg) may be necessary for individuals with existing cancer. There are no known side effects or drug interactions.

Prostate Cancer

The prostate is a single, doughnut-shaped gland about the size of a walnut that lies below the bladder and surrounds the urethra (the tube that connects the bladder to the tip of the penis). The prostate secretes a thin, milky, alkaline fluid that lubricates the urethra to prevent infection and increases the ability of sperm to move.

There are two main conditions that affect the prostate. One is prostate enlargement, also called benign prostatic hyperplasia (BPH). Almost every man will develop an enlarged prostate if he lives long enough. BPH is *not* cancer and is not life-threatening, but it can cause symptoms such as difficulty urinating and disturbed sleep. Treatment includes removing part or all of the prostate to improve urination.

The other condition, prostate cancer, is much more serious. It can cause symptoms similar to those in BPH, but it can also spread to other parts of the body and can be fatal. In men, prostate cancer is the second leading cause of death due to cancer. (Lung cancer is by far the first.) Prostate cancer is a hormone-sensitive cancer that will affect at least 1 out of every 6 men now living in the United States. Each year roughly 200,000 men are diagnosed with the disease in the United States, and more than 30,000 will die from it. Because prostate cancer is a very slow-growing disease, however, it is not always life-threatening. About 30 percent of men over 50 have signs of prostate cancer, but the disease is only fatal in about 3 percent of cases. Many men opt not to have treatment immediately after their diagnosis but rather to wait and see what happens. That's why it's often said that many men die *with* prostate cancer rather than *because* of it.

Risk Factors

Age: In the United States, prostate cancer is found mainly in men over age 55; more than 8 out of 10 men with prostate cancer are over 65. The average age of patients at the time of diagnosis is 70.

Family history of prostate (or breast) cancer: A man's risk for developing prostate cancer is increased twofold if his father has had the disease and fivefold if his brother has been affected. The risk increases twofold if both his mother and his sister have had breast cancer.

Race: Prostate cancer is roughly twice as common in black men than in white men. It is less common in Asian and American Indian men.

Hormones: Testosterone excess is thought to stimulate hormone-dependent prostate cancer in much the same way that estrogen stimulates breast cancer. Other hormones implicated are estrogen, prolactin, insulin, and IGF-1.

Vasectomy: Early studies found that prostate cancer develops up to twice as often in men who have had a vasectomy (surgery to make a man infertile), but more recent studies have found no difference in prostate cancer risk.

Diet: Current research indicates that diets high in red meat and saturated fat are associated with an increased risk of developing prostate cancer. Risks are also increased for those who have diets low in fruits, vegetables, phytoestrogens, selenium, vitamin E, lycopene, and other dietary antioxidants.

Male-pattern baldness: Men who gradually lose their hair at the front

The Bald Truth

According to a study of 4,000 men conducted by the National Institutes of Health (NIH), male-pattern baldness is associated with a higher risk of prostate cancer.[35] That's because both conditions involve the body's reaction to testosterone, the primary male hormone. Receptors for testosterone are found on hair follicles as well as the prostate. Male-pattern baldness has been linked to a higher risk for heart disease as well.

These findings do not mean that balding men will definitely get prostate cancer, only that they are at increased risk. Such men are advised to be more aggressive in following dietary and supplementation programs to reduce their risk of developing prostate cancer.

and/or crown of the head, beginning in their mid-twenties, are 50 percent more likely to develop prostate cancer (see the box above).

Detecting Prostate Cancer

Early prostate cancer often does not cause symptoms. When symptoms do occur, they include any or all of the following:

- A need to urinate frequently, especially at night
- Difficulty starting urination or holding back urine
- Inability to urinate
- Weak or interrupted flow of urine
- Painful or burning urination
- Difficulty in having an erection
- Painful ejaculation
- Blood in urine or semen
- Frequent pain or stiffness in the lower back, hips, or upper thighs

These symptoms are not specific to prostate cancer. The first four, especially, are also typically seen in cases of BPH. The latter symptoms can also result from prostate infections. If you are experiencing any of these symptoms, it is important to see a doctor immediately. The most important aspect in detecting prostate cancer for men over age 50 (for blacks, age 45) is seeing a physician for an annual physical exam that includes a digital rectal exam (DRE) and a blood test. During the DRE, the doctor inserts a lubricated, gloved finger into the rectum and feels the prostate through the rectal wall to check for hard or lumpy areas.

The blood test checks the level of a protein called prostate-specific antigen (PSA). Usually PSA is elevated in men who have prostate cancer, but approximately 35 percent of men with diagnosed prostate cancer will have a "normal" PSA (less than 4). Currently experts are debating whether this normal level should be lowered. Until more research is done, our recommendation at this time is to have the test done annually and watch for a change.

A newer test that measures the activity of an enzyme called telomerase, found in the semen, may be more sensitive as a screening tool for prostate cancer. At this time, the test is still being developed, but if research continues to prove its value, it may be available within a few years. Telomeres are like a "tail" on DNA. Each division of the cell shortens the telomere, and when it reaches a certain size the cell will no longer divide. Cancer cells bypass this control by using telomerase, which prevents the shortening of the telomeres and allows a cell to undergo unlimited divisions.

Lifestyle

While prostate cancer is associated with many of the same lifestyle factors associated with other cancers, the connections are not as strong or consistent as they are for breast or lung cancer. Nonetheless, it is important to engage in a healthy lifestyle by avoiding tobacco smoke and excessive intake of alcohol, while engaging in a regular exercise program in order to reduce the risk of prostate cancer.

Diet

There is so much convincing evidence on the role of diet in prostate cancer that William Fair and his colleagues from the Memorial Sloan-Kettering Cancer Center suggest that prostate cancer may be considered a "nutritional disease."[36] The prime suspects are diets that are

- high in animal foods, particularly grilled and broiled meats (which are high in heterocyclic amines); saturated fat; and dairy products
- low in protective nutrients, such as lycopene; selenium; vitamin E; soy isoflavonoids and other dietary phytoestrogens; omega-3 fatty acids (particularly those from fish); and isothiacyanates from cabbage family vegetables

As is true of breast cancer, these dietary factors are known to affect sex hormone levels, detoxification mechanisms, and antioxidant status. The following are some additional points to be aware of.

Supplementation Support

LYCOPENE

One of the most important anticancer nutrients is lycopene, a carotene that provides the red color to tomato products. Lycopene is one of the major carotenes in the diet of North Americans and Europeans. More than 80 percent of lycopene consumed in the United States comes from tomatoes, although apricots, papaya, pink grapefruit, guava, and watermelon also contribute.

The amount of lycopene in tomatoes can vary significantly, depending on the type of tomato and how ripe it is. In the reddest strains, lycopene concentration is close to 50 mg per kilogram (mg/kg), compared with only 5 mg/kg in the yellow strains. Lycopene appears to be relatively stable during cooking and food processing. In fact, you actually absorb up to 5 times as much lycopene from tomato paste or juice than you do from raw tomatoes, because processing "liberates" more lycopene from the plant's cells. Eating a lycopene source with oil, such as olive oil, can also improve its absorption. That's one reason why a Mediterranean diet (such as the Italian diet) has so many healthful properties.

Because lycopene is a more potent scavenger of oxygen radicals than other major dietary carotenes, it exerts additional anticancer effects. Recently Harvard researchers discovered that of all the different types of carotenes, only lycopene was clearly linked to protection against prostate cancer.[37] The men who consumed the highest levels of lycopene (6.5 mg per day) in their diet showed a 21 percent decreased risk of prostate cancer compared with those eating the lowest levels. It was also found that the high-lycopene eaters had an 86 percent decreased risk of prostate cancer (although this did not reach statistical significance, because of the small number of cases). In a study of patients with existing prostate cancer, lycopene supplementation (30 mg per day) was shown to slow tumor growth, shrink the tumor, and lower the level of PSA (discussed in more detail below).[38]

In addition to prevention of prostate cancer, population-based studies also indicate that lycopene protects against cancers of the colon, cervix, lung, and breast. As a bonus, researchers have also found a statistically significant association between high dietary lycopene and a lower risk of heart disease.[39,40]

While lycopene has clear benefits, it is important to point out that in a test tube study it was found that lycopene alone was not very effective at stopping prostate cancer tumors from growing. However, adding alpha-tocopherol resulted in a 90 percent decrease in cell proliferation.[41] This result implies that lycopene works best (and perhaps only) if vitamin E levels are sufficient.

Increasing your intake of lycopene is a key goal in preventing many cancers. Although lycopene supplements are available in pill form, they are relatively expensive, especially when compared with food sources.

In short, the cheapest and healthiest way to boost lycopene levels is through diet. Foods rich in the important carotenes will also be high in vitamin C and other antioxidants, but if you are at high risk for or currently have prostate cancer, then we definitely recommend supplementing your diet with an additional 30 mg of lycopene daily.

Lycopene supplementation appears to have therapeutic potential in prostate cancer. Twenty-six men with newly diagnosed, clinically localized prostate cancer were randomly assigned to receive 15 mg of lycopene twice daily or no supplementation for 3 weeks before surgical removal of the prostate. Blood levels of PSA decreased by 18 percent in the lycopene group, whereas they increased by 14 percent in the control group not receiving lycopene. These results suggest that lycopene supplementation (30 mg daily) may decrease the growth of prostate cancer.

FAT INTAKE, BLACK MEN, AND PROSTATE CANCER | Black men develop prostate cancer twice as frequently as white men. Although genetics play a role, dietary differences also are involved. In a study conducted by the National Cancer Institute of men who had been newly diagnosed with biopsy-proven prostate cancer and matched controls without prostate cancer, it was shown that increased consumption of foods high in animal fat was more often linked to prostate cancer (independent of intake of other calories) in black men than in white. The higher the intake of animal fat, the greater the risk for advanced prostate cancer.[42] Reducing fat from animal sources in the diet could lead to substantially decreased incidence and mortality rates for prostate cancer, particularly among American blacks.

SOY | The isoflavones of soy, genistein, and daidzein exert significant protection against prostate cancer, according to population-based studies. Test tube and animal studies have confirmed that soy isoflavonoids significantly inhibit growth of prostate cancer cells.[43] Since both testosterone-dependent and testosterone-independent prostate cancer cells are inhibited, it appears that soy isoflavonoids act against cancer in several ways. As is the case with breast cancer, the high intake of soy may be one of the key protective factors accounting for the low rate of prostate cancer in Japan and China compared with other parts of the world. Studies show that the blood and urine concentrations (an indicator of intake) of soy isoflavonoids were found to be 7 to 110 times higher in Japanese men consuming a traditional Japanese diet compared with Finnish men consuming a typical Western diet. A study of 12,395 male Seventh-Day Adventists (who generally eat a healthy diet and abstain from alcohol) found that those who drank soymilk had a 70 percent reduction of the risk of prostate cancer.[44] All together, studies conducted in 42 countries confirm that soy is one of the most important dietary factors for protection against prostate cancer.

OMEGA-3 FATTY ACIDS AND PROSTATE CANCER | Considerable evidence indicates that the risk of prostate cancer is reduced with higher intakes of the omega-3 fatty acids eicosapentaenoic acid (EPA) and do-cosahexaenoic acid (DHA), both derived from fish. To more accurately determine the degree of protection, researchers in New Zealand measured the level of EPA and DHA in red blood cells in a population-based study.[45] A high content of EPA and DHA was associated with a significantly reduced prostate cancer risk. This study confirmed findings from previous population-based and lab studies showing that these omega-3 fatty acids inhibit prostate cancer cells from growing. In addition to eating at least two servings of cold-water fish per week, we recommend taking enough capsules of a fish oil product to provide at least 120 to 360 mg of EPA and 80 to 240 mg of DHA per day for anyone at risk for prostate cancer.

FLAK ABOUT FLAXSEED | While the evidence clearly indicates that the risk of prostate cancer is reduced with the intake of EPA and DHA, there is conflicting evidence with alpha-linolenic acid (ALA)—the omega-3 fatty acid found in flaxseed oil. Some studies indicate that ALA may actually increase the risk of prostate cancer.[46-48] In some of these studies, however, ALA intake was used simply as a marker for meat intake. If no vegetable sources of ALA, such as flaxseed or canola oil, are consumed, the primary dietary source is from meat—the greater the meat intake, the higher the ALA tissue level. It is also possible that deficiencies of zinc or other nutrients involved in the conversion of ALA to EPA are ultimately responsible for the elevations in ALA noted in men with prostate cancer.

No one has actually looked at the effect of flaxseed oil in prostate cancer, but ground flaxseed appears to be quite helpful not only in preventing prostate cancer but also in men with existing prostate cancer (discussed in greater detail below). In addition to the phytoestrogen effect, flaxseed lignans bind to male hormone receptors and promote the elimination of testosterone.

Until the issue with ALA and prostate cancer is resolved by more careful studies, we recommend that men should avoid flaxseed oil and instead focus on consuming ground flaxseed and getting their omega-3 oils from fish and fish oil supplements.

Ground flaxseed also appears to be quite helpful not only in preventing prostate cancer but also in the treatment. In a study conducted at the Duke University Medical Center and Durham Veterans Affairs Medical

Center involving men with prostate cancer, a low-fat diet (in which fat represented no more than 20 percent of total calories) supplemented with 30 g of ground flaxseed (roughly 2 tablespoons) reduced serum testosterone by 15 percent, slowed the growth rate of cancer cells, and increased the death rate of cancer cells after only 34 days.[49]

VITAMIN E | Several population studies have suggested that vitamin E supplementation prevents prostate cancer. The same sort of protection has been demonstrated in clinical studies as well.

In the Alpha-Tocopherol, Beta-Carotene Cancer Prevention Study, more than 29,000 male smokers ages 50 to 69 from southwestern Finland were randomly assigned to receive vitamin E (50 mg), beta-carotene (20 mg), both nutrients, or a placebo daily for 5 to 8 years (median, 6.1 years). Researchers found 246 new cases of prostate cancer and 62 deaths from the disease during the follow-up period. A 32 percent decrease in the incidence of prostate cancer was observed among the subjects receiving vitamin E compared with the men who did not receive it. Mortality from prostate cancer was 41 percent lower among men receiving vitamin E. In the subjects receiving beta-carotene alone, rates of prostate cancer incidence and mortality were 23 and 15 percent *higher,* respectively, compared with the group that did not receive this treatment. These findings are consistent with the study's other main finding: that lung cancer rates were higher in the group receiving beta-carotene alone (see page 73).[50]

The main point is that antioxidants must be taken as a group—not singly—so that they can work together. Taking vitamin E alone for cancer prevention is not wise. It should be taken with the other important antioxidant nutrients, such as vitamin C, selenium, and zinc. That is why we stress the importance of taking a high-quality multiple vitamin and mineral formula.

In a study conducted in Washington County, Maryland, nearly 10,500 male residents donated blood and toenail samples for a specimen bank. Toenail and plasma samples were assayed to measure selenium, alpha-tocopherol, and gamma-tocopherol in a total of 117 of 145 men who developed prostate cancer and 233 matched control subjects. Researchers found that the higher the concentrations of alpha-tocopherol, the lower the risk of prostate cancer. Men whose levels of gamma-tocopherol were in the top 20 percent had one-fifth the risk of prostate cancer of the men in the bottom 20 percent. Selenium was also found to be protective. The highest level of protection, however, was found among those men who had high levels of *all three compounds*.[51] The conclusion: To achieve the greatest degree of protection, use natural mixed tocopherols that include both alpha- and gamma-tocopherol, not alpha-tocopherol alone. And take selenium as well as the other anticancer nutrients, according to the guidelines given on pages 312 and 313.

SELENIUM | Selenium supplementation appears to be critically important in reducing prostate cancer risk. In a double-blind study of 974 men, selenium supplementation produced a significant (63 percent) reduction in the development of prostate cancer compared with the placebo group.[52] Because the results from this study and other preliminary studies with vitamin E and selenium were so convincing, various follow-up studies with larger groups of men are now in progress. For example, the SELECT Prostate Cancer Prevention Trial—the largest trial of its kind to date—began enrolling patients in July 2001. SELECT (which stands for *Sel*enium and vitamin *E C*ancer Prevention *T*rial) will determine whether these two dietary supplements can protect against prostate cancer. Sponsored by the National Cancer Institute, the study will recruit more than 32,000 men over the age of 55 at more than 400 study sites in the United States, Puerto Rico, and Canada.

It will be many years before the results from this large study are available, but we believe that the existing evidence for supplementing the diet with these nutrients already indicates that they are of value and should be used according to the guidelines given.

Colon Cancer

Cancer of the colon (large intestine and rectum) is the major cancer of the gastrointestinal tract. Colon cancer makes up only 15 percent of all cancers, but it's the number-two cause of cancer deaths in the United States. The American Cancer Society estimates that there will be nearly 140,000 new cases of colon cancer each year in the United States and that roughly 50,000 Americans will die from the disease. The good news is that the death rate from colorectal cancer has been going down for the past 20 years because of better early detection and improved treatment.

Risk Factors

The risk factors for colon cancer are very similar to those of the other cancers in this chapter.

Age: Colorectal cancer is more likely to occur as people get older. About 9 out of 10 people with colorectal cancer are age 50 or older, but the disease can occur in high-risk people in their twenties.

Family history: First-degree relatives (parents, siblings, children) of a person who has had colorectal cancer are somewhat more likely to develop colon cancer themselves, especially if the relative had the cancer before the age of 50.

Personal history of polyps: Polyps are overgrowths of cells on the inner wall of the colon and rectum. Some types of polyps increase the risk of colorectal cancer. A condition known as hereditary familial adenomatous polyposis leads to the development of thousands of polyps in the large intestine. There's a very high risk that one or more of these polyps will convert to a cancerous form.

Diet: Dietary factors are thought to be responsible for 80 to 90 percent of all colon cancer. A diet high in animal fats and heterocyclic amines from grilled or broiled meats can increase the risk of colon cancer. Most studies on the benefits of fruits, vegetables, and fiber show a protective benefit, but others do not. Multivitamins with folic acid, vitamin E, and calcium supplements appear to offer significant protection.

Inflammatory bowel disease: Ulcerative colitis or Crohn's colitis is characterized by severe inflammation of the colon over a long period of time and is associated with an increased risk for colon cancer. People who have chronic inflammatory bowel disease for 20 years or more have a colon cancer risk of almost 1 in 5.

History of prior pelvic irradiation: Those who have been treated with radiation to the large intestine (for conditions such as prostate cancer, for example) are at higher risk for colon cancer resulting from radiation damage to colon cells.

Smoking: Smokers are 30 to 40 percent more likely than nonsmokers to die of colon cancer.

Obesity: Being very overweight increases a person's colorectal cancer risk.

Detecting Colon Cancer

Colon cancer screening should be part of your annual physical if you are over age 40, have a family history of colon cancer, or have any symptom suggestive of colon cancer:

- A change in bowel habits
- Diarrhea, constipation, or feeling that the bowel does not empty completely
- Blood (either bright red or very dark) in the stool
- Stools that are narrower than usual
- General abdominal discomfort (frequent gas pains, bloating, fullness, and/or cramps)
- Weight loss with no known reason
- Constant tiredness
- Anemia (Any case of unexplained iron-deficiency anemia must be examined to rule out colon cancer.)
- Vomiting, especially if associated with lack of bowel movements, as this might suggest intestinal obstruction

Early detection of colon cancer usually includes one or more standard tests:

- A *fecal occult blood test (FOBT)* screens for hidden blood in the stool (feces). Sometimes cancers or polyps can bleed, and FOBT is used to detect small amounts of bleeding. FOBT can identify about 25 percent of patients with colorectal cancer.
- A *sigmoidoscopy* is an examination of the rectum and lower colon (sigmoid colon) using a lighted instrument called a flexible sigmoidoscope. The problem with this test is that the device does not examine the entire colon. Your large intestine is shaped like an upside-down U. A sigmoidoscope can't "see around the corner" into the upper part, so it misses any polyps or cancers in those regions, where approximately 30 percent of cancers occur. Flexible

sigmoidoscopy and FOBT, when used together and performed only once, will miss about a quarter of patients with precancerous colon polyps or invasive cancer. Combining FOBT with sigmoidoscopy identifies about 3 out of 4 patients with colorectal cancer.

- A *colonoscopy*, which uses a lighted instrument called a colonoscope, is more thorough because it can view the entire colon. It's the most sensitive screening test for colon cancer (that is, it is most likely to find cancer if it exists), but it's also the most expensive and invasive.
- A *dual-contrast barium exam* is also considered adequate for screening. The problem with this test is that any suspicious areas cannot be sampled for a biopsy, so a colonoscopy is ultimately needed anyway if a possible lesion is found.

We recommend that people who have any family history of colon cancer or who experience any symptom that suggests colon cancer get a colonoscopy. For people without risk factors who are age 50 or older, we recommend a yearly FOBT, a sigmoidoscopy every five years, and a colonoscopy every ten years.

Lifestyle

Lifestyle risk factors for other cancers apply to colon cancer as well, especially high alcohol intake. In regard to exercise, the association between low physical activity and colon cancer has become one of the most consistent findings in large population studies for this disease. Well over a dozen studies have now demonstrated this association.[53,54] In an evaluation of over 47,000 men enrolled in the Health Professionals Follow-up Study, regular exercise was associated with a nearly 50 percent reduction in colon cancer risk.[54]

Diet

Dietary factors are thought to be the underlying cause of colon cancer in nearly 9 out of 10 cases. Countries where people eat a Western diet have up to 10 times the rate of colorectal cancer compared with countries that follow an Asian diet. Not surprisingly, diets high in animal fats and heterocyclic amines are particularly dangerous, while diets high in fruits, vegetables, and fiber show a protective benefit in most (but not all) studies.[55]

Diet has both direct and indirect effects. By direct effects, we mean that cells of the colon can be damaged when they come into contact with components of meat, particularly heterocyclic amines and saturated fat. By the same token, the intestines can also receive direct protection by coming into contact with antioxidants.

Indirect effects are a sequence of events set in motion throughout the body by a poor diet or a malfunctioning digestive system. For example, incomplete protein digestion or poor intestinal absorption of protein leads to the formation of polyamines, compounds that can dramatically stimulate cancer cell growth. Be sure to take the self-evaluation on page 46 to determine whether you may be suffering from incomplete protein digestion.

Bacteria in the gut are thought to play a central role in colon cancer. Health-promoting bacteria, such as lactobacillus, bifidobacteria, and propionibacter species, increase your body's ability to produce substances that protect you against colon cancer. These include short-chain fatty acids (SCFA), such as acetic, proprionic, and butyric acid. When it comes to these compounds, the more the merrier: the higher the level of production, the greater the protection. For your body to produce these, three criteria must be met:

- There must be sufficient quantities of health-promoting bacteria in the gut.
- The diet must be low to moderate in terms of meat consumption.
- The diet must be sufficient in dietary fiber.

A diet consisting mainly of animal foods and refined sugars and lacking fiber will lead to the predominance of bacteria that break down proteins through a process called putrefaction. In contrast, a healthy diet (plenty of fruits and vegetables, minimal meat consumption, lots of fiber) will result in an abundance of the bacteria that specialize in the breakdown of fiber through fermentation.

The most important SCFA for protection against colon cancer is butyric acid (butyrate). Even at extremely low concentrations, butyrate profoundly suppresses cell proliferation in cancerous cells. In test tube studies, butyrate stops the growth of cancerous colon cells, promotes apoptosis, inhibits the effects of tumor promoters, and causes colon cancer cell lines to change back into normal cells.[56]

FIBER | Certain fibers appear to be more effective than others in increasing the levels of SCFAs in the colon. Pectins (from apple, citrus, guar gum, and other legume fibers) and vegetable-fiber isolates produce more SCFAs than wheat fiber, corn fiber, or oat bran. A recent study looking at fiber from fruits and vegetables found that people consuming more than two-and-a-half servings of fruits and vegetables daily reduced the risk of colon cancer by 65 percent compared with those who consumed less than one-and-a-half servings daily.[57] Such studies show that even small changes in diet can produce dramatic reductions in colon cancer risk.

For years scientists have believed that evidence overwhelmingly supported the notion that dietary fiber protects against colon cancer. Lately, however, researchers have discovered that a high-fiber diet isn't enough to overpower the negative effects of a diet high in animal products. In fact, the low rate of colon cancer among black Africans, originally thought to result from a high-fiber diet, now appears more likely to result from a low intake of animal products.[58]

MEAT | A number of large studies have found an association between meat consumption and colon cancer. In a study of more than 88,000 women, those who had the highest ratio of red meat to chicken and fish intake had a colon cancer risk two and a half times that of the group with the lowest ratio.[59] A study of nearly 50,000 men found that those who ate beef, pork, or lamb as a main dish on an almost daily basis had greater than three times the risk of colon cancer compared with those who ate such foods less than once a month.[60]

Heterocyclic amines—compounds produced during high-temperature cooking—have been suspected as the main carcinogens resulting from meat consumption.[61] A high-fiber diet isn't enough to counteract the damage from these compounds if meat intake remains high. The gut bacteria still have to digest the meat, and they release cancer-causing chemicals as a result. The story gets even more complicated, because some people have a genetic abnormality that affects their ability to metabolize heterocyclic amines. What happens is that these individuals have an imbalance between Phase I and Phase II detoxification reactions (see page 48 for more information). Such folks are more likely to develop colon cancer.

SUGAR | Several studies have shown a strong link between colon cancer and intake of simple carbohydrates, such as sugar. Studies in Uruguay, Italy, and the United States found that a high-sugar diet increases the risk of colon cancer by 50, 60, and 70 percent, respectively.[62] One problem is that people who get many of their calories from sugar do not eat a lot of other healthy protective foods, such as fruits, vegetables, and green teas. To make matters worse, sugar and the insulin your body releases to process sugar have both been shown to enhance the growth of a wide variety of cancer cell types.

FISH OIL: NO FISH STORY | Individuals with a high risk of colon cancer or who tend to form polyps may want to consider supplementation with fish oils. In a study conducted at the Cancer Research Institute of Harvard Medical School, fish oil supplementation prevented overgrowth of colon cells (hyperproliferation) and polyps in people who had a prior bout with colon cancer or who formed precancerous polyps.[63]

The subjects were given capsules containing either fish oil or a placebo. Blood samples measuring the fatty-acid profile and colon biopsy were performed at the start of the study and at 3 and 6 months. In addition, colon cells were also analyzed to determine their replication rate.

Before supplementation began, there were no significant differences between the two groups in the rates at which the cells replicated and in the ratio of omega-6 to omega-3 fatty acids (see page 40 for definition and food sources). The researchers discovered that patients whose colon cells showed rapid proliferation had a higher ratio of omega-6 to omega-3 fatty acids. The rate of hyperproliferation slowed in subjects who took fish oil (a source of omega-3 fatty acids) and who showed beneficial changes in the omega-6 to omega-3 ratio. In fact, in no subject in the fish oil group had a polyp grow during the yearlong study.

Supplementation Support

CURCUMIN | Evidence is mounting that aspirin and other nonsteroidal anti-inflammatory drugs (NSAIDs) may prevent colorectal cancer.[64] These drugs work by slowing down the activity of an enzyme called cyclo-oxygenase 2 (cox-2). Cox-2 produces prostaglandins (see page 40) that cause inflammation. These prostaglandins can also irritate colon cells, which causes them to grow. Prostaglandins also may be involved in changing a harmless colon polyp into a potentially life-threatening tumor.

There's a way you can curb cox-2 without having to take NSAIDs. We recommend that you take advantage of the natural cox-2 inhibitors found in two common spices, ginger and turmeric, and in green tea.

In animal studies, curcumin has been shown to inhibit all stages of colon cancer—from initiation to promotion and progression—more effectively than aspirin. Curcumin protects against the disease before, during, and after exposure to carcinogens.[65,66]

In addition to inhibiting prostaglandin formation, curcumin also exhibits potent antioxidant effects (in some experimental studies it was found to be up to 300 times more potent than vitamin E). Curcumin is one of the key natural cancer fighters discussed in Chapter 8.

In high-risk individuals, we recommend taking supplements containing curcumin, the yellow pigment of turmeric, at a dosage of 200 to 400 mg daily. It is also important to increase your intake of foods containing curry powder and ginger. And it is recommended that you trade your regular beverage for three or more cups of green tea or ginger tea a day.

FOLIC ACID | According to the Nurses' Health Study, taking multivitamin supplements for 15 years or more has been shown to decrease colon cancer by up to 75 percent, particularly if folate is among the nutrients ingested.[67] The study focused on nearly 90,000 cancer-free women who from 1980 to 1994 regularly answered detailed questions about their diets, including the use of multivitamins.

Results showed that the reduction in colon cancer risk was stronger for women (ages 55 to 69) who took supplemental forms of folate than for women who got their folate through diet alone. The reason may be that the form of folate found in vitamins is actually more easily absorbed and utilized than the form supplied by food, even by high-folate foods such as green leafy vegetables like kale, spinach, beet greens, and chard. When intake of vitamins A, C, D, and E and calcium was also controlled for, results were similar. Long-term use appears to be required to achieve significant protection, however. After four years, women who used multivitamins containing folic acid had no benefit with respect to colon cancer; there were insignificant risk reductions up to the fourteenth year. But after fifteen years of use, the results were quite significant.

CALCIUM, VITAMIN D, AND ANTIOXIDANT SUPPLEMENTS TO PREVENT POLYPS | Calcium is thought to offer protection against colon cancer by reducing the concentration of bile acids that tend to stimulate cellular proliferation. Clinical studies have shown that calcium supplements moderately reduce the risk of recurring polyp growth in the colon and appear to reduce the risk of colon cancer. In a study published in the *New England Journal of Medicine,* researchers reported that people who were prone to polyp formation and who took 1200 mg of calcium daily had a 24 percent decrease in the number of polyps and a 19 percent decrease in the risk of recurrence.[68] Another study found that use of calcium supplements by cancer patients increased survival times.[69] Such information suggests that calcium may be of value for more than just prevention.

Colon cancer rates are higher in areas of the United States that get less sunshine. That's significant, because sunshine converts chemicals in your skin into vitamin D, which your body needs to metabolize calcium. Taking vitamin D supplements along with calcium may provide added protection. Population studies have shown that higher levels of vitamin D may reduce the risk of colon cancer by approximately 60 percent.[70]

Some studies also suggest that antioxidant supplements may have a small effect in preventing against polyp formation (as well as new colon cancers).[71,72] Therefore, supplementing the diet with a multivitamin and mineral formula with sufficient levels of antioxidants, along with some extra calcium (total daily supplement intake of 1000 to 1500 mg), is a reasonable part of an overall strategy for protection against colon cancer, especially in individuals at high risk.

Final Comments

We've highlighted extra steps you can take to protect yourself against the four main types of cancer. Such measures may be of value if you are particularly at risk for these diseases, because of family history, genetics, or other risk factors. Many of the steps we've described—adequate exercise, a healthy diet, sensible use of supplements, avoiding known carcinogenic substances or behaviors—apply across the board as components of a complete program for protection against all forms of cancer and other chronic diseases. In fact, they're pretty good guidelines for good health.

To help you with adding the specific measures recommended in this chapter to your daily routine, we have included them in the guidelines given in Appendix A, Daily Plan for Preventing Cancer.

Chapter Five

Attitude, Emotions, and Lifestyle in Cancer Prevention

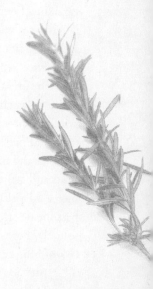

There is a growing appreciation within medicine of the tremendous interconnectedness of the mind and body. In fact, there is a whole new paradigm emerging. A paradigm is a model used to explain events. While the old medical paradigm viewed the body basically as a machine, the new paradigm focuses on the interconnectedness of body, mind, emotions, social factors, and the environment in determining the status of health. In this chapter, we will explore the roles of attitude, personality, emotions, lifestyle, stress reduction, exercise, and sleep in the prevention of cancer. Specifically, we will focus on the role of these factors in influencing the immune system. These factors play a significant role in cancer treatment as well.

In Chapter 1, we described the prototypical cancer personality as someone who suppresses anger, avoids conflicts, and has a tendency to feel helpless. The suppression and repression of emotions amplify the negative effects that stress produces on the immune system.[1,2]

The link between the brain, the emotions, and the immune system has led to a field of scientific research known as psychoneuroimmunology. What research in psychoneuroimmunology tells us is that every part of our immune system is connected to the brain in some way, be it via a direct nervous tissue connection or through the complex chemical language of chemical messengers and hormones.

What scientists are discovering is that every thought, emotion, and experience send a message to the immune system that will either enhance or impair its ability to function. A simplistic view is that positive emotions such as joy, happiness, and optimism tend to boost immune system function, whereas negative emotions such as depression, sadness, and pessimism tend to suppress immune function.

Since the immune system is so critical in preventing cancer, if emotions and attitude were risk factors for cancer we would expect to see an increased risk of cancer in people with long-standing depression or a pessimistic attitude. Does research support such an association? Absolutely. For example, smokers who are depressed have a much greater risk of lung cancer than smokers who are not depressed.[3]

Depression and the harboring of other negative unresolved emotions contribute to an increased risk of cancer in several ways. Most of the research has focused on the impact of depression and other negative emotions on white blood cells known as natural killer cells. These cells received their name because of their ability to destroy cells that have become cancerous or infected with viruses. They are the body's first line of defense against cancer development.

Considerable scientific evidence documents the link between negative emotions, stress, and a low level of activity of natural killer cells and an increased risk for cancer.[4] Studies have also shown that the classic cancer personality has lower natural killer cell activity compared with other personality types.[1,2] Negative emotions and stress paralyze many aspects of immune function and can cause natural killer cells literally to burst.[4,5] Furthermore, studies indicate that individuals with a personality type that is prone to cancer have an exaggerated response to stress, compounding the detrimental effects that stress has on natural killer cells and the entire immune system.[1,2]

Laugh Long and Often to Boost Your Immune System

Laughter is without question the most powerful immune enhancer available. Recent medical research has also confirmed that laughter enhances the blood flow to the body's extremities and improves cardiovascular function; plays an active part in the body's release of endorphins and other natural mood-elevating and painkilling chemicals; and improves the transfer of oxygen and nutrients to internal organs. Here are seven tips to help you have more laughter in your life.

1. Learn to laugh at yourself. Recognize how funny some of your behavior really is—especially your shortcomings or mistakes. We all have little idiosyncrasies or behaviors that are unique to us that we can recognize and enjoy. Don't take yourself too seriously.

2. Inject humor any time it is appropriate. People love to laugh. Get a joke book and learn how to tell a good joke. Humor and laughter really make life enjoyable.

3. Read the comics to find one that you think is funny and follow it every day or week.

4. Watch comedies on television. With modern cable systems, it is usually quite easy to find something funny on television.

5. Go see a funny movie with a friend. We laugh harder and more often when we are around others who are laughing. It is contagious, we feed off each other's laughter, and laughing together helps build good relationships.

6. Listen to comedy audiotapes in your car while driving. Check your local record store, bookstore, video store, or library for recorded comedy routines of your favorite comic.

7. Play with kids. Kids really know how to laugh and play. If you do not have kids of your own, spend time with your nieces, nephews, or neighborhood children with whose families you are friendly. Become a Big Brother or Sister. Investigate local Little Leagues. Help out at your church's Sunday school and children's events.

Interestingly, in one of the largest studies it was shown that regular exposure to stress situations actually appears to reduce the risk of cancer.[6] It seems that the regular exposure to stress dampens the stress response to major life events such as a death of a spouse, divorce, or loss of a child or parent. Major life events such as these are associated with a significantly increased risk for cancer in people who cannot externalize emotions and obtain appropriate help and counseling. When faced with a major life challenge, it is important to seek out the support and comfort of family and friends—and, if needed, the support of a counselor or a member of the clergy.

Depression and stress not only affect the immune system, they appear to hinder the cell's ability to repair damage to DNA as well. Most carcinogens cause cancer by directly damaging DNA in cells, thereby producing abnormal cells. One of the most important protective mechanisms against cancer in the cell's nucleus are enzymes responsible for the repair or destruction of damaged DNA. Several studies have shown that depression and stress alter these DNA repair mechanisms; for example, in one study, lymphocytes (a type of white blood cell) from depressed patients demonstrated impairment in their ability to repair cellular DNA damaged by exposure to x-rays.[7,8]

Developing the "Anticancer" Personality

Just as research has identified personality, emotional, and attitude traits that increase the risk of cancer, likewise the field of psychoneuroimmunology has identified traits to reduce your risk for cancer. This collection of "immune power" traits includes a positive mental attitude, an effective strategy for dealing with stress, and a capacity to openly admit traumas, challenges, and feelings to yourself and others.[4,9]

The Importance of a Positive Mental Attitude

The first step in developing the anticancer personality is expressing a positive mental attitude. As we have seen over and over in our patients' lives (and our own), it is not what happens in our lives that determines our direction; it is our *response* to those challenges that shapes the quality of our lives and determines to a very large degree our level of health. Surprisingly, it is often true that hardship, heartbreak, disappointment, and failure serve as the spark for joy, ecstasy, compassion, and success. The determining factor is whether we view these challenges as stepping stones or stumbling blocks.

Fortunately, according to Drs. Martin Seligman, the world's leading authority on attitude and explanatory style (the manner in which we explain the events in our lives), humans are optimists by nature. Optimism is not only a necessary step toward achieving optimal health, it is critical to happiness and a higher quality of life.

Detailed evidence supports the contention that optimists live longer, suffer from fewer and less severe diseases (including cancer), and are much healthier than pessimists. In a 30-year study conducted by researchers at the prestigious Mayo Clinic in Rochester, Minnesota, the survival rate among optimists was 19 percent greater than that of pessimists. All causes of death were reduced, including cancer.[10]

To determine your level of optimism, we encourage you to take the self-assessment developed by Dr. Seligman (see Appendix H, on page 346).

Learning Optimism

Our attitude is like our physical body: In order for it to be strong and positive it must be conditioned. Conditioning your attitude to be positive and optimistic means adopting specific healthy habits. Here are three key habits to help you develop a positive mental attitude:

- **Improve the way you talk to yourself.** We all conduct a constant running dialogue in our heads. In time, the things we say to ourselves percolate down into our subconscious minds. Those inner thoughts, in turn, affect the way we think and feel. Naturally, if you feed yourself a steady stream of negative thoughts, it will have a negative impact on your mood, immune system, and quality of life. The cure is to become aware of your self-talk and then consciously work to feed positive self-talk messages to your subconscious mind.

- **Ask better questions.** An expert in motivation, Anthony Robbins, believes that the quality of your life is equal to the quality of the questions you habitually ask yourself. For example, if you experience a setback, do you think, "Why am I so stupid?" or "Why do bad things always happen to me?" Or do you think, "Okay, what can I learn from this situation so that it never happens again?" or "What can I do to make the situation better?" Clearly, the latter response is healthier. Regardless of the situation, asking better questions is bound to improve your attitude. Here are some questions to start you off:
  - What am I most happy about in my life right now?
  - What am I most excited about in my life right now?
  - What am I most grateful for in my life right now?
  - What am I enjoying most in my life right now?
  - What am I committed to in my life right now?
  - Who do I love? Who loves me?
  - What must I do today to achieve my long-term goal?

- **Set positive goals.** Learning to set achievable goals is a powerful method for building a positive attitude and raising self-esteem. Achieving goals creates a success cycle: You feel better about yourself, and the better you feel about yourself, the more likely you are to succeed. Here are some guidelines for setting health goals:
  - State the goal in positive terms and in the present tense; avoid negative words. It's better to say, "I enjoy eating healthy, low-calorie, nutritious foods" than to say, "I will not eat sugar, candy, ice cream, and other fattening foods."
  - Make your goal attainable and realistic. Start out with goals that are easily attainable, like drinking six glasses of water a day and switching from white bread to whole-wheat. By initially choosing easily attainable goals, you create a success cycle that helps build a positive self-image. Little things add up to make a major difference in the way you feel about yourself.
  - Be specific. The more clearly you define your goal, the more likely you are to reach it. For example, if you want to lose weight, what is the weight you desire? What body fat percentage or measurements do you want to achieve?

Dealing with Stress

Stress can be devastating to immune function—that is why we are more susceptible to the common cold and the flu during stressful times. Usually the greater the stressor, the greater the negative impact. The stress response causes increases in adrenal gland hormones, including adrenaline and cortisol. Among other things, these hormones inhibit the formation and action of white blood cells and cause the main organ of the immune system—the thymus gland—to shrink (involute). Since stress seems to be an inevitable part of modern living, it is critical to develop effective methods to deal with stress.

Whether you are aware of it or not, you have developed a pattern for coping with stress. Unfortunately, most people have found patterns and methods that ultimately do not support good health. Negative coping patterns must be identified and replaced with positive ways of coping. Try to identify any negative or destructive coping patterns listed in Table 5-1 that you may have developed and replace the pattern with more positive measures for dealing with stress.

Calming the Mind and Body

Learning to calm the mind and body is extremely important in relieving stress. Among the easiest methods to quiet the body and mind are

Table 5-1.

NEGATIVE COPING PATTERNS	POSITIVE COPING STRATEGIES

Dependence on chemicals
  Drugs, legal and illicit
  Alcohol
  Smoking
	Calming the mind
	  Prayer
	  Meditation
	  Relaxation exercises

Escaping by distraction (e.g., watching television)	Physical exercise
Feelings of helplessness	Yoga or tai chi
Emotional outbursts	Constructive communication of feelings

Excessive behavior
  Overeating
  Overspending
	Supporting the body's ability to deal with stress by eating healthfully

relaxation exercises. The goal of relaxation techniques is to produce a physiological response known as *relaxation response*—a term coined by Harvard professor and cardiologist Herbert Benson in the early 1970s. Although an individual may relax by simply sleeping, watching television, or reading a book, relaxation techniques are designed specifically to produce the relaxation response.

Producing the relaxation response requires breathing with the diaphragm. By using the diaphragm to breathe, a person dramatically changes his or her physiology. It literally activates the relaxation centers in the brain. Here is a popular relaxation technique to breathe with your diaphragm.

- Find a comfortable and quiet place to lie down or sit.
- Place your feet slightly apart. Place one hand on your abdomen near your navel. Place the other hand on your chest.
- You will be inhaling through your nose and exhaling through your mouth.
- Concentrate on your breathing. Note which hand is rising and falling with each breath.
- Gently exhale most of the air in your lungs.
- Inhale while slowly counting to 4. As you inhale, slightly extend your abdomen, causing it to rise about 1 inch. Make sure that you are not moving your chest or shoulders.
- As you breathe in, imagine the warmed air flowing in. Imagine this warmth flowing to all parts of your body.
- Pause for 1 second, then slowly exhale to a count of 4. As you exhale, your abdomen should move inward.
- As the air flows out, imagine all your tension and stress leaving your body.
- Focus on relaxing your toes and progressively move up your body as you imagine the stress melting away.
- Repeat the process until a sense of deep relaxation is achieved.

Lifestyle

A healthy lifestyle not only reduces the risk of cancer, but also reduces the risk of heart disease and improves the quality of life. The key recommendations for an anticancer lifestyle are don't smoke, follow a regular exercise program, and make sure that you get enough sleep.

Don't Smoke

We have already stressed that smoking is a major risk factor for lung cancer as well as every other cancer. In fact, cigarette smoking is the single greatest cause of cancer death in the United States. Tobacco smoke contains more than 4,000 chemicals, of which more than 50 have been identified as carcinogens. Cigarette smokers have overall cancer death rates twice those of nonsmokers. The greater the number of cigarettes smoked, the greater the risk.

If you want good health and a lower risk for cancer, you absolutely must not smoke. How do you stop? Based on the results of published studies, it appears that the best strategy for quitting smoking is to just stop—to go "cold turkey." Nicotine-replacement therapy (using gum or the skin patch) is effective for about 13 percent of the people who try it. Behavioral modification (rewards and punishments) only works for about two people in every hundred. Acupuncture is only slightly better. Some people have been able to quit following hypnosis.

Exercise

Regular exercise is a powerful prescription for a positive mood. Tensions, depressions, feelings of inadequacy, and worries diminish greatly with regular exercise. Exercise alone has been demonstrated to have a tremendous impact on improving mood and the ability to handle stressful life situations.

Regular physical exercise is obviously a major key to good health, and its ability to prevent cardiovascular disease is well known, but can it prevent cancer? Yes! As mentioned in Chapter 1, increased physical activity, whether from structured exercise or physical labor, has been found to cut the overall cancer risk nearly in half. The preventive effects of exercise are seen even in people who have other risk factors, such as poor diet, excess body weight, and smoking.[11,12]

The benefits of regular exercise in the battle against cancer may be

Ten Tips to Stop Smoking

1. List all the reasons why you want to quit smoking and review them daily.
2. Set a specific day to quit, tell at least ten friends that you are going to quit smoking, and then DO IT!
3. Use substitutes. Instead of smoking, chew on raw vegetables, fruits, or gum. If your fingers seem empty, play with a pencil.
4. Avoid situations that you associate with smoking.
5. When you need to relax, perform deep-breathing exercises rather than reaching for a cigarette.
6. Realize that 40 million Americans have quit. If they can do it, so can you!
7. Visualize yourself as a nonsmoker with more available money, pleasant breath, unstained teeth, and the satisfaction that comes from being in control of your life.
8. Join a support group. Call the local American Cancer Society and ask for referrals. You are not alone.
9. Each day, reward yourself in a positive way. Buy yourself something with the money you've saved, or plan a special reward as a celebration for quitting.
10. Take one day at a time.

due to its effects on the immune system. For example, some studies have shown that regular exercise leads to a significant increase (up to 100 percent) in natural killer cell activity.[13] Although more strenuous exercise is required to benefit the cardiovascular system, light to moderate exercise may be best for the immune system. The research thus far suggests that light to moderate exercise stimulates the immune system, while intense exercise (e.g., training for the Olympics) can have the opposite effect.[14] In other words, walking, yoga, and stretching exercises may actually provide greater benefit to immune function than aerobics.

In fact, the best exercise for boosting immune function may be tai chi—a martial arts technique that features the movement from one posture to the next in a flowing motion that resembles dance. Studies have found that immune function, including natural killer cells, was significantly increased by the practice of tai chi exercises.[15] Tai chi is described in more detail on page 209.

So why does engaging in regular strenuous exercise damage the immune system? Because it is associated with increased generation of free radicals and other reactive compounds that can cause tissue damage.[16] The underlying factor appears to be depletion of antioxidants. Although some studies have shown that supplementation with individual antioxidants (mostly vitamin E) have some benefit in offsetting some of this damage, unfortunately, there have been no clinical studies with a comprehensive antioxidant program.[17] The use of any single antioxidant (like vitamin E) is not recommended, because each antioxidant requires partner nutrients in its battle against free radicals. Therefore, the studies that have been conducted suffer from a serious flaw. The bottom line is that individuals who train heavily need to bolster their defenses by following the dietary and supplement recommendations given in Chapters 2 and 3.

While the immediate effect of exercise is stress on the body, with regular exercise the body adapts; it becomes stronger, functions more efficiently, and has greater endurance. The entire body benefits from regular exercise, largely as a result of improved cardiovascular and respiratory function. Exercise enhances the transport of oxygen and nutrients into cells. At the same time, exercise enhances the transport of carbon dioxide and waste products from the tissues of the body to the bloodstream and ultimately to the eliminative organs. As a result, regular exercise increases stamina and energy levels.

Benefits of Exercise

MUSCULOSKELETAL SYSTEM

Increases muscle strength

Increases flexibility of muscles and range of joint motion

Produces stronger bones, ligaments, and tendons

Lessens chance of injury

Enhances posture, poise, and physique

Prevents osteoporosis

HEART AND BLOOD VESSELS

Lowers resting heart rate

Strengthens heart function

Lowers blood pressure

Improves oxygen delivery throughout the body

Increases blood supply to muscles

Enlarges the arteries to the heart

Reduces heart disease risk

Helps lower blood cholesterol and triglyceride levels

Raises levels of HDL, the "good" cholesterol

BODILY PROCESSES

Improves immune function

Aids digestion and elimination

Increases endurance and energy levels

Promotes lean body mass and burns fat

MENTAL PROCESSES

Provides a natural release from pent-up feelings

Helps reduce tension and anxiety

Improves mental outlook

Helps relieve moderate depression

Improves the ability to handle stress

Stimulates improved mental function

Induces relaxation and improves sleep

Increases self-esteem

CREATE A REGULAR EXERCISE ROUTINE | Exercise is clearly one of the most powerful medicines available. The time you spend exercising is a valuable investment in your good health. To help you develop a successful exercise program, see Appendix I, on page 356.

The Importance of Sleep

Sleep is the period of time that the body and mind are recharged. Sleep is also the time the most potent activators of the immune system are released. Evidence is emerging that failure to get a good night's sleep increases the risk of cancer.[18] Every cell of the body is compromised and will be running on less than all cylinders, leaving the cell more susceptible to damage, with a reduced capacity to heal. In one study, healthy male volunteers were deprived of four hours of sleep for a single night. The next day, the activity of certain immune cells—their natural killer cells—fell by as much as 30 percent. Fortunately, a single good night's sleep restored the cells to their normal level of functioning.[19]

In a study of women at risk for cervical cancer because of an abnormal result on a Pap smear, sleep quality was shown to be directly related to immune function—the higher the quality of sleep achieved, the better the immune function. The evidence was so significant that the researchers concluded it was "important to systematically screen for and manage sleep disturbance in women at high risk for cervical cancer."[18] We would extend that recommendation to everyone.

The group most susceptible to sleep disturbances are shift workers—those whose job hours change over the course of weeks or months. Night shift workers have more trouble falling asleep and staying asleep. Poor sleep quality is probably the factor explaining why shift workers have a greater risk for cancer, suffer more illnesses, have more accidents, and die younger than do people with more stable schedules.[20] Inside our brain is a kind of master clock that coordinates the timing of many physiological functions. One important role of sleep is to help orchestrate these various biological rhythms. We achieve optimal health if we keep our rhythms in sync. If you are a shift worker, we recommend taking 3 mg of melatonin at bedtime and 3 mg of a special form of vitamin B_{12} known as methylcobalamin (available at health food stores) upon arising.

Melatonin is a hormone secreted by the pineal gland, a small pea-sized gland at the base of the brain. The exact function of melatonin is still poorly understood, but it is critically involved in regulating the natural biorhythm of hormone secretion referred to as the circadian rhythm as well as the control of sleep/wake cycles. Release of melatonin is stimulated by darkness and suppressed by light. Shift work tends to disrupt melatonin secretion and as a result disrupt the circadian rhythm. If melatonin is taken before going to sleep, it can help reset the biological clock and promote a good night's sleep.

Several studies have shown that methylcobalamin—a special form of vitamin B_{12}—is an effective treatment to improve sleep in shift workers as well as in people with excessive daytime sleepiness, restless nights, and frequent nighttime awakenings.[21] The subjects taking methylcobalamin experienced improved sleep quality and increased daytime alertness and concentration, and in some cases they also reported improved mood. Much of the benefit appears to be a result of methylcobalamin's influence on melatonin secretion and resetting the biological clock. Specifically, methylcobalamin causes a significant decrease in daytime melatonin levels while increasing nighttime levels.

Here are some additional tips for improving sleep quality:

1. Avoid sleep inhibitors such as sources of caffeine and alcohol.
2. If you eat bedtime snacks, choose whole-grain cereals and breads to keep blood sugar levels steady throughout the night and to increase serotonin levels within the brain.
3. Get regular exercise, but avoid exercising two hours or less before bedtime.
4. Consider nutritional and supplemental strategies to improve sleep:
   - Melatonin can help promote sleep at a dosage of 3 mg at bedtime.
   - Some people benefit by taking herbal products known to promote sleep, such as valerian (150 to 300 mg of dry powdered extract), 45 minutes before bedtime.
   - If you have muscle cramps or "restless legs" that disturb sleep, try taking magnesium (250 mg at night) and vitamin E (400 to 800 IU a day).

Part Two

Treating Cancer with

Natural Medicine

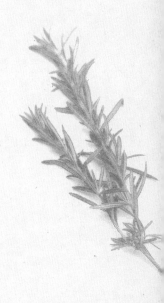

Chapter Six

You've Been Diagnosed: Now What?

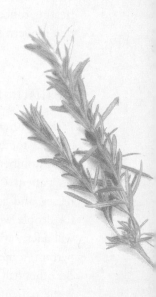

As physicians, caregivers, and human beings, we fervently hope for the day when the perfect cancer treatment becomes available—one that's effective, predictable, and without side effects. But despite years of research and an aggressive "war" on cancer, scientists have yet to figure out how to conquer this terrible disease once and for all.

Until they do, people with cancer must make difficult choices. Depending on the nature of their diagnosis, they have to select from among a bewildering array of conventional treatments: surgery, drugs, radiation. Their task is made more difficult because they must make their choices under stressful circumstances while navigating a complex and confusing health care system. And advice flows at them from all directions: doctors, nurses, friends, neighbors, fellow patients, the media.

What is the most rational approach to this disease? How do you chart a course of treatment that combines the practical and the personal, that balances the physical and the philosophical? When your body is under attack, how can you best draw on the resources of the mind and the spirit as allies in your fight to become whole again?

Our goal is to help you answer these and other essential questions. To do so we'll draw on our years of collective experience in the field of treating cancer through natural healing strategies that support the best that modern medicine has to offer.

Realistic Expectations

Patients often ask tough questions about their expected life span, chances for cure, risk for recurrence, and so on. As we've discussed, those numbers only apply to large groups, not to individuals. Each cancer patient is unique, with different characteristics, strengths, weaknesses, and genes. Physicians talk with patients about *average* survival for people with their particular type and stage of cancer. Often, they will refer to the five-year survival rate. If the five-year survival rate is 50 percent, it means that half of the patients will die within five years while the other half will live more than five years. On one end of the spectrum is the patient with rapid disease progression and early death. On the other end is the patient that enjoys complete cure, long-term remission, or many years of disease-free survival. Most patients will fall somewhere in the middle between these two extremes. Our job as caregivers is to try our best to move each patient as far to the positive end of the spectrum as possible, to include them among the other long-term survivors.

To do so, we encourage them to make all the lifestyle changes necessary and to use the natural medicines we discuss throughout this book. At the same time we encourage them to take advantage of the appropriate conventional therapies for their condition. With this integrated approach, we maximize their chances, not just for longevity—a greater number of years—but for an increased *quality* of life during those years.

As we've noted, cancer treatments attack and destroy cancerous cells, but they have the unfortunate downside of killing many healthy cells in the process. That's a pretty big tradeoff, and sometimes the destruction of bad cells comes at too high a cost, in terms of the number of healthy cells destroyed.

For this reason, we sometimes work with patients not so much to focus on the need to eliminate *all* detectable cancer but more to accept the fact that the cancer is present. The goal then shifts to achieving an acceptable balance between cancerous and healthy cells in the rest of the body.

In this revolutionary approach, the ultimate idea is to think of cancer as a long-term manageable disease, somewhat like diabetes or arthritis. Treatment is then designed to minimize symptoms and control the damage from the disease process. As we've noted, some cancers, such as prostate cancer, tend to be slow-growing. Making lifestyle changes to assure that they *stay* slow-growing and noninvasive may be better for some men than undergoing aggressive therapy with multiple side effects. The effectiveness of this approach can be estimated by looking at prostate cancer incidence and mortality around the world. When the prostates of elderly Japanese men are examined during autopsy, they are found to have prostate cancer about as often as men in the United States. The difference is that their cancer is microscopic, causes no symptoms, and is only discovered as an incidental finding during routine autopsy. The rate of prostate cancer deaths in the two countries varies by a factor of 20.[1] As we interpret this finding, diet, lifestyle, and genetics can be harnessed to keep existing cancer in a quiescent, noninvasive form.

The classic question after learning about a diagnosis of cancer is, "How long have I got?" No one—whether a health care practitioner, Nobel Prize–winning researcher, religious leader, or counselor—can predict exactly how long another person will live. When time runs out is really up to God, but we urge our patients to remember the old saying "God helps those who help themselves." We stress that the more changes they make in their way of living to keep themselves strong and healthy, the better their chances that they'll be one of the lucky ones who migrate to the right end of the bell curve for long-term survival.

Expectations have much to do with our experience of reality. By that we mean that our bodies often make real the things we expect to have happen. This is the basis of the so-called placebo effect and the power behind positive visualization. When people expect an outcome, it will often occur, not because they *imagined* it but because they *expected* it. As a result of their powerful expectation, their body went to work manufacturing the enzymes, neurotransmitters, and blood chemicals to make that expected outcome a reality. If you *expect* to have a positive outcome from your cancer treatment, it is more likely to occur. By the same token, if you expect the worst, then that's what you're likely to get. We're not necessarily saying you can think your way out of cancer. But we strongly believe you can certainly point out the right direction to your body and trust that the magnificent healing machine inside you will go to work trying to make that outcome real.

Goals of Treatment with Natural Medicine

We believe that natural medicine should play a central role in the rational approach to cancer. Cancer reflects the presence of imbalance and loss of control (dysregulation) in the body. Natural medicine focuses on bringing balance back into the system, making it less vulnerable to cancer. The big goals in the utilization of natural medicine in the rational approach to cancer are to:

- **Support the whole person.** You are not your disease. You are an individual who happens to have been diagnosed with a particular illness called cancer. Chapter 5 describes important guidelines to employ the tremendous healing power of the human mind and spirit.
- **Take away any factors that support cancer development.** It is important to eliminate harmful dietary, lifestyle, and other practices that promote cancer. For example, a recent study found that the recurrence rate for colon cancer was one-tenth as high in women who had low levels of insulin than it was in those with high insulin.[2] Insulin is a hormone whose output can be reduced by improvements in diet and exercise. The message? Eat right and stay active and you lower your risk of recurrence. The importance of dietary factors, exercise levels, maintaining healthy weight, avoidance of pesticides and radiation, and many more changes cannot be underestimated in their ability to contribute to a successful treatment outcome.

- **Utilize natural medicines to treat cancer and prevent recurrence.** Regardless of the form or location of cancer, appropriate natural medicines can be used to inhibit tumor growth, boost the immune system, promote natural death of cancer cells, and boost the effect of conventional therapies while reducing their side effects.

Manage Your Response to the Diagnosis

The diagnosis of cancer poses a daunting challenge to the psyche and the human spirit. Many of our patients tell us that the worst part of the whole process of overcoming cancer is the time right after the diagnosis. After hearing the words "You have cancer," most people naturally experience a flood of powerful feelings as they absorb the shock and adjust to their new reality. Among these emotions are:

- Denial ("The tests were wrong." "It can't be true.")
- Anger ("Why did I get cancer?" "Why couldn't it have been someone else?")
- Guilt ("Why did I smoke?" "Why didn't I take better care of myself?")
- Depression ("It's hopeless." "I might as well give up.")
- Fear ("There's nothing ahead for me but pain and suffering." "I'm going to die.")

These emotions are to be expected and are in fact a normal human reaction. But they are just the starting point, step one of the healing process. The next stage in managing your response to the diagnosis usually involves accepting your new reality and deciding on a course of action. The fact that you are reading this chapter—either for yourself or on behalf of someone you love—suggests that you have reached this important stage. And that's great news, because you're taking positive action to regain control over your life. Many challenges still lie ahead. But you are laying a solid groundwork for making empowering, correct decisions.

These decisions must be right *for you*. That's essential, because each of us responds to the challenges of life in different ways. Some people like to charge ahead, daring life to stop them. Others proceed slowly, gathering information along the way. Still others look inward and depend on their own intuition for guidance. The truth is, most of us draw on all of these strategies, but at different times and to different degrees. There's no one right way.

Whatever the strategy, the goal is the same: to overcome cancer. You have the best shot at achieving that goal if you:

- establish a strong system of support—emotional, physical, and spiritual
- build good relationships with your physicians and other caregivers
- understand your particular form of cancer
- follow the recommendations in this book to maximize your odds of beating cancer

Take Control

After they receive a diagnosis of cancer, many patients feel they have lost control—of their bodies, their lives, their destinies. No doubt much of that feeling arises from the disease itself, since cancer seems to take control of the body. But much of it also results from having to deal with the health care system. Patients must submit themselves to a series of invasive tests and procedures. In the course of treatment, they come into contact with a bewildering assortment of health care professionals, some of whom they see once and then never meet again. Decisions must be made quickly, often under the most emotional and trying circumstances. At the same time, family members and friends may appear on the scene, offering advice that's well meaning—but often conflicting or just plain wrong.

One of the most important things you can do to help your fight against cancer is to regain as much control as you feel you want to handle. We urge you to take control of your health care decisions, your choice of treatment, and the steps needed to promote your recovery. We believe that taking control improves your chances in three main ways:

- You'll make better treatment choices—choices that are best for you, your body, your circumstances.
- You'll get better results.

- And you'll gain a psychological edge, an inner source of strength and courage.

UNDERSTAND YOUR DISEASE | The first step in taking control is to fully understand the type of cancer you have—to "know thine enemy."

After first hearing about your disease from your doctor, you'll probably want to probe a little further. If you are comfortable working your computer, you can find a wealth of valuable information on the Internet. A good place to start is Cancernet (http://cancernet.nci.nih.gov). This site was developed to provide recent and accurate cancer information from the National Cancer Institute (NCI), the federal government's principal agency for cancer research. The site is designed to serve the needs of patients, caregivers, health care professionals, and researchers, among others. The information is the best of what is available from the conventional medical circle. Here you'll find links to information on virtually every type of cancer and its treatment, recent updates on clinical trials, and other useful information. If you can't locate the information you need or do not have access to the Internet, contact the NCI's Cancer Information Service, toll-free, 800-4-CANCER (800-422-6237), to speak with a trained information specialist. Another good source is the Web site of the American Cancer Society (http://www.cancer.org). The site has information for patients and their families, discussion groups, and tips for survivors.

Keep in mind that cancer is not really a single disease. There are dozens of different forms of cancer, each with its own personality. The worst ones are aggressive and invasive, wasting no time in spreading to other parts of the body. Others are more slow-growing and may never progress to the point where they become life-threatening. Some types of tumors cause symptoms (pain, bleeding, and so on); others do not.

Many cancers come in different varieties (or subtypes). Breast cancer, for example, takes several forms, depending on where it develops and other factors. Tumors that respond to the presence of hormones (estrogen) must be treated in a different way from those that are not hormone-sensitive. There are many other factors that come into play. The main point is that once all these individual factors have been determined, it becomes increasingly possible to size up the overall strengths and weaknesses of the particular cancer you're dealing with. This, in turn, allows you to make informed choices regarding treatment decisions.

Following are some of the key questions to ask in assessing your cancer and its potential treatment.

What type of cancer do I have?

The name of the cancer is based on the cell type and location. The major types of cancer are:

- carcinomas (arising in cells in the surface layer or lining of an organ)
- sarcomas (arising in connective tissue, bone, or muscle)
- leukemias or lymphomas (arising in blood cells or lymphatic tissue)

During diagnosis, the cancer is named according to the site in which it first arises. If the cancer spreads, it retains the name of the site where it originated. Thus breast cancer that has traveled to the liver is considered to be metastatic breast cancer (not liver cancer), and it would still be treated with drugs appropriate for breast cancer.

The pathology report on your tumor (based on diagnostic tests or biopsy) often includes other details, such as the presence of certain hormone receptors and other markers of abnormality. In prostate cancer, for example, the Gleason score defines how aggressive (how fast-growing and fast-spreading) a prostate cancer tumor is.

Where is it located, and what is the extent of the spread?

Cancer can be confined to a small primary site or can spread throughout the body. Smaller, well-contained tumors are often curable by surgery alone, but tumors that have spread into neighboring tissues or metastasized to different sites in the body indicate the need for more aggressive and systemic therapy.

What stage is my disease?

Staging is the process of evaluating the spread of a cancer. To stage cancer, doctors might order biopsies or imaging tests, such as computed tomography (CT or "CAT") scans or magnetic resonance imaging (MRI) scans. They're looking for enlarged lymph nodes, masses in different sites, or small areas called hot spots that might indicate the presence of microscopic cancerous cells.

Generally speaking, the following stages apply to most cancers:

- Stage 1: Tumor is small and localized (that is, it hasn't spread beyond its original location).
- Stage 2: Tumor is large but still localized.
- Stage 3: Tumor is pushing against, or penetrating into, adjacent tissues.
- Stage 4: Cancer cells have spread to tissues at other distant sites in the body.

Each tumor type has slightly different criteria for the determination of stages. In colon cancer, for example, the pathologist determines how deeply the tumor has penetrated the relatively thick wall of the large intestine.

Another way of describing tumors is the TNM system, which is a somewhat more precise way of noting the extent of the disease. The letters represent various facts about the tumor: T stands for primary tumor features; N means extent of lymph node involvement, and M indicates distant metastasis. The accompanying numbers provide additional information. For example, left breast infiltrating ductal carcinoma staged as T1,N0,M0 indicates that the tumor is small, has no involved lymph nodes, and has not metastasized.

What other characteristics does this tumor have?

The presence or absence of markers of cellular irregularity may predict how aggressive a cancer will be. The less a tumor resembles normal healthy tissue, the harder it is to treat and the more aggressive your treatment plan will need to be. These markers vary according to the cancer involved. Your doctors may want to evaluate as many of these variables as possible to fully understand the nature of your disease.

What are my treatment options?

Medicine is as much an art as a science, and nowhere is that more true than in the treatment of cancer. While there are certain clearly defined protocols that many physicians opt to use, there is no "one-size-fits-all" approach. Instead, the best strategy involves carefully tailoring the treatment plan to meet the individual patient's needs. Ask your oncologist about *all* treatment options available to you, including those that may be available through other caregivers or even through treatment centers in another city.

Choosing one approach to treatment often leads to other decisions that wouldn't arise after choosing a different approach. For example, a breast cancer patient may undergo a lumpectomy (removal of the tumor) and elect to have radiation therapy to destroy any lingering cancer cells that still may be present in the breast. A patient who has a mastectomy (complete removal of the breast) to remove a localized tumor that has not metastasized may not need to consider radiation if all the affected tissue was removed during the surgery.

And treatments require different strategies depending on various circumstances. For example, some courses of chemotherapy require weekly intervals; others are administered three times a week or once every three weeks. Radiation might be delivered in a few large doses, or it may be fractionated (involving the use of smaller doses given more frequently). In some cases, radiation is delivered directly to the tissue by means of internally implanted radioactive seeds. Each option has a different set of benefits and drawbacks. By asking your doctor to describe all your choices, as well as the pros and cons of each, you'll be better able to pick which approach offers the best combination of safety and efficacy for your situation.

Too often cancer patients decide for or against a proposed cancer treatment after hearing stories—usually told by well-meaning relatives or friends—who were treated years ago, when things were quite different, medically speaking, from what they are today. Once they hear those tales (many of which are "horror stories"), they get sidetracked in their effort to explore current treatment options and techniques. But no two cases of cancer are ever the same. And treatments are always being improved. Newer drugs and techniques and the addition of natural therapies can dramatically decrease the potential toxicity of conventional therapy and at the same time significantly improve its effectiveness.

Another way of looking at your treatment options is to consider what is fundamentally important to you in life and then to make your choice from that perspective. In general, younger people are frequently more willing to choose aggressive therapies with potentially severe side effects, since these often offer the best chance of significantly prolonging life. On the other hand, a man in his eighties may decide that he would rather spend quality time with friends and family than cope with the major side effects of surgery or radiation. Remember, both quality and quantity of life matter. So, too, do your plans for how you spend your remaining years. If there's a positive side to cancer, it's that it often helps you get your priorities straight.

Doctors are human, and so naturally they will have their own habitual preferences. Understandably, they will usually offer the type of treatment with which they have the most experience. Surgeons like to think that surgery is the best option, while radiation oncologists would naturally urge a choice involving radiation. It is often helpful when seeking information on choices to get a second opinion from another provider. (Of course, getting a second opinion that contradicts the first can make the choice that much more complex.) For more about bias and second opinions, see those sections below.

When you speak to doctors, be sure to ask them for information about the success rate for the treatment advised. Most treatments have been well studied, and their efficacy has been documented. Still, such statistics are really only valid for large groups. A treatment's past performance doesn't guarantee how it will work in the future for a given individual.

Conventional Cancer Treatments: A Quick Overview

Surgery

Surgery is often the first approach used in treating many kinds of cancer. Surgical removal of the tumor often results in a cure, especially if the tumor is small and localized.

New surgical techniques can also improve outcomes. During a lumpectomy, for example, sentinel node biopsies can be performed. These allow physicians to analyze one or two lymph nodes during the procedure to determine how far the disease has spread. Removing just the nodes involved avoids the more extensive axillary node dissection (removing a long section of nodes), thus reducing the risk of serious, sometimes debilitating side effects such as chronic lymphedema (swelling).

Radiation Therapy

New developments in radiation therapy equipment and techniques over the last few years have made it possible for physicians to deliver more radiation to smaller areas while causing less damage to healthy tissue. Drugs such as amifostine, newly available by prescription, help reduce the side effects from certain types of radiation treatment. Many natural therapies can also limit side effects while simultaneously improving response rates (for more information, see Chapter 12).

Advanced scanners and radiation technology make it possible for doctors to plan and administer treatments with a degree of precision never before achievable, increasing effectiveness while minimizing side effects. Such machines are not yet widely available, however, so patients desiring these treatments may need to travel to facilities with the most up-to-date equipment.

Chemotherapy

Chemotherapy is a general term covering scores of different cancer drugs, available in hundreds of different combinations that can be administered in many different ways. And the type and severity of side effects from those drugs will vary greatly, depending on the agent, its dosage, and its method of administration. Chemotherapy is probably the conventional cancer treatment that generates the most questions and concerns from patients. Opponents often deride chemotherapy as "toxic waste being pumped throughout your body." Such images would frighten anyone and, besides being inaccurate, are not helpful.

Not all chemotherapy regimens are alike. Therefore, questions about chemotherapy effectiveness and side effects need to be very specific to both the drugs being considered and the type of cancer being treated.

What are the likely side effects?

The problem with cancer is that it affects cells, and treatment that destroys unhealthy cells often destroys normal cells in the process. Military specialists refer to this as collateral damage, while doctors call these side effects. The potential benefits of any treatment—cure, increased survival time, and so on—must be weighed against the possible risks of treatment.

In making your choice, remember that there are many steps you and your caregivers can take to prevent side effects or at least minimize their impact. For example, many chemotherapy drugs cause nausea, but new antinausea medications have dramatically reduced the seriousness of this problem. Many natural therapies can also help to limit side effects such as fatigue and nerve damage. More information on this topic appears in Chapter 13.

If you read the package inserts that accompany cancer drugs (or any prescription medications, for that matter), you'll no doubt discover a seemingly endless list of potential adverse effects from the therapy. Please don't let this list alarm you or play a big role in your treatment decisions. Remember that these are *potential* side effects. They have been reported in a certain percentage of patients, and the drug manufacturer is required to list them. But most of the problems on those lists occur only rarely (that is, in less than 1 percent of cases). Just because a drug *may* cause an adverse reaction, doesn't mean it necessarily *will* in your case.

For peace of mind, be sure to ask your doctor, nurse, or pharmacist what problems are most likely to occur with a given therapy and what steps can be taken to minimize their impact.

What are the long-term risks of this treatment?

Some treatments carry long-term risks, such as the danger of heart damage or nerve damage from chemotherapy. Unfortunately, some treatments even increase the risk of developing another (secondary) cancer. Knowing about such risks may help you decide between two seemingly similar options, one of which may carry fewer or less serious long-term complications.

Remember in all this discussion that *the risks of the treatment must always be weighed against the risks of the disease itself and the cost of doing nothing,* which could include medical complications, unnecessary pain, and even death.

How do I know which treatment gives me my best chances?

Conventional medical doctors often refer to the outcomes of cancer treatment in terms of the percentage of patients who survive 5, 10, or more years after therapy. Such information can be highly valuable in helping you decide which course of treatment to follow. Here are the key questions to ask as you make your decision:

- What is the difference in survival rates among the various treatment options?
- What are the differences in risks of side effects and toxicity?
- What impact on my quality of life will each of the treatments have?
- What is the difference between response and survival rates? (Many tumors are called responsive because they get smaller with treatment, but that change may not result in improved survival times or enhanced quality of life.)
- What is my outlook if I choose to have no treatment at all?

In cancer care, as in all medicine, the risks of treatment must be weighed against the possible benefits. Here's an example of what this means.

Mary, a 55-year old woman, learns that, in her case, surgery alone will give her a 70 percent chance of living another 5 years and a 50 percent chance of living 10 years. If she also undergoes radiation and chemotherapy, her odds improve a little: Her chances of five-year survival rise to 80 percent and her ten-year chances to 60 percent. In her case, she decides that the possible adverse effects of additional therapy aren't worth the small increase in her odds. John, a 40-year-old man, has a different scenario. In his case, surgery will give him a 50 percent shot at five-year survival and a 30 percent chance of living another ten years. Having radiation and chemotherapy increases his chances to 80 and 60 percent, respectively. Clearly, it's in his best interests to go for all three forms of treatment.

Of course, it's worth keeping in mind that the survival rates your physician will discuss with you probably do not take into account the potential benefits of alternative and complementary therapies. We believe that appropriate use of these modalities will significantly improve the outcome, in terms of longevity, quality of life, and reduced risk of recurrence.

How can I best prepare for this treatment?
Having access to a full and balanced care team allows you to draw on the expertise of many providers and viewpoints. This team might include your oncologist; the nursing staff; your naturopathic doctor, acupuncturist, and nutritionist; and trusted friends.

Consult with the team to learn how best to pre-treat yourself to reduce the likelihood of potential complications. Such strategies, discussed in more depth in Part 3 of this book, can include improved diet, prescription medications to control nausea, stress reduction, lifestyle and job changes, getting adequate rest and exercise, and steps taken to improve your overall health and spiritual sense of well-being.

Because cancer therapy can reduce your immune function, oral infections are a common consequence of treatment. For this reason, we urge our patients to visit their dentists for a complete checkup and, if time permits, to have any dental work completed before treatment begins.

Are there support groups or information services available for my type of cancer?

Absolutely. Most hospitals and oncology offices have support groups for cancer patients. These groups are invaluable in helping you to understand the bewildering medical whirlwind you're caught up in. They allow you to meet others who have been through the same process and who have valuable experiences and insights to share. Several years ago a breakthrough study conducted at Stanford University's School of Medicine convincingly showed that cancer patients (in this case, breast-cancer patients) who attended regular weekly support groups *doubled* their chances of survival.[3] Subsequent studies have shown that group psychotherapy not only increases survival but also significantly improves the quality of life.[4]

In addition to general cancer support groups, there are groups for specific cancers such as breast cancer, prostate cancer, bone marrow transplant patients, and so on. These targeted groups often lead to strong bonds among members, because everyone present has had similar experiences and problems. They may also be able to offer more specific and helpful suggestions than those provided by a "mixed" group of cancer survivors.

There are even support groups for family members and care providers to help them find better ways to help their loved ones and to emphasize the importance of taking care of themselves during the treatment process.

In addition to support groups, many patients have found it helpful to set up a "caring circle" of four to six close friends who agree to help you during your treatment. Such help could be in the form of driving you to appointments, helping with housework, preparing meals, walking the dog, or running errands. Putting such a system in place before you begin treatment makes it easier for you to ask for help and provides a welcome outlet for the love and concern those around you feel at this time.

Are there any new drugs or treatments available for people with my type of cancer?

In this country, drugs are approved by the federal government for use in specific conditions. The purpose of the drug, called its indication, is listed in the prescribing information that comes in the package. Often, however, researchers discover that a certain drug may offer some benefits for conditions that are not specifically listed on the package insert. These are known as off-label indications. Doctors have the right to use their judgment in prescribing any medication for any reason they see fit. Sometimes patients have benefited greatly from receiving such treatments, which have gone on to become standard therapy for those conditions. We encourage you to ask your doctor whether other treatments are available.

One approach is to consider taking part in clinical trials—scientific studies designed to evaluate the safety and efficacy of new drugs or to see if previously approved drugs might offer some benefit in different indications. Of course, many drugs tested in such trials end up offering no benefit, or they turn out to be unsafe. Reasons for taking part in clinical trials range from being a willing volunteer to see if a treatment works to grasping at any straw that might offer hope of a cure. Whether you decide to participate in a clinical trial is a difficult and personal issue.

Where should I go to get the best treatment?

Many cancers can be adequately treated in local oncology centers. In more advanced cases, or in rare cancers, there may be a particular "center of excellence" offering a higher degree of expertise in your illness. Your doctor may refer you to one of these sites or you may find out about it by researching Cancernet (http://cancernet.nci.nih.gov). There may also be newer procedures or equipment that produce greater efficacy with a lower risk of adverse effects and that are only available in a few centers around the country. An example is high dose rate (HDR) brachytherapy for prostate cancer. The procedure uses brief exposure to higher doses of radiation inside the prostate rather than lower doses administered over a longer time through the use of permanently implanted radioactive seeds. Sometimes your caregivers know about treatment options available in your area but may not be aware of valid therapies available in more distant care centers. You may need to be more aggressive in your research to find out about the latest treatments and where they can be obtained. Organizations such as the National Cancer Institute can be helpful in this regard.

Surgery is another situation that calls for doing a little homework. Studies have shown that the rate of complications—for example, impotence and incontinence after prostate surgery—is lower at university centers where more of these procedures are performed. It is only reasonable to expect that doctors who do high numbers of certain procedures will have more practice and get better at it. Ask your doctors to refer you to the surgeon or the center that *they* would go to if they had this illness.

Get a Second Opinion

In most cases, you'll want to get a second opinion, both about your diagnosis and about your treatment options. Confirming the diagnosis is essential, since cancer—a wily disease that appears in many forms and whose nature can change rapidly in just a short time—can often mislead even the most highly trained professionals. For example, one of the deadliest forms of cancer, malignant melanoma, can look just like some noncancerous conditions, such as moles or pigmented lesions. Unfortunately, misdiagnosis does occur, and delays in identifying the disease correctly can prevent patients from receiving timely, appropriate care.

In some cases, getting a second opinion might mean speaking to a physician in the same general field of medicine as the one who provided your initial diagnosis. Or it might mean seeking guidance from someone who can add new information to the mix, such as a naturopathic physician or other alternative medicine provider. Ideally, you'll consider both strategies. Whatever your approach, the goal is to broaden your perspective concerning your disease and the choices available to you.

Making Your Choice

After asking all these questions, you'll ultimately come to the moment when you need to make some decisions about treatments. In many cases there is no "right" decision. You may have to choose from among a bewildering array of options. And you'll probably have to make some choices based on technical medical data, much of which may be confusing—and a little scary.

For many people, the hardest part of the decision is realizing that there are very few absolutes. Your doctors usually won't be able to promise that they "got it all" or that there's "no chance" you'll experience a certain side effect. Realistically, the best your doctors and advisers can do is talk about statistics and percentages. Trouble is, these statistics don't really apply to an individual. There might be only a 1 percent chance that you'll experience Adverse Effect X—but if you're the 1 out of 100 who has that side effect, the fact that a treatment is "99 percent side-effect-free" won't mean much to you.

There are several strategies we urge our patients to use to help with their decision making.

Majority rules: In this technique the patient seeks a second, third, and sometimes even fourth opinion from experts. If everyone agrees on a single treatment, the patient will go forward with that. If one gets as many opinions as consultations, then there is obviously no "best" answer, and other strategies may need to be considered.

Self-awareness: Many people have long-held opinions or feelings about themselves or a certain treatment, and such opinions may affect their decisions. For example, some women would agree to any form of drug or radiation treatment to avoid losing a breast through mastectomy. Some men would do the same to avoid the risk of impotence following surgery for prostate cancer. As long as there is an equally viable treatment to choose from, basing decisions on your awareness of your needs and priorities is a solid way to make decisions. Just be sure that you don't rule out the treatment most likely to save your life because of old preconceptions or fears.

Intuition: Trusting to intuition is a way to get in touch with your inner feelings and may help clear the way to making a decision. People do this in various ways. For you it may mean keeping a journal of your feelings, writing down your dreams, meditating on a question, or actively seeking out your own innate knowledge. Each of these is a way to filter through and sort out the information you are collecting. Sometimes one path will just resonate as the right one to take. It often pays to listen to these gut feelings. But we urge our patients to be sure that the answers that come to you address your highest good—and that you're not just giving yourself an easy answer, the one you wanted most to hear. Sometimes the hardest path to follow is the one that provides the greatest rewards at the end.

Regret minimalization: One of our patients told us about this technique. It involves looking forward into the future, seeing all the possible outcomes of each decision, and experiencing the emotions you would feel if that particular outcome were to become a reality. In her case, she knew she'd found the right decision when she imagined an outcome that might have been less than ideal but that still allowed her to feel she'd made the right decision based on what she knew at the time.

Imagine success: Once you've made your decision, there's another step to take that we believe is essential for achieving the optimal outcome. Simply put, that step is to *imagine success.* Prepare yourself to be as healthy as possible and go forward trusting in the ability of your body and your spirit to survive with the help of your caregivers and your loved ones. Remember that you are always in control at all stages of this process. In most cases, if the initial plan isn't working, you can revisit the decision and make another choice.

It is also helpful to realize that with most cancers, you have some time to educate yourself as thoroughly as you wish about your illness and treatment choices. Although receiving a diagnosis often leads to a sense of urgency—and in some cases there truly is an urgent need to act—the reality is that by the time a cancer has been diagnosed, it has probably been present in the body for several years.

Unless the tumor is causing acute symptoms, taking a few weeks to allow time for learning, introspection, and decision making will actually improve your chances. You'll have a better grasp on your options and will make smarter choices. This learning time can also allow you to come to terms with emotional issues such as sadness about possible loss of body function, fears about mortality, and so on.

Time spent in such preparation is not wasted. For one thing, it helps you achieve a greater sense of emotional balance. That helps your immune system function better—remember that your immune system is a vital link to the process of healing from cancer and its treatment. Having a good understanding of what is to come, and having taken an active part in the decision process, is itself therapeutic. This is also the time to improve your dietary and lifestyle habits to physically prepare for treatment.

Choose the Physician Who's Right for You

Even in this era of managed care, most cancer patients have some control over whom they go to for care. Unfortunately, in some cases patients get stuck working with doctors who are not a good match for them on a personal level.

By reading this book, you are making a strong statement that you are interested in using natural medicine to help you fight cancer. If you find that your physicians believe that you should not use these strategies, then you may need to keep looking. It's probably easier to find a doctor who supports you than to try to change someone's mind on the subject.

Fortunately the situation is improving. Today many conventional oncologists recognize that natural medicine does have its place in conventional cancer care. This book is written as much for them as it is for you.

Build a Good Relationship with Your Caregivers

To get the most out of your treatment, it's necessary to develop a relationship of trust and confidence with your caregivers—physicians, nurses and staff, therapists, and others. That may seem like a difficult task, but it can be done.

Try to be as organized as possible. Time is as valuable to your doctors as it is to you. There are only so many hours in a day, and the health care system today puts pressure on physicians to keep visits as short as possible.

You can make your experience more valuable by bringing with you a list of questions or issues that you want to discuss. If the list is long, schedule a longer consultation visit so that there will be time to fully understand the answers.

Take notes or even tape-record your session. Keeping track of such information during the visit can help bring all the members of your support network up to date.

We encourage you to bring someone with you to doctor appointments, chemotherapy treatments, and hospital visits. Such a person acts as your advocate—someone who is there to support you and help take action on your behalf. Advocates are useful for several reasons. People coping with illness often find it hard to absorb everything that happens to them during a medical visit. There are so many questions to be answered, facts to learn, choices to be made. It's hard to grasp all the details. An advocate helps ensure that you get all you need from these encounters. Having a second set of ears to listen, take notes, and review the visit with you afterward means you're less likely to miss some important point because of information overload.

It is especially important to have a knowledgeable and informed advocate available during a stay in the hospital. At the very least, having an advocate can make a trip to the hospital seem less frightening and overwhelming. This person can help assure that you receive the best care and can reduce the possibility of complications and mistakes. Because of budget constraints, hospitals today have fewer nurses on staff. Many services are provided by overworked paraprofessionals. Sad to say, such a situation can lead to mistakes in medications or provision of care. Your stay will be more pleasant and you will recover more quickly with fewer complications if your advocate is there to verify that your medications are given at the right time, that it is the medication you should be taking, and that your safety and comfort needs are being met.

We urge our patients to nominate one, or at most two, people as advocates. Having the same person involved when needed at different steps along the way helps provide consistency and oversight concerning your medical care. What's more, a regular advocate is more likely to notice changes in treatments, such as different medications or dosing, and confirm with health caregivers that such a change is intended.

Watch for Bias

You might have heard the old expression "When the only tool you have is a hammer, then every problem looks like a nail." Applied to the medical profession, this means that specialists offer the solutions that reflect their particular area of expertise. That's certainly understandable. Doctors are like all of us: If we're not up on something, we tend to be down on it. Historically, all that they ever learned in medical school about complementary medicine was to instruct patients to stay away from it.

As a result, there has been an inherent bias against the use of natural approaches to cancer and other diseases. Many experts refuse to consider or incorporate promising strategies that lie outside their immediate realm of experience. As a patient coping with today's complex health care system, it is your responsibility to carefully weigh the advice you're given. There's another old expression that applies here: "When given advice, consider the source."

Use Natural Medicines

Currently, standard approaches to cancer treatment produce a cure only about 50 percent of the time. Anything that we can do to enhance success rates, without increasing the risk of side effects, is clearly needed. As naturopathic physicians, we recommend to our cancer patients a wide spectrum of natural products to help them win the battle.

The ultimate aim of both natural and conventional medicine is the same: to treat and cure cancer. But the approach we prefer to take as naturopathic physicians is different. Instead of trying to destroy cancer cells directly by toxic means such as chemotherapy agents or radiation alone, our main strategy is to strengthen and activate the body's own natural cancer-fighting mechanisms as well.

The main strategies of natural medicine are to:

- **Support immune function.** A healthy immune system is better able to recognize cancer cells as abnormal and destroy them before they produce tumors.
- **Inhibit tumor growth.** Tumors cells are abnormal because they do not respond to signals that regulate their growth, the way healthy cells do. Many natural compounds partially restore cell responsiveness, thereby slowing the uncontrolled growth of a tumor.
- **Support normal cell differentiation.** Normal mature cells have features that make them look and act differently from immature cells. Scientists refer to cancer cells as *undifferentiated* because they

lack these mature features. Lack of differentiation makes it possible for cancer cells to evade the signals that normally control growth. Some natural medicines promote the differentiation of cancer cells into more normal cell types.

- **Promote programmed cell death (apoptosis).** By restoring the normal function of important cellular regulators, we can enhance the cell's natural ability to destroy itself if it becomes damaged or cancerous.

- **Inhibit the spread of cancer.** By preventing the tumor from spreading (metastasizing), we help the immune system deal more effectively with the primary tumor instead of having to combat cancer at multiple sites.

- **Inhibit formation of new blood vessels.** Unless they have blood vessels to supply them with nourishment, tumors cannot grow much larger than a sesame seed. Tumor cells are capable of stimulating the growth of new blood vessels, a process known as angiogenesis. Compounds that inhibit such growth are called anti-angiogenics and are some of the most exciting and promising in cancer research. Through this strategy, the goal is not to kill cells directly but to starve them and keep the tumor from growing larger. Natural medicine can help achieve this important goal.

- **Reduce the likelihood of recurrence or future mutations.** Unfortunately, many conventional cancer treatments can actually cause new cancers to occur. Our goal with natural medicine is to avoid this tragic complication.

Discuss Natural Medicines with Your Doctor

The fact is, most of the 2.5 million patients diagnosed with cancer each year will use some form of alternative therapy. Despite this, roughly 70 percent of these patients never tell their oncologist about the alternative and complementary therapies they may be using. Such secrecy is at best unfortunate and at worst downright dangerous because of potential interactions—but it's also understandable. Many of our patients have told us that conventional physicians and oncologists have reacted negatively when they hear that their patients are using these other approaches. These doctors make derogatory comments or deride advice from health care professionals who may have another valuable perspective to bring to bear on the treatment of cancer. Such reactions only confuse the picture.

The negative reaction arises in large part from the wild, unsubstantiated claims of cancer cures made over the years by unqualified alternative-therapy enthusiasts. Such claims have made many physicians reluctant to consider whether natural measures that are rational and well supported by data from scientific research might play a role in a complete strategy for fighting cancer.

Nonetheless, it is essential that you talk to all members of your cancer care team about the alternative strategies you are using. Here are some guidelines for discussing with your physician the use of natural medicine in conjunction with conventional care:

- Do your research and be prepared.
- Be open and nonconfrontational.
- Make sure that your advocate is present.
- Stress that you are not choosing an "alternative" to conventional care, but rather tell your physician, "I want to allow conventional care to work more effectively for me while reducing side effects by following the guidelines of *How to Prevent and Treat Cancer with Natural Medicine.*"
- Take this book with you to your appointment and show your physician the letter from the authors of this book (see Appendix F).
- Be sure to tell them that your goal is identical to theirs—you want an excellent treatment outcome—and you would do nothing to jeopardize that goal. Emphasize that it's important to you that you both must be on the same team.

Breaking the News

For many people, one of the hardest parts of dealing with a diagnosis of cancer is having to share the news with their loved ones, especially children. But telling them about your situation is a crucial step in enlisting their support and their prayers. We recommend being as direct and honest with spouses and adult loved ones as possible. Allow them to share your emotions and offer you the support you deserve.

Telling Children

Many parents wonder if they should keep the news of their illness from their children. That's an understandable impulse. Children are so innocent and vulnerable. We want to protect them from fear and worry as much as possible.

But the truth is, children are more perceptive than we may think. When bad news strikes, children will sense the tension in the house. They know that something is wrong. Our advice is to tell children what's happening. Presenting them with simple facts builds their sense of trust in you. Opening a channel of communication with them helps prevent their active imaginations from picturing something worse. Just as important, it gives them a chance to show you the love you truly need right now.

Exactly what to tell children will vary with their age and developmental level. Young children in particular often have a difficult time when a parent is sick. Besides worrying about losing the parent, they may resent the lack of attention, and they may be confused by changes in routine. To help them overcome these feelings, you may want to consider asking family members or trusted friends to devote time and attention to younger children while you are ill. For example, occasional trips to parks or amusement places can provide welcome diversion. Even bringing the kids along on errands can become an adventure. Simply having play dates at home can be both diverting and reassuring.

We recommend that you speak with people you trust—physicians, nurses or other caregivers, therapists, religious advisers—about the best way to handle your particular situation. Family counseling may be appropriate. There are also a number of books available to help children understand when a parent has cancer. Among the ones we recommend are:

For children 4 to 7 years of age:

- *Tickles Tabitha's Cancer-tankerous Mommy,* by Amelia Frahm and Elizabeth Schultz. Nutcracker Publishing Co., 2001.
- *Becky and the Worry Cup: A Children's Book About a Parent's Cancer,* by Wendy Schlessel Harpham. HarperCollins, 1997.
- *Once Upon a Hopeful Night,* by Risa S. Yaffe and Troy Cramer. Oncology Nursing Press, 1998.

For children ages 7 and older:

- *Cancer in the Family: Helping Children Cope with a Parent's Illness,* by Sue P. Heiney, Joan F. Hermann, Katherine V. Bruss, and Joy L. Fincannon. American Cancer Society.

For parents:

- *When a Parent Has Cancer: A Guide to Caring for Your Children,* by Wendy Schlessel Harpham. HarperCollins, 1997.

Telling Others

What you choose to tell friends, neighbors, and coworkers will vary with how close you are to them. Only you can determine what makes you comfortable. Some patients complete their cancer treatment without revealing anything about their illness to coworkers, while others are far more open about the situation. Generally, though, we recommend letting others know so that you can continue to develop your support network. Many people we know who at first were reluctant to tell others about their condition have been pleasantly surprised by the concern and caring that these people show for their well-being.

Often, when people find out you're sick, they say, "Let me know if there's anything I can do." In our experience, they mean what they say. They are willing to donate a little time and effort to help you in your moment of need. Don't hesitate to take advantage of their offer. Let people know what kind of help you need most. That might mean asking someone to sit with you while you recover from surgery or chemotherapy. Other times it might mean having someone prepare meals, run errands, take the kids to school, help with housework, or make small home repairs. Some patients have developed deep friendships with those who became close during their illness. You may feel reluctant to ask for help or to "impose" on others. Just keep in mind that by getting better, you'll be around to repay their kindness with your ongoing friendship.

While in treatment, most cancer patients prefer to maintain their normal routines to the greatest extent possible. If for you this means going to work, then by all means do so. Feeling useful and productive can be an essential aspect of healing. But don't feel you have to push yourself. Remember, you are dealing with a serious illness, and you need to make recovery your priority. Speak to your employer about options. Being forthright with your boss can be especially important if you need to take time away and need others to share your responsibilities in your absence. Explore creative solutions to the situation. Consider working half-time, taking different shifts, or scheduling time off to bounce back from chemotherapy or radiation treatments.

Many patients have told us that the experience of cancer was a great teacher. It enabled them to figure out what is most important in their lives, and it showed them who their true friends were. They felt as if they were stronger and happier people because of the changes they made while fighting to get better.

Many people have found it useful to ask one person to be the central point of contact during cancer therapy. Those who are concerned can call that person to get the latest updates. This approach reduces stress on the patient while making information available to concerned friends and family.

Having cancer can be a very isolating experience. But remember: you are not alone. Thousands of patients have come before you and found some solutions that have worked for them. You can benefit from their expertise. Use as many resources as possible to prevent that sense of being alone in a scary and confusing world. Support groups, family and friends, and church groups all can help keep your spirits up when the situation becomes stressful. Contact the American Cancer Society (800-227-2345; www.cancer.org) and the National Coalition for Cancer Survivorship (310-650-8868; www.canceradvocacy.org) for information about all the stages of your illness and treatment, and about what coping strategies have worked for others.

Workplace Issues

During some phases of treatment, such as surgery or radiation, it is unavoidable that you will miss some work. At other times, such as during chemotherapy, you may feel too weak or tired to work full-time. A successful recovery demands that you avoid becoming exhausted. We frequently suggest that our patients consider working part-time during active treatment. Depending on company policy, this strategy usually allows them to maintain insurance benefits while getting adequate rest. Some patients find that if they take their chemotherapy on Friday, they can rest over the weekend and will feel up to working the rest of the week. Other patients feel that going to work helps to preserve a sense of living normally. They enjoy their job and coworkers and feel that the contact is beneficial.

One concern about working is potential exposure to infections from coworkers or the public. When your white blood counts are low because of chemotherapy or radiation, you will be more susceptible to infections and need to take more precautions. Wash your hands regularly (especially if you handle materials such as money). Urge coworkers who are ill to stay away from your work area, and try to minimize contact with the public when your white counts are low.

Another concern in the workplace is potential exposure to harmful chemicals. If your job involves working with strong chemicals, pesticides, or solvents, you may find yourself more sensitive to these compounds during treatment. Sometimes even benign substances such as perfumes can trigger nausea. Certain compounds may overwork your liver's detoxification system, which is already working hard to process all your medications and chemotherapy. At worst, organic chemicals may increase your risk for certain cancers, especially non-Hodgkin's lymphomas and breast cancer. Consider asking for a transfer to a position with less exposure to these compounds.

Many people, when dealing with cancer, claim that one of the valuable lessons they learn is the importance of making every day of their lives as fulfilling as possible. Often during treatment patients realize that their jobs may not be as meaningful as they might wish. But they feel trapped, because they depend on their insurance benefits to pay for their treatment. We urge our patients in this situation to use the opportunity to begin considering other scenarios: explore new job options, take classes to learn new skills and to prepare for a career change, or explore other careers within the same company.

During economic downturns many companies offer early retirement options. One advantage of this is that your insurance benefits will often continue when you retire, and there is frequently a buyout package of cash and incentives that may be especially appreciated with all the medical bills associated with cancer therapy. Talk to your Human Resources department to find out if this is an option for you.

Under federal law, most employers cannot discriminate against workers with handicaps (and a chronic illness such as cancer can be considered a handicap). The Americans with Disabilities Act of 1990 and the Federal Rehabilitation Act of 1973 offer you protection from unreasonable job actions based on your illness. To find out more about your rights, contact the Equal Employment Opportunity Commission at 800-669-3362 or visit their Web site: www.eeoc.gov.

Final Comment

In dealing with cancer, the most rational strategy is to use every method available that carries with it some hope of achieving the desired results. Reasonable people may disagree about what that means. From our perspective, it means taking steps to integrate natural medicine and conventional therapies to provide the optimal outcome. Doing so requires some effort, since it involves taking steps to understand your disease, working with caregivers to explore all avenues of treatment and recovery, and becoming your own best ally in determining the course of action you want to take. But the reward—a longer, healthier life—is worth it.

Chapter Seven

Battling Cancer
Through Diet

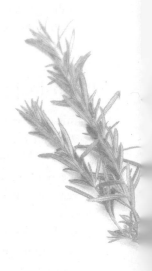

Here's a shocking statistic: Even when the right conventional medical treatment is used—whether it's surgery, chemotherapy, or radiation, or some combination—half of all people with cancer will eventually die from their disease. To our way of thinking, that cold fact is reason enough to make us want to explore all avenues for helping our patients get well.

But there are plenty of other reasons. For example, studies show that in women who had surgery for breast cancer who were less than 50 years old, chemotherapy added only an extra ten months of life compared with women who did not receive chemotherapy.[1,2] For women over 50, the added survival is about seven months. That's not a lot, especially when that precious extra time is often spoiled by the toxic side effects of therapy. We know many people who opted not to undergo treatment because they were afraid of side effects. For them, the cure seemed worse than the disease. But we counsel them that natural therapies are known to lessen the impact of side effects, while at the same time allowing conventional treatment to work. In most cases, natural therapies can actually increase the benefits from other therapies, working synergistically to improve the outcome. When given that perspective, many patients are more willing to undergo conventional treatments—and thus improve their chances of getting better.

In our clinical practice, we have met people who had tried all the conventional treatments for their cancer, but nothing worked. Told their disease was terminal, they figured they had nothing to lose by exploring a broader, more integrated approach to care. They heard about our philosophy and came to talk to us about their options. A few years later, many of these people were disease-free.

It's worth remembering the flip side of the statistic we used earlier: Fifty percent of cancer patients *survive* their disease, and many are completely cured. No one can predict exactly who will recover completely from cancer. And no physician can guarantee a cure. But we believe that you'll increase your odds of survival and have a higher quality of life if you take advantage of the whole spectrum of therapies, including those that harness the healing power of nature.

In this chapter we describe some of the general strategies that offer benefit to just about everyone who is coping with cancer.

Diet and Nutrition

The importance of high-quality nutrition in the battle against cancer cannot be overstated. Cancer patients who have higher nutritional status are not only more likely to fight off infections and recover from their illness, they're also better able to tolerate therapy and its side effects. In previous chapters we offered some general dietary guidelines that help protect your body against the onset of cancer. Many of those same principles apply to people who are undergoing treatment for the disease. Following are some additional dietary steps that cancer patients can take to minimize the negative effects of their condition, especially if they are on any chemotherapy drugs.

For someone with good energy levels, appetite, and nutritional status, following the recommendations given in the daily plan provided in Appendix A may be all that is necessary to provide them optimal nutrition. But many people with advanced cancers and most people going through chemotherapy will usually be challenged with such things as low energy levels, loss of appetite, and nausea (and possibly even vomiting).

Nausea and vomiting are among the most troubling complications of cancer. The problem sometimes results from the cancer itself, but often it's an adverse effect of chemotherapy or radiation. If nothing is done to control nausea and vomiting, patients may lose their appetite. (The technical term for this condition is *anorexia*.) When they stop eating a healthy balanced diet, patients may gradually lose a severe amount of weight. This wasting away, called *cachexia*, is a sign that the body has started to use up all of its energy reserves. After it burns all the energy stored in fat cells, it begins using the muscle cells. Rapid weight loss is one of the most serious signs of trouble for a cancer patient.

Often anorexia and cachexia are two sides of the same coin: If you don't eat, your body may waste away. Cachexia, however, can also occur in people who are eating enough—their bodies are so ravaged by disease that they cannot properly absorb the nutrients. In some cases, tumors produce large amounts of cell proteins called *cytokines*. (The word means "cell activators.") Cytokines act on the body by revving up the metabolism, thus burning more cells, accelerating tissue breakdown, and speeding up the wasting process of cachexia. By some estimates, approximately 40 percent of cancer fatalities result not from the disease itself but from malnutrition.

Patients with anorexia or cachexia may find it necessary to suspend healthy eating habits and focus on eating the things that appeal to them. That is fine for the short term, but we cannot stress enough the importance of high-quality nutrition to effectively fight cancer. You will find dietary suggestions that can help improve nutritional status in cancer patients experiencing anorexia or cachexia in Appendix B on page 308.

Enteral/Parenteral Support

Sometimes it just may not be possible for cancer patients to get the nutrition and fluids they need through eating and drinking. They may need additional measures, such as enteral nutrition (feeding via a tube directly into the stomach) or parenteral nutrition (infusion through a vein). These methods are helpful when

- upper gastrointestinal blockage prevents eating or drinking
- side effects of treatment limit eating or drinking (e.g., burns or irritation to the throat resulting from radiation therapy to the esophagus)
- anorexia or other problems such as severe depression, confusion, or disorientation keep the patient from eating or drinking sufficiently
- pain makes it difficult to chew or swallow
- surgery has involved removal of part of the gastrointestinal tract
- the patient has difficulty maintaining adequate body weight and muscle mass

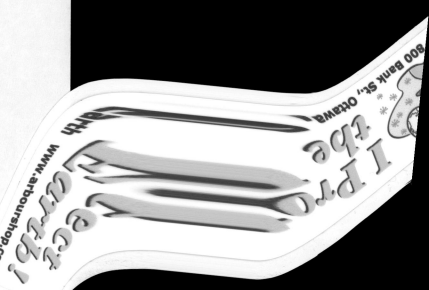

High-Protein Smoothies

Often we find that cancer patients need to increase their intake of protein, especially if they are showing signs of cachexia or they are on chemotherapy. Protein is especially important for many of the functions necessary for your recovery. It helps maintain muscle mass, nourishes the lining of the gastrointestinal tract, boosts blood counts, heals tissues, and boosts the immune system to help fight cancer and prevent infections. On the other hand, inadequate protein intake slows recovery from illness and decreases resistance to infection. Undergoing conventional cancer therapy may require as much as 50 percent more protein than usual.

Smoothies are an ideal—and delicious—way for people with cancer to consume lots of high-quality protein. There are plenty of great-tasting protein powders on the market. You can mix them with water, juice, nonfat milk, or soymilk to make your own great-tasting smoothie. Several delicious recipes are given in Appendix B.

Not only is the protein quality higher in these powders, but these smoothies are much easier and more palatable for the cancer patient to consume than fish, chicken, or red meat.

The highest-quality protein powder comes from whey, a natural by-product of the cheesemaking process. Cow's milk has about 6.25 percent protein. Of that, 80 percent is casein and the remaining 20 percent is whey. Cheese uses the casein molecules and leaves the whey. During processing, the lactose, fats, and minerals are filtered out. What's left behind is pure whey protein.

Whey is called a complete protein because it contains all essential and nonessential amino acids. (Amino acids are the building blocks of protein that are released during digestion and later used to make the thousands of different kinds of protein your body needs.) Whey protein, when processed properly, also has the highest biological value (BV) of all proteins. BV is a measure that indicates how much of the protein you eat is actually absorbed, retained, and used in the body (as opposed to the amount that passes out of the body unused). One reason the BV of whey protein is so high is that it has the highest concentrations of glutamine (an amino acid) and branched-chain amino acids (BCAAs) found in nature. Glutamine and branched-chain amino acids are critical to cellular health and protein synthesis.

Glutamine, the most abundant amino acid in the body, is involved in more metabolic processes than any other amino acid. Glutamine is especially important as a source of fuel for white blood cells, and for cells that divide rapidly, such as those that line the intestine. It has become an important component of intravenous feeding mixes in hospitals, since double-blind studies have shown that it dramatically increases survival in critically ill subjects.[3-5] Glutamine also prevents the mouth ulcers (stomatitis) and suppression of the immune system in cancer patients receiving chemotherapy. It also heals peptic ulcers, enhances energy levels, boosts immune functions, and fights infections.[5-7]

We recommend that patients obtain their glutamine by taking daily doses of 20 to 30 g of whey-protein concentrate twice a day. We believe that acquiring glutamine from whey protein provides additional benefit over simply taking glutamine. Whey protein is more beneficial because it contains other compounds (called fractions and peptides) that are known to improve immune function and boost glutathione concentrations.[8-10] If for some reason (e.g., allergy) you cannot take whey protein, then you can take glutamine supplements, 3 to 10 g daily.

Whey protein and/or glutamine can be used to support recovery from surgery, radiation therapy, and chemotherapy. If you have trouble keeping your weight up, then we would recommend using one of the whey-based weight-gain products on the marketplace.

Whey protein comes in premeasured individual serving packets and bulk canisters and is available in many different flavors—chocolate, vanilla, strawberry, pina colada, orange, and so on—from many different manufacturers. For many of the products, just mixing the whey protein with 8 to 12 ounces of water, juice, nonfat milk, or soymilk and a few ice cubes is all that is needed to make a delicious shake. You can also add some frozen or fresh fruit, ½ to 1 cup, to make it even more nutritious and higher in calories. Smoothies are also a great way to add flaxseed oil or ground flaxseed to your diet. We provide a few smoothie recipes to try in Appendix B, Daily Plan for Beating Cancer.

Reducing Tumor Cell Glutathione Levels with Whey Protein

Glutathione is a powerful antioxidant that also helps enzymes rid the body of toxic substances. Ironically, some studies show that the concentration of glutathione is higher in tumor cells than in neighboring normal cells. This difference in glutathione status might explain why some cancer cells are resistant to chemotherapy—they've "recruited" glutathione to protect them.

If that's true, then it would make therapeutic sense to try to reduce the levels of glutathione in tumor cells. Whey protein might be the answer. Studies indicate that whey protein selectively depletes cancer cells of their glutathione, thus making them more susceptible to cancer treatment, and inhibits cancer cell growth, thus reducing the tumor burden.[8-10] At the same time, it increases glutathione in normal cells and increases their growth. These benefits were not seen with other proteins. The researchers concluded: "Selective depletion of tumor cell glutathione may in fact render cancer cells more vulnerable to the action of chemotherapy and eventually protect normal tissue against the deleterious effects of chemotherapy."[9]

How does whey accomplish this neat trick? Scientists aren't sure. We do know that glutathione production is self-regulated—that is, when levels are high enough, the cell switches off production. Perhaps whey protein "fixes" this feedback mechanism in tumor cells, causing them to shut down their overproduction of glutathione.

Hydration

For optimal health, it's important for everyone to take in adequate fluid. For people with cancer—especially those undergoing chemotherapy—it's absolutely essential to maintain good hydration. Without adequate water your body cannot detoxify the drugs and remove them from your system. The buildup of these toxins will lead to further symptoms and discomfort. You also need fluid to remove the metabolic by-products of your fight against cancer, including the debris from dead cells.

Lack of adequate water can cause a range of medical complications, including cystitis, excess calcium buildup, electrolyte disturbances, fatigue, muscle spasms, and irregular heartbeat. The risk of dehydration is higher if chemotherapy causes vomiting and diarrhea.

Here are some tips to maintain good hydration:

- Drink bottled, filtered, or purified water.
- Prepare herbal ice teas and keep a glass at your side throughout the day. If you sip just 4 to 6 ounces every hour, you'll reach your daily quota for fluids.
- Avoid caffeine and alcohol. These act as diuretics, which means they draw water from your cells and cause you to urinate more fluid than you are consuming.
- Eat more soups, stews, and other "watery" foods. These are often easier to digest. They're also easy to reheat when you are tired, and they increase your total water intake with each serving.
- Freeze ice pops made with weak fruit juice and water or seltzer and suck on them when your mouth is sore.
- Drink most of your fluids between meals to leave more room to take in nutritious food when you eat.
- Avoid drinking large amounts of fluids all at once, since that can cause nausea and perhaps aggravate the dehydration. Instead sip several ounces, wait about 15 minutes, and sip some more.
- Eat more fresh fruits, especially juicy ones. Watermelon is a particularly good choice.
- Choose sorbets and ices for dessert.
- If you are extremely tired, keep an ice chest by your chair or bedside to make it easier to reach fluids throughout the day.

Suggestions for Dealing with Dehydration

Electrolytes (such as potassium, calcium, and sodium) are chemicals your cells need to function. Dehydration can cause an electrolyte imbalance. If you are dehydrated because of vomiting or diarrhea, it is important to drink fluids that replenish electrolytes, such as Gatorade or other sports drinks. You can make your own electrolyte drink by combining 1 quart water, 4 tablespoons honey, 1 teaspoon salt, and 1 teaspoon baking soda. For milder dehydration, fruit juices and teas are adequate (and they taste better).

For severe dehydration, intravenous fluid replacement may be necessary. This can be done at your doctor's office or with the assistance of a visiting home nurse. Replacement of fluids can often lead to an immediate return of well-being and reduction of nausea. Be sure to notify your doctor if you are unable to drink fluids, if you have severe diarrhea or vomiting, or if you experience a rapid weight loss within several days. Other signs of dehydration include dry lips, dark urine, or getting dizzy or lightheaded upon standing.

Get a Juicer!

Juicing provides an easy and effective way to meet many needs of the cancer patient. It is a great way to get pure, clean water into your system, and it is a very efficient way to dramatically increase your intake of cancer-fighting phytochemicals.

One of the most consistent experiences of cancer patients who start drinking fresh fruit juice and vegetable juice is a tremendous increase in energy levels. Juicing helps the body's digestive process and allows for quick absorption of high-quality nutrition. The result: increased energy levels.

Of course, you will need a juice extractor to prepare the juice yourself. Any department store or store that sells small kitchen appliances should have juicers for sale. The Juiceman models from Salton are the most popular and are very affordable ($59 to $189, depending on the model).

We recommend that you drink 18 to 24 ounces of fresh fruit or vegetable juice daily, but don't drink your allotment of fresh juice all at once; break it up into 8- to 12-ounce dosages throughout the day. Note that if you do not want to invest in a juice extractor, you will need to double up on your green drinks (see Chapter 3, page 63) to provide your body with higher levels of phytochemicals. Take two servings of the green drinks daily.

Carrot juice is perhaps the most popular juice prepared on home juice extractors. Its flavor and sweetness blend well with other vegetables. Juicing four carrots along with one apple can mask many of the stronger vegetables such as broccoli or kale. Carrots should be fresh-looking, firm, smooth, and vibrantly colored. Avoid carrots that have cracks, are bruised, or have mold growing on them and be sure to wash and scrub with a vegetable brush before juicing. The same guidelines apply to any of the other produce that you use.

Pineapple juice also makes a good juice base for the cancer patient. Believe it or not, juicing kale, spinach, or other greens with pineapple juice is delicious, as is mixing a green drink mix. If your juicer can handle it, you can juice pineapple skin and all (be sure to wash and scrub thoroughly with a biodegradable produce wash before juicing). For a delicious treat, juice ½ pineapple along with 1 cup fresh blueberries, raspberries, or cherries (remove pits before juicing).

With juicing, the best recommendation is to let your taste be your guide. It is pretty much anything goes. We provide several recipes in Appendix B, Daily Plan for Beating Cancer, to help you get started.

Ginger for Loss of Appetite, Nausea, and Vomiting

Ginger is an extremely valuable ally for the cancer patient as it exerts significant benefits in alleviating nausea. Ginger acts directly on the gastrointestinal system as well as areas in the brain that control nausea. In addition to studies in preventing motion sickness and nausea and vomiting during pregnancy, several double-blind studies have shown that ginger reduces nausea after surgery and the nausea caused by chemotherapy.[11–13]

Ginger is available in dried ginger, freeze-dried, and tincture—and in various extracts, mostly in capsule or tablet form. Although most studies have used powdered gingerroot, fresh (or possibly freeze-dried) gingerroot or extracts might yield even better results, because they might deliver higher levels of active components.

The typical dosage used in studies has been 1 to 2 g of powdered dried ginger. This dosage would be equivalent to approximately 10 g, or ⅓ ounce, of fresh gingerroot, roughly a ¼-inch slice of an average-sized-root. If you have a juicer, fresh ginger can be added to any fresh juice recipe to give it a little zing as well as greater health benefit. Here is a juice recipe that is quite soothing to the stomach and intestinal tract:

Tummy Tonic

Juice the following:

¼ slice ginger
½ handful fresh peppermint or spearmint
½ small fennel
2 apples, cut into wedges

Ginger tea can be made by adding slices of fresh ginger to hot water and steeping for 6 to 8 minutes. The longer it is steeped, the stronger the flavor. A squeeze of fresh lemon and a spoonful of honey can be added if desired.

Ginger rice can also be eaten to try to reduce nausea. It also provides some good nutrition. Cook either brown or white rice as you normally would, but add 1 piece peeled fresh ginger (1 inch long by about 1 inch in diameter), and cut into thin slices for each 1-cup serving of rice.

Homemade ginger ale can be made with your juice extractor. Juice a ¼-inch slice of an average size root, 1 lemon wedge, and 1 green apple and add it to 4 ounces sparkling mineral water. Stevia, a natural sweetener available at your local health food store, can be used to sweeten, if needed.

Soy in Cancer Treatment

Increasing the intake of soy foods appears to be helpful in most cancers. The possible exception is in women who have estrogen-sensitive breast tumors. While studies in test tubes and in animals show that the isoflavone genistein stimulates the growth of estrogen-receptor positive tumors, it inhibits growth of breast cancer cells that lack estrogen receptors as well as most other cancer cells. It appears that for most cancers, especially prostate and lung cancers, there is some benefit to increasing the consumption of the soy foods, such as tofu, tempeh, and miso, and "second-generation" soy foods that simulate traditional meat and dairy products, such as soymilk, soy hot dogs, soy sausage, soy cheese, and soy frozen desserts, found at the grocery store.

Soy isoflavonoids prevent the formation of new blood vessels, thus preventing tumors from obtaining a blood supply necessary for continued growth. They also prevent tumor cells from dividing and growing by inhibiting enzymes involved in cell replication.[14]

We encourage you to consume at least one serving of soy per day unless you have a history of estrogen-positive breast cancer, in which case we encourage you to limit soy consumption to no more than four servings per week. Remember that you can use soymilk as the base for your whey-protein smoothies.

Basic Nutritional Supplementation for the Cancer Patient

Nutritional supplementation is absolutely essential in order to give the body the tools that it needs to fight cancer. While the five key dietary supplement recommendations given in Chapter 3 would still offer some benefit to the cancer patient, more intensive support is needed. Here is the supplement program that we recommend for basic support to the cancer patient (NOTE: additional recommendations are given in Chapter 8. The Super Eight, and Appendix B, Daily Plan for Beating Cancer):

- Use a high-potency multiple vitamin and mineral formula according to the guidelines given on page 312.
- Take extra vitamin C—a total of 500 to 1000 mg three times a day.
- Make sure that your vitamin E intake is in the 400-to-800 mg range.
- Take green tea extract—enough to provide 300 to 400 mg of polyphenols daily.
- Consume one to two servings of a green drink daily (see page 63 for description).
- Take a probiotic supplement that provides 5 to 10 billion live lactobacillus species, bifidobacteria species, and/or propionibacterium freudenrichi daily.

- Use fish oil supplements at a dosage to provide 700 to 1200 mg of EPA and 400 to 800 mg of DHA per day.

If you have cancer, then green tea extract definitely becomes your appropriate flavonoid-rich extract. Green tea polyphenols not only exert significant protective action against cancer, but according to preliminary studies they exert significant therapeutic effects as well and can be safely used with conventional chemotherapy.[15–19]

If you have breast or prostate cancer, we would also add the following:

- Ground flaxseed or flax meal—2 tablespoons daily
- Indole-3 carbinol—300 to 400 mg daily
- Lycopene—30 mg daily
- Calcium d-glucarate—400 mg daily

These supplements were discussed in Chapter 4, Special Steps for Preventing Lung, Breast, Prostate, and Colon Cancers. These supplements appear to be particularly important for hormone-sensitive cancers like breast and prostate, but they might be shown to be of benefit in other forms of cancer as well. In addition to a protective effect against breast and prostate cancers, these natural compounds have shown some therapeutic benefits as well. For example, in a study of 30 women with precancerous lesions of the cervix (CIN stages II and III), indole-3 carbinol (I3C) at a dosage of 200 or 400 mg daily showed impressive results.[20] While no subject in the placebo group had complete regression of CIN, about 50 percent of the women (4 of 8 patients in the 200 mg/day arm and 4 of 9 patients in the 400 mg/day arm) had complete regression of their precancerous lesions based on their 12-week biopsy.

I3C may have benefit in nonhormone-related cancers as well. The basis for this statement is the result in the treatment of 18 patients prone to recurrent respiratory papillomas—precancerous lesions of the lungs and airways.[21] Thirty-three percent (6 of 18) of the study patients had a cessation of their papilloma growth, six patients had reduced papilloma growth rate, and six (33 percent) patients showed no clinical response to indole-3-carbinol. No side effects were noted in any of the trials with I3C.

Anxiety About Antioxidants During Chemotherapy and Radiation

One of the main areas of controversy about natural medicine and cancer involves the role of antioxidants during chemotherapy and radiation. The concern is that the antioxidants will protect the tumor cells and negate the benefits of treatment, but just the opposite appears to happen. It seems that when cancerous cells are exposed to the appropriate levels of antioxidants that we are recommending, they increase the rate at which they destroy themselves through apoptosis (cellular suicide) and become less able to switch on the gene that tells them to grow.[22–25]

As we've noted elsewhere, the big drawback of cancer therapy is that while treatment destroys the bad cells, it also destroys many healthy cells and normal tissues. Use of appropriate antioxidant therapy, fortunately, can protect healthy cells from damage and so reduce the severity of side effects from chemotherapy and radiation.

An inappropriate use of an antioxidant would be taking enormous dosages far beyond the levels that we recommend. When animals have been given huge dosages of an antioxidant that far exceed the amount corresponding to normal human use, as well as in vitro (test tube) studies that used concentrations of antioxidants not achievable in living systems, antioxidants have been shown to inhibit the cancer-killing effects of radiation and chemotherapy. For example, when vitamin E is given to mice at dosages equivalent to greater than 35,000 IU in humans, it can definitely reduce the effectiveness of radiation therapy.[26] Other studies have shown that lower amounts of vitamin E given before, during, and after radiation actually increased the effectiveness of the radiation in killing cancer cells while blocking the effect in normal cells.[22–25] Of course, 35,000 IU of vitamin E is a dosage not easily obtained through supplementation and is certainly well beyond the 400 to 800 IU that we recommend to cancer patients.

The bottom line in the whole discussion about antioxidants with conventional therapies is that there is considerable evidence in animal studies showing benefit, and emerging evidence suggests that people who use antioxidants at appropriate levels during chemotherapy survive longer. For example, in one study involving people with small-cell lung

Vitamin C and Cancer

Perhaps the most controversial use of vitamin C supplementation is in the treatment of cancer. In 1976, Linus Pauling, a two-time Nobel Prize winner (1954 Chemistry; 1962 Peace), brought vitamin C into the limelight by reporting the results of a groundbreaking study. Pauling and his colleague Ewan Cameron gave 100 terminally ill cancer patients 10 g of vitamin C per day. Sixteen of these patients survived more than one year. Such results may not seem significant—until you realize that in the control group (1,000 terminally ill patients who did not receive vitamin C), only three survived at least a year. Thus the survival rate with vitamin C was 16 percent among treated patients, compared with just 0.3 percent of those who did not get treatment. Another way of stating the results is that the survival rate was 53 times higher among the vitamin C group.[28,29]

Cameron conducted another study and reported similarly impressive results. The study included 1,826 "incurable" patients. Of these patients, 294 received high doses (10 g per day) of vitamin C. The remaining 1,532 patients served as controls. In analyzing the data, the researchers found that the treated patients had an overall survival time almost double that of the controls (343 days compared with 180 days).[30] Japanese researchers also published similar results from two uncontrolled trials conducted at two different hospitals in Japan during the 1970s.[31,32]

These studies had some flaws. They were not double-blind (that is, they were not set up so as to prevent the researchers and the patients from knowing who was getting vitamin C). Since the patients knew the purpose of the experiment, a placebo response might have affected the results. Other scientists who later conducted double-blind studies to test (some say disprove) Pauling's contentions have not found that vitamin C is better than a placebo.[33,34]

In our opinion, while vitamin C alone may not be a strong enough intervention in the treatment of most active cancers, we believe that vitamin C is appropriate for cancer patients (who typically have very low vitamin C levels anyway), because it appears to enhance their immune function, improve quality of life, and extend survival time.[28] Our dosage recommendation is 500 to 1000 mg three times daily.

cancer who used several chemotherapy drugs and underwent radiation therapy, the group that used supplements (antioxidants, vitamins, trace elements, and fatty acids) lived longer compared with most published combination chemotherapy treatment regimens alone.[27]

The Importance of Fish Oil Supplements (Again)

We cannot stress enough the importance of utilizing fish oil supplements rich in the omega-3 fatty acids EPA and DHA in cancer patients. Fish oil supplements not only address many of the underlying biochemical features of cancer but also have been shown to address quite effectively the underlying features that contribute to cancer cachexia. This benefit has now been documented by several clinical studies, including studies of patients with cancers associated with severe cachexia.[35-38] Fish oil supplementation along with vitamin E has also been shown to produce favorable effects on immune status and the survival of cancer patients.[39]

Fish oil supplementation is very much indicated in anyone taking chemotherapy, especially anyone receiving the drug doxorubicin. Not only has it increased survival time in humans and animals taking the drug, but there is considerable evidence in test tube studies that fish oils (especially DHA) increase the effectiveness of the drug.[40-43]

Use fish oil supplements at a daily dosage of 700 to 1000 mg of EPA and 400 to 800 mg of DHA.

Chapter Eight

The Super Eight: Fighting Cancer Through Key Natural Products

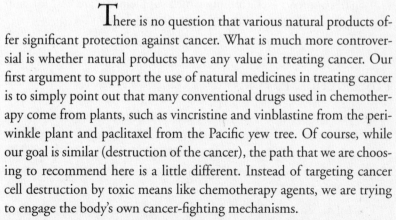

There is no question that various natural products offer significant protection against cancer. What is much more controversial is whether natural products have any value in treating cancer. Our first argument to support the use of natural medicines in treating cancer is to simply point out that many conventional drugs used in chemotherapy come from plants, such as vincristine and vinblastine from the periwinkle plant and paclitaxel from the Pacific yew tree. Of course, while our goal is similar (destruction of the cancer), the path that we are choosing to recommend here is a little different. Instead of targeting cancer cell destruction by toxic means like chemotherapy agents, we are trying to engage the body's own cancer-fighting mechanisms.

We have chosen eight cancer-fighting natural products that we are calling the Super Eight. These are listed in what we believe is their order of overall effectiveness. We based our ranking on five key criteria:

- clinical evidence of effectiveness
- scientific rationale
- safety
- compatibility with conventional therapies
- our own clinical experience

The Super-Eight Natural Medicines for Cancer Treatment

1. Proteolytic enzymes
2. Curcumin (from *Curcuma longa*)
3. Quercetin
4. Maitake D- or MD-fraction
5. PSK/PSP
6. Polyerga
7. Modified citrus pectin
8. Ip6 (inositol hexaphosphate)

While these Super Eight are important, they certainly do not represent the only products that we recommend. Also, it is not necessary in most cases to take all eight. For example, most patients won't need to take both curcumin and quercetin, or both maitake MD-fraction and PSK. The choice will depend on the type of cancer they have or the conventional treatment. Determining which supplements are best for your needs is discussed in Appendix B, Daily Plan for Beating Cancer.

Proteolytic Enzymes

Proteolytic enzymes (or proteases) refer to the various enzymes that digest (break down into smaller units) protein. These enzymes include the pancreatic proteases chymotrypsin and trypsin, bromelain (pineapple enzyme), papain (papaya enzyme), fungal proteases, and Serratia peptidase (the "silkworm" enzyme).

Proteolytic enzymes have a long history of use in cancer treatment.[1]

In 1906, John Beard, a Scottish embryologist, reported in his book *The Enzyme Treatment of Cancer and Its Scientific Basis* on the successful treatment of cancer using a pancreatic extract. Proteolytic enzymes have been promoted by numerous alternative cancer practitioners for many years, but most recently by Nicholas Gonzalez.

More than two decades ago, while attending Cornell University Medical College, Dr. Gonzalez began researching the use of oral proteolytic enzyme therapy as a treatment for cancer. At that time, he met William Donald Kelley, a Texas dentist who for twenty years had been treating cancer patients with proteolytic enzymes. Eventually, what began as a student project developed into a two-year formal research effort that Dr. Gonzalez pursued during his formal training in immunology.

Dr. Gonzalez reviewed records of nearly 10,000 cancer patients who had received proteolytic enzymes. He further interviewed and evaluated over 500 patients with appropriately diagnosed advanced cancer. In 1986, he summarized his findings in a monograph, describing in detail 50 patients whose prognoses were poor but who enjoyed long-term survival or apparent regression while following their nutritional regimen. The report met with skepticism by many in the medical community.

Dr. Gonzalez moved to New York, where he continued his investigations. In July 1993, the National Cancer Institute, as part of its effort to evaluate nontraditional cancer therapies, invited Dr. Gonzalez to conduct a pilot study involving treatment with proteolytic enzymes. He chose patients who had inoperable adenocarcinoma of the pancreas. Of the 11 patients followed in the trial, 9 of 11 (81 percent) lived longer than one year, 5 of 11 (45 percent) lived two years, 4 of 11 lived longer than three years (36 percent), and 2 lived longer than four years. In comparison, in a recent trial of the newly approved drug gemcitabine, of 126 patients with pancreatic cancer, not one lived longer than 19 months.[2]

As a result of the pilot study, the NCI and the National Center for Complementary and Alternative Medicine approved funding for a large-scale clinical trial at Columbia Presbyterian Medical Center in New York, comparing Dr. Gonzalez's protocol against gemcitabine in the treatment of inoperable pancreatic cancer. Interested patients can learn more about the study and its objectives by visiting the Web site www.dr-gonzalez.com.

The Power of Proteolytics

Proteolytic enzymes appear to have a number of valuable anticancer effects. In addition to increasing the manufacture of cancer-blocking antiproteases, they also inhibit angiogenesis and metastasis, enhance the immune response, and promote differentiation of cancer cells.[1]

Clinical studies have included patients with cancers of the breast, lung, stomach, head and neck, ovaries, cervix, and colon, and lymphomas and multiple myeloma. Results suggest that treatment improves the general condition of patients and their quality of life and produces slight-to-modest increases in life expectancy.[1] Since the patients were also undergoing conventional treatment, it appears that proteolytic enzymes can be used as adjunctive (additional) therapy. They are especially helpful in fighting against viral infections as a result of chemotherapy-induced immune suppression.[3] Table 8-1 summarizes the results of several studies that used the following combination of enzymes:

ENZYME	DOSE
Pancreatin (8X)	100 mg
Papain	60 mg
Chymotrypsin	1 mg
Bromelain	45 mg
Trypsin	24 mg
Rutin	50 mg

Table 8-1. Proteolytic Enzyme Studies[1]
Patients Receiving Chemotherapy

CANCER	STUDY DESIGN	TREATMENT (# PATIENTS)	DURATION OF THERAPY	EFFECTS OF ENZYME THERAPY
Lung (inoperable)	Prospective randomized	Fluorouracil, vinblastine, cyclophosphamide with (25) vs. without enzymes (26)	12 months	• Improvement in general condition and quality of life • Some improvement in life expectancy • Fewer side effects

CANCER	STUDY DESIGN	TREATMENT (# PATIENTS)	DURATION OF THERAPY	EFFECTS OF ENZYME THERAPY
Gastric	Prospective open	Mitomycin, fluorouracil, cytarabine (76) vs. picibanil (80) vs. picibanil plus enzymes (89)	6–12 months	Increase in the ratio of T lymphocytes to total lymphocytes
Ovarian	Prospective, randomized, placebo-controlled	Carboplatin, epirubicin, prednimustine with (36) vs. without enzymes (23)	6 months	More rapid fall in tumor enzymes
Multiple myeloma	Retrospective parallel group cohort	Multicombination chemotherapy with (166) vs. without enzymes (99)	At least 6 months	In patients with stage II multiple myeloma, survival increased by 36 months
Colon	Prospective, randomized, double-blind, placebo-controlled	Fluorouracil plus levamisole with (30) vs. without (30) plus enzymes	2–45 months	• Reduction in adverse effects of chemotherapy • Fewer metastases • More patients survived >42 months
Colon	Retrospective parallel group cohort	Combination chemotherapy with (166) vs. without enzymes (99)	Up to 83 months	3-year increase in survival time in patients with stage III colon cancer

For years, experts opposed to the use of orally administered proteolytic enzymes claimed that these products got digested before they could be absorbed in the body or that the molecules were too large to be absorbed at all. More recent research has shown, however, that these enzymes are indeed absorbed intact.

Table 8-1. Proteolytic Enzyme Studies *(Continued)*
Patients Receiving Radiation Therapy

CANCER	STUDY DESIGN	NUMBER OF PATIENTS (ENZYMES VS. PLACEBO)	DURATION OF THERAPY	EFFECTS OF ENZYME THERAPY
Abdominal	Prospective randomized	32 vs. 25	2–44 weeks	Delay in appearance of metastases; reduction in tumor size
Oral	Open randomized	20 vs. 19	5 weeks	Shorter duration of radiation side effects
Head and neck	Prospective randomized	47 vs. 53	7+ weeks	Significant reduction in mouth sores, difficulty in swallowing, and skin reactions
Cervical	Prospective randomized	60 vs. 60	>10 weeks	Significant reductions in radiation-induced side effects

How to Pick an Effective Product

To get the most out of proteolytic enzymes, the first step is to use a high-quality product, and the second step is to take an adequate dosage. To judge the quality of an enzyme preparation, it is vital that you know what you are looking for. Most of the proteolytic enzymes have well-established guidelines developed by the United States Pharmacopoeia (USP) or the Food Chemical Codex (FCC). We recommend avoiding products whose potency is not listed.

Proteolytic enzyme products are often "enteric-coated"—meaning that the pill has a coating around it to prevent the pill from being broken down in the stomach, where the acid would destroy the enzyme. An enteric-coated pill passes into the small intestine, where because of the pH change it will break down there. Non-enteric-coated enzyme preparations appear to be acceptable to use if they are taken prior to a meal (for digestive purposes) or on an empty stomach (for anticancer or anti-inflammatory effects).

Because the animal- and vegetarian-derived enzymes have slightly different effects, we recommend using a combination of enzymes similar to the mixture used in the clinical studies for maximum benefit such as Wobenzyme (Naturally Vitamins) or Zymactive (Natural Factors).

Proteolytic enzymes have an excellent safety profile, but there are situations in which they should not be used. For example, do not use proteolytic enzymes two to three days before or after surgery, because they might increase the risk of bleeding. Afterward, proteolytic enzymes are very important and may be helpful against lymphedema (discussed on page 223).[4]

Also, because the effects of proteolytic enzymes during pregnancy and lactation have not been sufficiently evaluated, do not use them during these times unless directed to do so by a physician.

Although no significant side effects have been noted with any of the proteolytic enzymes, allergic reactions might occur (as they can with most therapeutic agents). Pancreatic enzymes should not be used by anyone allergic to pork; bromelain should not be used by anyone allergic to pineapple; and papain should not be used by anyone sensitive to papaya.

Dosages for Individual Proteolytic Enzymes*

ENZYME	DOSAGE	NOTES
Pancreatin	300–900 mg 3x/day	Dosage is for full-strength product (8X USP)
Chymotrypsin	180–540 mg 3x/day	1 mg = 1000 USP units
Trypsin	3–9 mg 3x/day	1 mg = 25,000 USP units
Bromelain	250–750 mg 3x/day	1200–1800 mcu or gdu
Fungal proteases	15,000–45,000 USP 3x/day	
Papain	50–150 mg 3x/day	1 mg = 30,000 USP units
Serratia peptidase	50–150 mg 3x/day	200,000 Serratia peptidase units per g

*We recommend using combination products like Wobenzyme or Zymactive to provide a broader range of activity compared to any single proteolytic enzyme.

A Closer Look at the Proteases

PANCREATIN | Pancreatin is an enzyme prepared from fresh hog pancreas. The two primary proteases of pancreatin are chymotrypsin and trypsin (also available from ox bile). These proteases are also available separately.

The USP has set a strict definition for activity levels of pancreatin. Each mg of a 1X pancreatin product has at least

- 25 USP units of amylase activity
- 2 USP units of lipase activity and
- 25 USP units of protease activity

Higher-potency pancreatin is given a whole-number multiple indicating its strength. For example, a pancreatic extract that is 4 times more active than the 1X USP standard is labeled 4X USP. We recommend that our patients take only the full-strength product (8X), however. That's because lower-potency products (1X or 4X) are often diluted with salt, lactose, or galactose. These products can still be effective, but you will need to increase the dosage.

BROMELAIN | Bromelain refers to a group of sulfur-containing proteases obtained from the pineapple plant *(Ananas comusus)*. Commercial bromelain is usually derived from the stem, which differs from the bromelain found in the fruit. Bromelain has shown anticancer effects in test tube and animal studies.[5] Human research indicates that it might augment standard chemotherapy treatment and might also directly activate key immune functions often deficient in cancer patients.[6]

The activity of bromelain is defined according to two methods: milk-clotting units (mcu) and gelatin-digesting units (gdu). Both numerical values are virtually the same (that is, mcu = gdu), and either method is acceptable. For most indications, the recommended mcu or gdu of bromelain range is 1200 to 1800.

FUNGAL PROTEASES | *Aspergillus oryzae* is a mold (fungus) that produces enzymes important in the production of fermented soy foods such as soy sauce, tamari, and miso. These same enzymes are also used for medicinal purposes. Proteolytic enzymes derived from *A. oryzae* offer an advantage over other fungal proteases in that they demonstrate an unusually high stability and activity under a broader range of pH conditions. For example, pepsin is active only below a pH of about 4.5, while pancreatin has digestive activity only in an alkaline medium (pH above 7). In contrast, some preparations of *A. oryzae* enzymes are stable and active at pH levels ranging from 2 through 12.

PAPAIN | Papain is a mixture of protein-digesting enzymes derived from the green, unripe papaya and is used commercially in many meat tenderizers. Papain activity is measured in USP and FCC papain units. (Some products also use the same units as bromelain—mcu and gdu.) We recommend using papain standardized to provide 30,000 USP per mg.

SERRATIA PEPTIDASE | Serratia peptidase is an enzyme naturally present in the intestine of the silkworm. Its role is to help the emerging moth to dissolve its cocoon. Scientists have figured out how to produce the enzyme commercially by enlisting the help of a bacterium called Serratia species E15. Serratia peptidase has been used in Europe and Asia as a medicine for more than a quarter of century. In fact, it is regarded as the most powerful of the proteolytic enzymes. In clinical trials it has been shown to ease pain from sprains, torn ligaments, and other traumatic injuries, and it relieves postoperative inflammation. It also has been shown to improve sinusitis, upper respiratory tract infections, asthma, and chronic obstructive pulmonary disease as a result of its ability to improve the quality of fluid that lines our airways. Serratia peptidase exerts more powerful effects than chymotryspin and trypsin in all of these applications.

Higher quality products are standardized to provide 200,000 Serratia peptidase units per gram.

Curcumin

Curcumin is the yellow pigment of turmeric *(Curcuma longa)*, the chief ingredient in curry. In experimental and clinical studies, curcumin has demonstrated significant anti-inflammatory and anticancer effects.

The benefits of turmeric and curcumin have been demonstrated at all stages of cancer formation: initiation, promotion, and progression.[7–11] Evidence also suggests that curcumin causes cancer to regress—that is, to grow smaller. Some of curcumin's benefits come from its known activity as an antioxidant. Curcumin also

- inhibits the formation of cancer-causing nitrosamines
- enhances the body's production of cancer-fighting compounds such as glutathione
- promotes the liver's proper detoxification of cancer-causing compounds
- prevents overproduction of cyclooxygenase 2 (cox-2), an enzyme that can contribute to the development of tumors

Curcumin has also been shown to inhibit tumor growth in several ways:

- *Inhibiting epidermal growth factor (EGF) receptor sites.* EGF stimulates cells to proliferate by connecting to a receptor on the cell surface. About two-thirds of all cancers produce an abundance of these receptors, which make them highly sensitive to EGF. By reducing the number of EGF receptors, curcumin decreases the cell's tendency to proliferate.[10]
- *Inhibiting angiogenesis.* Fibroblast growth factor is a protein that promotes the formation of new blood vessels to feed the growing tumor. Curcumin inhibits production of this growth factor.[11]
- *Inhibiting nuclear factor kappa beta (NF-kb).* This is a protein that many cancers produce to block the signals commanding it to stop proliferating.[10]
- *Increasing the expression of the nuclear p53 protein.* This protein is essential for apoptosis, the normal process of cell "suicide."[10]
- *Inhibiting growth-promoting enzymes* (see discussion of tyrosine kinase in the section on quercetin, below).[10]

Experimental (test-tube) studies have found that curcumin fights tumors arising from prostate, breast, skin, colon, stomach, and liver cancers.[12–17] These benefits have also been seen in a human study involving 62 patients who had either ulcerating oral cancer or skin cancer and who had not responded to the standard treatments.[18] Patients received either an ethanol extract of turmeric (for oral cancers) or an ointment containing 0.5 percent curcumin in petroleum jelly. The ointment or extract was applied to the affected area three times daily. After 18 months, the treatment had effectively reduced the smell of the lesion (90 percent), itching and oozing (70 percent), pain (50 percent), and the size of the lesion (10 percent). These may not seem like spectacular results—but remember, standard treatments had not worked for these patients.

While more human studies are needed on the use of curcumin in cancer treatment, the experimental and preliminary evidence is quite encouraging.

What forms of cancer can be treated with curcumin?

Curcumin appears to be useful in virtually all types of cancer, because of its fundamental mechanisms of actions against cancer progression. In particular, preliminary studies suggest that curcumin is likely to inhibit prostate, breast, skin, colon, stomach, and liver cancers and is suitable for use in conjunction with chemotherapy.[12-19]

What is the proper dosage for curcumin?

The recommended dosage for curcumin is 200 to 400 mg one to three times a day. The body does not absorb curcumin all that well. To enhance absorption we recommend taking curcumin along with proteolytic enzymes (discussed above). This combination is best taken on an empty stomach 15 to 20 minutes before meals or between meals.

Is curcumin safe?

Curcumin has an excellent safety profile. In fact, no lethal dose has been reached in animal studies.[20] Curcumin at a dosage of 2.5 g/kg fed to mice, rats, guinea pigs, and monkeys produced no mortality or genetic mutations in offspring.

Quercetin

Quercetin is the most common flavonoid in the human diet. The estimated average daily intake in the United States is 25 mg. It's also the most active of the flavonoids. Many medicinal plants owe much of their activity to their high quercetin levels.

Many flavonoids have been shown to inhibit tumor formation, but quercetin has consistently proved itself the most effective.[21,22] Quercetin doesn't attack tumors directly. Instead, it works by keeping cancer cells from dividing. Here's one example. In human breast cancer cells, the presence of mutant p53 protein—a common cancer mutation—leads to uncontrolled cell growth and cancer. But quercetin suppresses the production of mutant p53 protein to nearly undetectable levels.[23]

Quercetin also works by inhibiting a family of enzymes known as tyrosine kinases. These proteins are located in or near the cell membrane. When activated, tyrosine kinases send powerful signals to the nucleus telling cancer cells it's time to divide. In one study, intravenous administration of quercetin inhibited tyrosine kinase in 9 out of 11 patients with advanced cancers. The effects were still being seen up to 16 hours after administration.[24] Drugs targeting tyrosine kinase activity (tyrophostins) are thought to represent a new approach to chemotherapy. They inhibit cancer growth, but because they don't actually kill cells (including healthy cells), they appear to be free of toxic effects. Quercetin was the first tyrosine kinase-inhibiting compound tested in a human trial. Further research is needed to determine which types of cancer are most likely to benefit from this nontoxic therapy.

As a possible treatment for breast cancer, quercetin appears to work in a unique way. It causes cancer cells to produce type II estrogen receptors (ER II), and then it binds (attaches) to those receptors. By blocking ER II receptors, quercetin stops growth signals from being generated, thereby keeping the cell from dividing. The more ER II the cell produces in response to quercetin, the more sites there are for quercetin to attach itself to, and the greater the degree of tumor suppression.[25]

What forms of cancer can be treated with quercetin?

In experimental models, quercetin has demonstrated significant antitumor activity against a wide range of cancers, including those of the breast, lung, skin, ovaries, colon, rectum, and brain, and also enhances the effects of chemotherapy while reducing its side effects.[26–39] In humans, ER II sites are found in normal tissue and on many tumors, including those just mentioned, and in leukemias and melanomas. This suggests that quercetin may be helpful against these cancers as well.

What is the proper dosage for quercetin?

The recommended dosage for quercetin is 200 to 400 mg one to three times a day. We recommend talking it with proteolytic enzymes to enhance absorption.

Is quercetin safe?

Human studies have not shown any adverse effects associated with oral administration of quercetin in a single dose of up to 4 g or after one month of 500 mg twice daily.[40,41]

Maitake D-fraction and MD-fraction

The maitake mushroom *(Grifola frondosa)* is the source of immune-enhancing compounds that offer significant health benefits. In the early 1980s, Hiroaki Nanba of Japan discovered that maitake extracts demonstrated more pronounced antitumor activity in animal tests than other mushroom extracts.[42] One of maitake extract's key benefits is that it can be taken by mouth, while other mushroom extracts (such as shiitake) are only effective when injected into the bloodstream.

In 1984, Dr. Nanba identified a specific component of the mushroom (which he called maitake D-fraction) that possessed a significant ability to stimulate white blood cells known as macrophages (whose name translates literally as "big eaters"). These specialized white blood cells engulf foreign particles, including cancer cells, bacteria, and cellular debris. Further purification produced a more potent version called the MD-fraction.[43] The MD-fraction appears to be about 30 percent more active than the D-fraction.

Maitake fractions consist of complex sugar compounds (polysaccharides known as beta-glucans) and protein. Beta-glucans appear in many forms. Those in the maitake fractions have a unique and complex structure that makes them different from the glucans found in other foods. The biggest difference is a greater number of branching side chains. Scientists believe that the more branches the beta-glucan molecule has, the better the chance that it will reach and activate a greater number of immune cells. The unique branching pattern of maitake MD-fraction makes it the ideal beta-glucan source. In contrast, beta-glucans from other foods, such as oats and barley, tend to form a viscous gel. When consumed with a meal, beta-glucans from oats and barley act as a good source of soluble fiber in lowering cholesterol and blood sugar levels, but they really don't have much of an impact on the immune system. Purified beta-glucans from common baker's yeast *(Saccharomyces cerevisiae)* possess benefits similar to those of maitake fractions but may not be as well absorbed.

Researchers have identified four primary mechanisms by which maitake fights cancer:[43–46]

- By protecting healthy cells from becoming cancerous
- By enhancing the immune system's ability to seek out and destroy cancer cells
- By helping the cell regain control of cell division and programmed cell death (apoptosis)
- By helping to prevent the spreading (metastasis) of cancer

Because maitake MD-fraction is purer than its D-fraction cousin, it is more likely to provide superior results. In a study described in the patent application for the product, both fraction forms were administered to mice who had carcinomas.[43] Tumors in the group receiving the MD-fraction showed significantly more inhibition growth than the tumors in the group given the D-fraction. The researchers also found that MD-fraction had greater effects on white blood cells (macrophage and killer T-cell activity) and on immune system potentiation. Both the D- and MD-fractions are considered to have low toxicity and high safety.[44–47]

Maitake fractions exert profound effects on immune function. In a nutshell, it appears that the beta-glucans in the MD-fraction bind to receptors on the outer membranes of macrophages and other white blood cells, including natural killer (NK) cells and cytotoxic T cells.[44–47] These immune cells are very important in protecting against and fighting cancer because they can attack tumor cells directly. Like a key inserted in a lock, the binding of the beta-glucan literally turns white blood cells on, triggering a chain reaction that ultimately results in increased immune activity. Macrophages are better able to engulf and destroy cancer cells, microbes, and other foreign cells. Immune cells step up production of important signaling proteins such as interleukin-1, interleukin-2, and lymphokines. In a kind of chain reaction, these immune activators further ramp up your body's defenses by activating other parts of the immune system.

Beta-glucans from maitake also stimulate the production of white blood cells within bone marrow, where most of your white blood cells are produced. Increased bone marrow production means higher white cell counts and better protection against infection and cancer. This beneficial effect of the beta-glucan can be put to good use in cancer patients undergoing radiation therapy or chemotherapy—treatments that often destroy white blood cell production.

What forms of cancer can be treated with maitake fractions?

Preliminary studies in animal models have shown that maitake fractions inhibit the growth of tumors in the colon, lungs, stomach, liver, prostate, cervix, bladder, and brain, as well as inhibiting leukemia. Whether similar results occur in humans is not clear at this time.

In 1994, Chinese scientists conducted a pilot study on 63 cancer patients. They reported a total regression rate against solid tumors at higher than 95 percent and a regression rate against leukemia higher than 90 percent.[45] In a preliminary study conducted by Dr. Nanba, it was reported that 165 patients with advanced cancer experienced significant improvement in symptoms or regression of tumors: 73 percent of patients with breast cancer, 67 percent with lung cancer, and 47 percent with liver cancer.[48] In contrast to the high response rates reported in the Chinese study, in Dr. Nanba's study less than 50 percent of the leukemias and cancers of the prostate, brain, stomach, and bone seemed to respond.

These preliminary studies need to be followed up by larger, better-controlled studies. In 1998 the FDA approved an Investigational New Drug Application for researchers to conduct a more detailed pilot study on maitake D-fraction's potential effects on advanced breast and prostate cancers.

What is the proper dosage for maitake D- or MD-fraction?

The dosage of maitake extracts is based on the level of the D- or MD-fraction and is calculated based on body weight: 0.5 to 1.0 mg for every 1 kg (2 pounds) of body weight per day. That translates to a dosage of approximately 35 to 70 mg of the D- or MD-fraction. For best results, take 20 minutes before meals or on an empty stomach.

What about the safety of maitake D- or MD-fraction?
The safety of maitake is well established, as it has been used as food in Japan for hundreds of years, in amounts up to several hundred grams per day, without significant adverse effects.

PSK/PSP

PSK (also known as Krestin) and PSP are closely related protein-bound polysaccharides from the cloud fungus mushroom *(Coriolus veriscolor)*. They are among the products most widely used by cancer patients in Japan and China.[49,50] As in maitake D- and MD-fractions, the active components of PSK and PSP are beta-glucans that significantly enhance immune function.

It is not necessary to take both PSK/PSP and maitake MD-fraction— one or the other can be used. We rank maitake MD-fraction over PSK/ PSP because it has shown greater immune-enhancing effects over PSK and PSP in animal studies, but there is a mountain of evidence on PSK/PSP—more than 400 scientific studies, including several clinical studies—confirming their benefits.

In one of the human studies, 111 colon cancer patients who were treated with surgery alone were given PSK or a placebo.[51] The patients were followed for the next ten years. Compared with the placebo group, the number of patients in remission (or disease-free) was twice as high in the PSK group. Their survival rate—the number of patients still alive after a decade—was more than double. In addition, white blood cells in the PSK-treated patients showed remarkably greater activity, such as the ability to move and engulf foreign materials.

What forms of cancer can be treated with PSK/PSP?
Preliminary animal studies show that, like other immune-enhancing compounds containing beta-glucans, PSK/PSP can inhibit the growth of virtually every type of tumor.[49,50] Clinical studies have also shown that PSK/PSP enhances the positive effects of chemotherapy while reducing their side effects.[51–56]

What is the proper dosage for PSK/PSP?
The typical dosage for PSK and PSP is 1 to 3 g per day.

Is PSK/PSP safe?

No side effects have been reported with PSK or PSP.

Polyerga

Polyerga is a highly purified extract of peptides (small proteins) obtained from the spleens of pigs. The discovery that these proteins might have medicinal value came about as the result of a happy accident. Prior to the late 1980s, the only source for therapeutic insulin (a hormone secreted by the pancreas and used in the treatment of diabetes) was from pigs. But in Germany after World War II, there was a shortage of pigs and consequently of insulin. Scientists scrambling to find new sources for the hormone studied other organs, including the spleen. A medical doctor and researcher, Walter Kuhlmey, found that pig spleen extract did have some insulin-like activity. But the substance also boosted energy and enhanced a person's general sense of well-being. He began selling the product, which he called Polyerga (from Latin words meaning "multiple" and "power"), as a kind of tonic.[57]

But in 1951 the situation changed. An oncologist named Heinrich Pophanken was treating his patient, Julia Meir, for advanced pancreatic cancer—a condition that usually has a very poor prognosis. Her case was considered hopeless, and she was expected to die any day. To ease her suffering, Dr. Pophanken gave her injections of Polyerga. The results astounded the physician: Her pain abated, her fatigue lifted, and she felt alive again. She received three to six injections a week for two months, then two per month after that. The patient lived for another three years and died from causes unrelated to cancer. At autopsy, pathologists discovered that the pancreatic tumor—once the size of an egg—had disappeared entirely. This case stimulated interest in Polyerga as a possible cancer treatment.

Since then, Polyerga has been evaluated in several clinical studies involving cancer patients.[57–61] In one of the largest trials, 158 breast cancer patients were divided into two groups.[58] The women in the Polyerga group received injections three times per week while the women in the control group received placebo injections. The Polyerga group showed significant improvements in the percentage of white blood cells, various measures of immune function, body weight, and general sense of well-being compared with the control group.

Polyerga contains substances that bind to receptors on white blood cells.[62–64] In response, the white cells release chemical messengers that stimulate other immune responses. Messages to the bone marrow, for example, trigger the production of more white cells—an important effect in the fight against cancer, particularly if a person is taking chemotherapy drugs that suppress white blood cell formation.

Many of the effects of Polyerga are thought to result from increased output of a protein called gamma-interferon.[65] This chemical acts as a communications link between the macrophages and lymphocytes. A low gamma-interferon level—a common problem among cancer patients—significantly impairs immune function. Polyerga may also have other beneficial effects, such as

- preventing some of the side effects of chemotherapy[66]
- enhancing the effectiveness of conventional chemotherapy and radiation treatment
- preventing metastasis
- enhancing the general sense of well-being, improving energy levels, and preventing weight loss
- increasing both the quality of life and the survival time of cancer patients.

What forms of cancer can be treated with Polyerga?

According to a study of 248 cancer patients, the best results were obtained in breast cancer patients and patients suffering from colon and other carcinomas.[60] In contrast, lung cancer patients and patients with metastases did not seem to respond as well to Polyerga. In patients with breast cancer and colon cancer, Polyerga given orally for four months improved appetite, reduced pain, increased energy and activity levels, and improved the general sense of well-being.

What is the proper dosage for Polyerga?

Each Polyerga tablet contains 100 mg of polypeptides. People who weigh under 140 pounds should take one tablet three times a day. For every additional 40 pounds of body weight, add an additional tablet. For example, a 220-pound person would take five tablets daily at even intervals. There is no toxicity with Polyerga, so there is no concern about overdosage, but taking more than recommended does not necessarily produce more effect. For best results, take Polyerga on an empty stomach before meals. Also, do not take Polyerga at the same time you take digestive enzymes like pancreatin, bromelain, or papain.

We recommend starting treatment with Polyerga as soon as possible after a diagnosis of cancer. Continue using it as directed, especially if you are also taking chemotherapy or undergoing radiation therapy.

Is Polyerga safe?

Since the "mad cow" scare hit the headlines, some of our patients are concerned about taking products derived from animal tissue. We reassure these people that no mad-cow-like diseases have ever been found in pigs. Polyerga has been used for over 50 years. During this time, no adverse side effect has ever been reported with use of either the injectable or the oral preparation. No allergic reactions have been reported, because all potentially allergenic proteins are removed during manufacture.[67]

Modified Citrus Pectin

Modified citrus pectin (MCP), also known as fractionated pectin, is a complex sugar (polysaccharide) obtained from the peel and pulp of citrus fruits. Modified citrus pectin is rich in short, nonbranched, galactose-rich carbohydrate chains. These shorter chains dissolve more readily in water and are better absorbed and utilized by the body than ordinary, long-chain pectins.

MCP appears to reduce the risk of metastasis—the spread of cancerous cells from one tumor to other sites in the body.[68–70] For metastasis to occur, cancer cells must first clump together. Protein molecules called galectins appear on the surface of cancer cells. The more galectins present, the easier it is for the cancer cells to clump together and metastasize. According to preliminary research, MCP binds to the galectins. By doing so, it blocks the cancer cell's ability to clump and spread.

Although MCP has no significant direct anticancer effect, we feel that it can be an important natural anticancer strategy.

What forms of cancer can be treated with modified citrus pectin?

Lab studies suggest that MCP is best used in preventing the metastasis of breast cancer, prostate cancer, lung cancer, and melanoma. There is not a lot of human data available yet. In one of the few human studies, MCP was shown to decrease the cancer growth rate in 4 of 7 men with prostate cancer as measured by a reduced rate of increase in PSA levels (a sign of prostate cancer severity).[71]

What is the proper dosage for modified citrus pectin?
The typical dosage recommendation for adults ranges between 6 and 30 g daily in divided doses (e.g., 6 g one to five times daily). The MCP powder is usually dissolved by blending in water or juice.

What about the safety of modified citrus pectin?
MCP is regarded as exceptionally safe. As with any dietary fiber, MCP at high doses may result in mild cases of loose stool, but this is usually only a temporary inconvenience.

Ip6 (Inositol Hexaphosphate)

For years experts have recommended eating a high-fiber diet as a way of protecting the body against cancer. It now appears that a component of fiber, called Ip6, may be responsible for the protective effects.[72,73]

Ip6 is found mainly in the fiber from whole grains and legumes. It might be better, however, to take supplements containing purified Ip6 plus inositol. The supplement form offers several advantages. First of all, in grains and beans, Ip6 binds to molecules of protein and minerals such as calcium, magnesium, or potassium to form a salt. The body has trouble absorbing this complex. Studies have shown that pure Ip6 is significantly more bioavailable than the Ip6 found in foods.[72]

Taking Ip6 along with additional inositol may actually enhance its cancer-fighting properties. To help you understand why, here's a quick chemistry lesson. Inositol is a vitamin-like substance that forms the "backbone" of the Ip6 molecule. Each of the six carbon atoms in a molecule of inositol can bind with another molecule called a phosphate. When all six carbons are "occupied" by phosphates, Ip6 is the result. But phosphates don't like to feel too crowded. When there are extra inositol molecules in the neighborhood, the phosphates make room for themselves: Three of them leave the Ip6 and attach to the inositol molecule, thus yielding two new molecules (now called Ip3). As reported by A.K.M. Shamsuddin, of the University of Maryland, it appears that Ip3 is better able to make its way into cancer cells and immune cells, where it exerts its beneficial properties. To ensure optimum Ip3 formation, Dr. Shamsuddin recommends a ratio of 4:1 of Ip6 to inositol.[72]

Ip3 plays an important role inside the cells of our bodies. When Ip3 levels are low (as they are in cancer cells), the cells replicate out of control. But when cancer cells are bathed in a broth with Ip3, they literally turn themselves off.

The combination of Ip6 and inositol has also been shown to be an effective antioxidant and immune function booster. The combination is especially helpful in stimulating the activity of white blood cells known as natural killer (NK) cells, so called because they literally kill cancer cells, viruses, and other infecting organisms. Adding Ip6 and inositol enhances the NK cells' killer instincts.

What forms of cancer can be treated with Ip6?
Lab studies show that the combination of Ip6 and inositol exerts anticancer effects against virtually all types of cancers, including cancers of the breast, prostate, lung, skin, and brain, as well as lymphomas and leukemia.[73-74] Unfortunately, at this time there are no results available from human studies.

What is the proper dosage of Ip6?
In patients who have cancer or who are at high risk for cancer, the recommended daily dose is 4800 to 7200 mg of Ip6 along with 1200 to 1800 mg of inositol. To ensure the best absorption, Ip6 and inositol should be taken on an empty stomach.

Is Ip6 safe?
Ip6 is extremely safe, according to extensive animal testing. Even in high doses, there are no reported significant negative effects on body weight, mineral content, or any internal organ. High doses have been given intravenously to humans without causing adverse effects.

Can Ip6 and inositol be used along with conventional cancer treatments?
Yes. Animal studies confirm that this combination can be used in combination with conventional cancer treatments such as radiation and

chemotherapy.[72,73] In fact, according to these studies, Ip6 has been shown to enhance the effects of these therapies.

Final Comment

The Super Eight should in no circumstance be used as "magic bullets" to fight cancer. Although these compounds exert significant benefits on their own, they are best utilized in the context of a truly comprehensive approach to cancer that includes the other components of Part 2 of this book along with the recommendations given in Part 3 as well.

Chapter Nine

The Mind-Body Connection

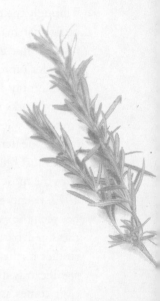

Complete treatment of cancer requires approaches from many directions. Conventional strategies, in combination with natural medicines, provide the body with the physical tools it needs to defeat the disease. Especially important are strategies that harness the spiritual and emotional powers of healing. In some cases, these methods serve to orchestrate the body's response to illness. In others, the benefits may be less direct—a greater sense of well-being, an enhanced feeling of calm in the face of calamity, or a more profound focus on the truly important things in life. We encourage you to draw on your body's own innate healing presence and the healing power of the mind and human spirit.

The Link Between the Mind and the Immune System

As discussed in Chapter 5, psychoneuroimmunology is a relatively new field of research dedicated to understanding the interactions among the emotional state, nervous system function, and the immune system. Through their scientific studies, researchers have documented something that many people innately knew: The human mind has a profound influence on one's state of health. In particular, our moods and attitudes profoundly affect the ability of the immune system to function. Simply stated, when we are happy and optimistic, our immune system works much better. Conversely, when we respond negatively to stress, the system tends to break down.

The greater the stress, the greater the impact on the immune system. Here's just one example: For many people, the loss of a spouse is perhaps the most stressful of life's events. In a landmark study published in 1977, twenty-six bereaved spouses were documented to have a clear link between the extent of grief and significantly lower immune function, as measured by the reduced activity of natural killer cells.[1] Subsequent studies further demonstrated that bereavement, depression, and stress significantly diminish important immune functions.[2,3]

It comes as no surprise that a diagnosis of cancer, and the stress of dealing with a life-threatening chronic disease, can pack a huge emotional wallop. Still, it is possible to boost immune function by consciously creating positive emotional states. In perhaps a sign of things to come, several cancer treatment centers have developed specialized psychoneuroimmunology programs for cancer patients and their families. Elements of these programs include:

- Relaxation and imagery training
- Spiritual meditation
- Stress management
- Support groups for patients, women, and families
- Individual, couples, and family counseling
- Psychoeducational groups
- Educational resources
- Humor therapy

Prayer

One of the most powerful healing techniques known costs nothing, has no negative side effects, and fits perfectly into any treatment plan. No matter what faith you embrace, you can use the power of prayer to lead you to better health—of body, mind, and soul.

Some people reading this book may be surprised to learn that prayer can be considered an alternative medicine. Indeed, many practitioners of conventional medicine cling to the notion that spirituality lies outside the scope of medical care. They believe that faith is not amenable to serious scrutiny, that at best it's merely a relic from less-enlightened ages, a crutch for the unscientifically minded.

The fact is, faith and the power of prayer are powerful healing forces. They've even been validated by several rigorous scientific studies. And today many patients innately feel that addressing their spiritual needs must be an essential part of their healing process. In a recent poll of 1,000 U.S. adults, 79 percent of the respondents endorsed the belief that spiritual faith and prayer can help people recover from disease, and 63 percent agreed that physicians should talk to patients about spiritual faith and prayer. Indeed, we would argue that *not* to include a spiritual dimension to a patient's plan for treatment and recovery is to be medically irresponsible.

One of the leaders in bringing the healing power of prayer to the forefront is Larry Dossey, author of the best-selling books *Healing Words: The Power of Prayer and the Practice of Medicine* (HarperCollins, 1993) and *Prayer Is Good Medicine* (HarperCollins, 1996). In these books, Dr. Dossey provides a thorough review of the scientific evidence. Not surprisingly, he found that prayer has received relatively little attention by the research community. His systematic analysis of more than 4.3 million published reports indexed on Medline (the U.S. government's medical database) from 1980 to 1996 revealed only 364 studies that included faith, religion, or prayer as one of the treatment parameters. The numbers are small, but the conclusion is huge: The data show that prayer and religious commitment promote good health and healing.

Scientific investigation into the healing power of prayer has shown that it can affect physical processes in a variety of organisms. Specifically, studies have explored the effects of prayer on humans and on non-human subjects, including water, enzymes, bacteria, fungi, yeast, red blood cells, cancer cells, pacemaker cells, seeds, plants, algae, moth larvae, mice, and chicks. In these studies, prayer affected the manner in which these organisms grew or functioned. What scientists discovered—no doubt to their amazement—is that prayer affected a number of biological processes, including

- Enzyme activity
- Growth rates of leukemic white blood cells
- Mutation rates of bacteria
- Germination and growth rates of various seeds
- Firing rates of pacemaker cells
- Healing rates of wounds
- Size of goiters and tumors
- Time required to awaken from anesthesia
- Autonomic effects such as electrodermal activity of the skin
- Hemoglobin levels

In our opinion, given the scientific support of prayer's beneficial effects, *not* praying for the best possible outcome may be the equivalent of deliberately withholding an effective drug or a surgical procedure.

If praying is good for others, can we do it for ourselves? Absolutely. Herbert Benson, another pioneer in mind-body medicine, has studied the physiological changes that prayer sets in motion. He found that patients who prayed or meditated evoked their body's relaxation response. This response—the exact opposite of the stress response, the "fight-or-flight" reaction that we feel during tense situations—includes decreases in heart rate, breathing rate, muscle tension, and sometimes even blood pressure. The medical implications of the relaxation response are enormous and may serve as the underlying basis for most mind-body techniques, such as guided imagery (discussed below) and meditation.[4] The relaxation response has been shown to produce useful effects in a variety of different disease states. It can also help cancer patients better tolerate chemotherapy, radiation, and surgical procedures. For example, cancer patients who undergo chemotherapy treatment and learn to evoke the relaxation response are significantly less likely to experience nausea and fatigue.[5,6]

Creating the Relaxation Response

Here is a simple exercise we use with many of our cancer patients to help them achieve the relaxation response and program white blood cells to destroy tumors. The exercise will improve your ability to breathe from the diaphragm, achieve the relaxation response, and reduce stress. Practice the following for at least 5 minutes, twice a day.

- Find a quiet, comfortable place to sit or lie down.
- Place your feet slightly apart and find a comfortable position for your arms.
- Inhale through your nose and exhale through your mouth.
- Concentrate on your breathing.
- Inhale while slowly counting to four. Notice with each breath you take that you are breathing effortlessly by using your diaphragm. You should feel as if the air is first expanding into your abdomen and then up into your lungs, then extending warmth to all parts of your body.
- Pause for one second, then slowly exhale to a count of four. As you exhale, your abdomen should move inward. As the air flows out, feel the tension and stress leaving your body.
- As you begin to relax, clear your mind of any distractions by imagining a peaceful, healing environment. Bathe yourself in the feeling of love.
- Begin to focus on the location of the cancer. Imagine that your white blood cells are flowing into the area and eating the cancer away like the little Pac-Men they are.
- Repeat the process for 5 to 10 minutes or until you achieve a sense of deep relaxation.

If you find yourself having trouble learning how to relax or perform visualization exercises, we recommend contacting the Academy for Guided Imagery (800-726-2070) or visiting their Web site (www. interactiveimagery.com) to find a practitioner who specializes in guided imagery. You can also ask your doctor for a referral. Taking a yoga class is also a great way to learn how to breathe with your diaphragm and learn how to relax.

Effective Prayer

Spindrift Research is a publicly supported foundation that since 1969 has been dedicated to the scientific research of healing through prayer. The experts at Spindrift have identified two main types of prayer: directed prayer, in which prayers state a specific goal, image, or outcome, and undirected prayer, in which no specific outcome is requested. Surprisingly, perhaps, the researchers found that while both types of prayer produced results, the undirected approach was quantitatively more effective, frequently yielding results twice as great, or more, as those arising from the directed approach.[7]

Undirected prayer involves letting go of any preconceived outcome. It is a simple affirmation of trust and faith in God that is at once a source of release, peace, and hope. Embracing the concept "Thy will be done," such prayer is thought to confer its own immediate blessing, regardless of physiological outcome. Through undirected prayer, a new perspective can be achieved, one in which cancer can be seen less as an

For further information on the role of faith and prayer in healing, contact:

International Center for the Integration of Health and Spirituality (ICIHS)
6110 Executive Boulevard Suite 680
Rockville, MD 20852
www.nihr.com

Bastyr University
Department of Spirituality in Health and Medicine
14500 Juanita Drive
Kenmore, WA 98028
www.bastyr.edu

Spindrift
2407 La Jolla Drive NW
Salem, OR 97304
home.xnet.com/~spindrif/index.htm

enemy and more as a powerful teacher leading a person to the doorway to spiritual awakening. In the words of Paramahansa Yogananda, "Your trials did not come to punish you, but to awaken you—to make you realize that you are a part of Spirit and that just behind the spark of your life is the Flame of Infinity."

Guided Imagery

As we've just learned, prayer is thought to be most effective when it's undirected—not focused on any specific goal or outcome. In contrast, the best way we know to harness the healing power of the mind is through a technique known as guided imagery. This method enhances well-being through the use of relaxation and mental visualization.

Carl Simonton is one of the leading pioneers in the practice of using guided imagery and visualization in cancer therapy. After earning his medical degree from the University of Oregon Medical School, Dr. Simonton completed a three-year residency in radiation oncology. It was during that time that he became convinced that a patient's state of mind could influence the ability to survive cancer.

In a pilot study conducted from 1974 to 1981, Dr. Simonton assessed the impact of the technique. First he taught patients to visualize their cancer cells or tumors as accurately as possible. He explained that cancer cells are weak, mixed up, disorganized. He instilled in his patients the confidence that their bodies could naturally and normally defend against cancer. He also encouraged patients to visualize their treatment as powerful and effective, capable of producing the desired outcome. Most important, he asked patients to visualize their white blood cells as a numerous and powerful army, attacking and destroying the cancer. At the end of the study, he discovered that the technique increased survival time and improved quality of life. He published his results in *Getting Well Again: A Step-by-Step Self-Help Guide to Overcoming Cancer for Patients and Their Families* (Bantam, 1978).

Predictably, the medical community was slow to accept Dr. Simonton's findings. Gradually the situation changed, and now many oncologists, hospitals, and cancer treatment centers offer his program or similar visualization techniques for their patients. In 1997 the American

Medical Association honored Dr. Simonton's video *Affirmations for Getting Well Again* (Touchstar Productions, 1997) as the best wellness film of the year.

Dr. Simonton's books and tapes are available at most major bookstores and through online outlets. We also recommend several other books and audiotapes for learning how to employ guided imagery against cancer, including those written by Petrea King or Belleruth Neparstak and available through Innervisions Studio (www. innervisionstudioinc.com).

For children we recommend *Healing Images for Children: Teaching Relaxation and Guided Imagery to Children Facing Cancer and Other Serious Illnesses* by Nancy C. Klein.

Exercise

Understandably, many people with cancer feel that they have to give up their regular exercise while coping with their disease and its treatment. Stress, strain, and fatigue can deplete the body's precious supply of energy. We would make the case, however, that exercise is never more important than when trying to help your body recover from cancer. Physical movement keeps the body in optimal working condition, which in turn helps your cells defeat the disease and allows your body to respond better to conventional treatments. Exercise also offers psychological and emotional benefits.

Your exercise program needn't be grueling or exhausting. In fact, tai chi (described in Chapter 10, Other Alternative Medical Therapies) or yoga may be the most beneficial. Even something as simple as walking 20 to 30 minutes most days of the week can be helpful. Ask your health care team to design a program that's right for you.

There is plenty of scientific evidence that exercise provides benefits. In studies in women with breast cancer, for example, women who exercise report having higher self-esteem, improved body image, less nausea during chemotherapy treatment, and less fatigue, depression, and insomnia.[8–10] The exercise does not have to be strenuous: One study showed that women who walked at their own pace for 20 to 30 minutes 4 or 5 times per week reported feeling less fatigued and less emotionally distressed and had an improved physical performance level.[8] One of the other benefits of regular exercise in breast cancer patients is that exercise helps prevent weight gain. Weight gain is a troublesome and potentially serious problem for breast cancer patients undergoing chemotherapy. Women who gain more weight during chemotherapy treatment are more likely to have breast cancer recurrences and are more likely to die of their breast cancer than patients who gain less weight.[10]

Chapter Ten

Other Alternative
Medical Therapies

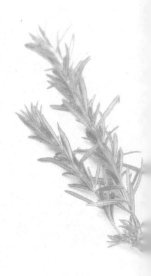

The field of alternative medicine is eclectic and diverse. Many types of treatment are available that may offer benefit to cancer patients, either by boosting the body's ability to deal with the cancer or by helping it cope with conventional medical therapies. In this chapter we explore three key alternative therapies you might want to consider including in your plan for cancer recovery:

- Hydrotherapy
- Traditional Chinese medicine (including acupuncture, qi gong, and tai chi)
- Reiki therapy

Hydrotherapy

We define hydrotherapy as the application of water in any form for the treatment of disease and the maintenance of health. In its broadest sense, the term includes both internal and external uses of water. Hydrotherapy is often recommended for cancer patients because it is a gentle treatment that can produce powerful benefits to the immune system.

The history of hydrotherapy goes back to the earliest recorded times. The Egyptians, the Chinese, and the Greeks all used it. Hippocrates, the Father of Modern Medicine, wrote about the use of hot and cold applications for the treatment of various illnesses. Modern hydrotherapy began with the publication in 1697 of the book *The History of Cold Bathing,* by an Englishman, Sir John Floyer. The popularity of the technique increased in the eighteenth century thanks to the work of such famous hydrotherapists as Vincent Preissnitz (1799–1852) and Father Sebastian Kneipp (1821–1897). People from around the world flocked to clinics in Europe seeking water cures. The founders of naturopathic medicine, Benedict Lust and Henry Lindlahr, were also advocates of hydrotherapy as a powerful healing agent. J. H. Kellogg, a medical doctor and founder of the Kellogg's cereal company, published a detailed scientific study, entitled *Rational Hydrotherapy,* that discussed various techniques and their indications. In the early 1900s, naturopathic physician O. G. Carrol opened a hydrotherapy clinic in Spokane, Washington, which ran continuously until his death in 1962.

The underlying principle of hydrotherapy is to support the inherent healing power of the body. Internal hydrotherapy does this by stimulating the elimination of metabolic waste products. External hydrotherapy works by stimulating reflexive changes in the flow of blood and lymphatic fluid to increase the ability of your cells to absorb oxygen and nutrients.

Many conventional physicians tend to discount the healing power of hydrotherapy. But research clearly supports some of the claims made by proponents. For example, studies indicate that hydrotherapy treatments can boost immune function, eliminate excess fluid, and reduce the frequency of colds and flu by over 50 percent.[1]

Internal Hydrotherapy

Internal hydrotherapy involves any internal use of water and fluids, including drinking bottled, filtered, or purified water; using water or teas as enemas or douches; and breathing steam inhalations.

Most people today do not drink enough water. We strongly encourage our cancer patients to increase their consumption of fluids to facilitate elimination of metabolic wastes from the cells. As tumors break down, they release large amounts of dead tissue that needs to be carried out of the body. Adequate hydration can be particularly important during chemotherapy, especially when taking agents that can damage the bladder or kidney. Extra water helps to dilute and flush those chemicals out of the body after they have done their job, thus reducing the risk and severity of long-term side effects.

As a general rule we suggest drinking approximately eight glasses (48 to 64 ounces) of water daily in the form of plain, spring, bottled, filtered, or purified water of any sort. Tap water is less desirable because it often contains chlorine, fluoride, and other undesirable chemicals. In addition to plain water, we recommend drinking fresh vegetable juices, green drinks (see page 63), and herbal teas, which can count toward the total fluid intake and which can also offer anticancer benefits of their own.

The other internal hydrotherapy techniques are more specific and should be used only under the guidance of trained physicians. For example, some alternative health providers recommend that cancer patients take coffee enemas. This technique may have some value in controlling pain and in helping the liver and gall bladder release wastes. As a rule, however, we do not recommend this technique. Coffee enemas can lower your electrolyte levels. Electrolytes are chemicals that facilitate electrical signals in nerves, muscles, and other tissues. Low electrolytes can induce cardiac arrhythmia, muscle cramping, and weakness. If you use enemas of any sort, be sure to have regular blood tests to evaluate electrolytes.

External Hydrotherapy

External hydrotherapy uses applications of hot and cold water to stimulate the flow of blood and lymphatic fluid. Methods can be as simple

as a foot bath or a sitz bath, or they may involve more complex procedures. In all cases, the effect of treatment depends on regulating such
variables as temperature, duration, and site of application. Hydrotherapy can be used to draw blood to an area, to direct blood flow away
from a congested area, or to alternate blood inflow and drainage.

External hydrotherapy treatments have been shown to produce profound effects on immune function. In particular, applications of hot
water have been shown to boost the number and activity of natural
killer cells—key white blood cells in the fight against cancer.[2]

External hydrotherapy should be provided by someone knowledgeable in the technique and its uses, such as a naturopathic physician. But
there's one simple external hydrotherapy treatment that just about any-
body can use, involving the use of alternating hot and cold water after a
shower. This technique is a good way to stimulate overall vitality and
immune function:

Step 1. Begin by taking a 5-minute comfortably warm to hot shower.
Step 2. After 5 minutes of hot water, turn the water to cool for 20 to 30
seconds.
Step 3. Return to hot water for 1 to 2 minutes.
Step 4. Reapply cool for 20 to 30 seconds.
Step 5. Return to hot for 1 to 2 minutes.
Step 6. Finish with cool for 5 to 30 seconds.

The above can be modified by slowly increasing the coldness of the water to increase the contrast between hot and cold over several weeks. You
can also begin with a shorter duration of cold until you build up your
tolerance.

There are several guidelines generally applicable to almost all external hydrotherapy:

- Always begin with warm-to-hot applications.
- Always use less cold than hot.
- Always finish with a cold application.

Among the advantages of hydrotherapy for cancer patients are its
simplicity and low cost. It's helpful to have a powerful yet inexpensive

> **Warning**
>
> Use external hydrotherapy only under supervision if you have heart disease, are debilitated, or have nerve damage that affects your ability to judge temperature.

technique that facilitates recovery from illness or treatment. Ask your health care provider about other individualized hydrotherapy treatments that might be right for you.

Traditional Chinese Medicine

Traditional Chinese medicine (TCM) is a complete medical system developed and refined over the past 5,000 years. The first book on acupuncture, *The Yellow Emperor's Classic of Internal Medicine,* appeared approximately 2697 B.C. and was attributed to the emperor Huang Ti. This text discusses many of the principles that still guide TCM today.

To derive the full benefit of TCM, it helps to understand something of its language, concepts, and philosophy.

One essential difference between TCM and Western medicine lies in the primary emphasis in diagnosis and treatment. Western medicine tends to focus on matter and on material changes in body chemistry. Western doctors use lab tests, fluid samples, and other concrete materials to determine how best to prescribe medications, which of course are other types of physical matter. In contrast, a Chinese medical practitioner analyzes a patient's energy, looking for signs of excess or deficiency, for indications that something is blocking energy flow, or for clues that there is an imbalance between the main types of energy in the body—the yin and the yang.

In our view, there is no fundamental clash between Western medicine and TCM. Like the black and white keys on a piano, both can co-exist happily. There are many ways of approaching a health problem, especially one as complicated and stubborn as cancer. Just as a beam of light can exist as both particles and waves, health problems can affect both chemical balance and energy balance. TCM and Western medicine analyze and treat the same illness via two distinct but not necessarily contradictory processes. Remember, TCM has been practiced for millennia, longer than any other medical system. There must be something valuable in it!

The main underlying concept of Chinese medicine is *qi* (pronounced "chee"; also spelled *chi*). Qi is the fundamental life force that guides and controls all life processes, from breathing and the beating of the heart to digestion and sleep. Qi is produced by the metabolism of food and the intake of breath. Qi serves many functions throughout the body and exists in various types, such as protective qi and food qi. Practitioners of TCM evaluate the adequacy of a patient's qi and determine whether something is disrupting its smooth flow throughout the body. Too much or too little qi can lead to imbalance and illness, as can stagnation or blockage of qi. The goal of diagnosis in TCM is to identify the state of one's qi and then decide on steps to correct any disharmony.

Another fundamental concept is that of *yin* and *yang*. These terms represent the primary opposing and counterbalancing forces that operate in the universe and, consequently, within each individual. Yin and yang are not merely opposites, like black and white. Instead, taken together, they represent a complete dynamic equilibrium, a constantly changing balance. Yin and yang are expressed in many ways: hot and cold, inner and outer, moist and dry, dark and light, male and female. When there is a balance between the qualities of yin and yang, harmony and good health exist. If either becomes too predominant, then disharmony exists. Illness may result. Here's a simple example: One yin quality is moisture. If too much is present, the body may experience edema (swelling) or diarrhea. But if dryness (yang) predominates, a person may experience dry mucous membranes, dry skin, or internal dryness leading to constipation. It isn't a question of which is better, yin or yang. Both are necessary. What's important for good health is the balance between the two. An analogy is that of an engine: the yin is gasoline and the yang is the spark. Without either one, the engine can't operate. Neither is more important than the other until one is missing.

The system of TCM is based on the existence of 14 major channels for the flow of energy. These channels are called meridians. Qi flowing smoothly through the meridians results in health. Excessive, deficient, or blocked qi leads to illness. Each meridian regulates one or more organs and has other associated qualities, such as emotions.

In the Chinese view, the body has five major organs (see box). Bear in mind, however, that these aren't necessarily the same organs we would identify on a Western anatomical diagram. What a Chinese doctor calls a "spleen" is what a Western doctor would identify as the pancreas. The important thing to understand is that in TCM, organ names more generally refer to energetic complexes that regulate a wide variety of body processes, emotions, and functions. In similar fashion, when we in the West say that people have "heart," what we're talking about are their emotions, compassion, courage, and love.

Organ Recital

The five major yin organs in TCM are the lungs, kidneys, liver, heart, and spleen. To the Chinese way of thinking, the organs are complexes that include the organ's function as well as associated emotions, seasons, foods, flavors, and predilections. Each of the organs has an associated paired organ as well as an element; these associations help explain the relationships among the various organ systems.

Lungs
The lungs serve the function of breathing and absorbing air qi. They are associated with the immune function and the skin and are paired with the large intestine meridian. The lung energy can be damaged by too much dryness and also by excess grief. Signs of weakness in the lungs include frequent colds and flu, asthma, chest tightness, and skin rashes as well as chronic melancholy. The yang organ associated with the lungs is the large intestine. The lung element is metal, and the lungs feed the kidneys, whose element is water.

Kidneys
The kidneys are considered the root of life. They hold the Jing, which is the essence or spark of life. Through their action on the Jing, the kidneys determine the strength of a person's constitution. The kidneys gov-

ern the fluids in the body and support the nerves, brain, and bone marrow. Signs of kidney imbalance can include slow growth or early degeneration, infertility, back pain, and edema. The yang organ associated with the kidneys is the bladder. The kidney element is water, and the kidneys feed the liver, whose element is wood.

Liver

The function of the liver is to store blood and to regulate the free flow of qi and blood throughout the body. The associated yang organ is the gallbladder. The emotion associated with liver imbalance is anger. Symptoms of liver disharmony can include breast tenderness, PMS, high blood pressure, headaches, and red eyes. Emotional signs of liver blockage or congestion include frustration, irritability, and rage. The liver element is wood, and the liver feeds the heart, whose element is fire.

Heart

The heart's role is to move the blood. In the world of TCM, the heart is also the regulator of the spirit as well as the other organs. The paired yang organ of the heart is the small intestine. Symptoms of heart meridian imbalance include chest pain, confusion, anxiety, and severe depression. The heart element is fire, and the heart feeds the spleen, whose element is earth.

Spleen

The function of the spleen in TCM is to form blood and qi. The spleen is sometimes referred to as the transformer and transporter. Other functions of the spleen include assimilation of information, holding the abdominal organs in place, and maintaining the muscles. Signs of spleen weakness include fatigue, obesity or wasting diseases, digestive problems, prolapse of organs, diarrhea, and obsessive thinking. The associated yang organ to the spleen is the stomach. The element for the spleen is earth, and the spleen feeds into the lungs, whose element is metal.

There are other concepts that reflect the difference in perspective between East and West. For example, a TCM practitioner might decide that a patient has a diagnosis of "wind." This doesn't necessarily mean excess stomach gas (although it might). Instead, wind symptoms have to do more generally with things that are moving, changing, and sudden in onset, such as a sudden cold. Western medicine has no equivalent concept.

As we see it, the advantage of Western medicine is that it does an excellent job of treating infectious disease, surgical problems, and traumatic illness, whereas TCM is better at helping patients manage pain, chronic illness, and nonspecific diseases. In particular, cancer patients seem to respond quite well to the various elements of TCM, especially acupuncture (discussed below).

The main branches of Chinese medicine are acupuncture, herbal medicine, qi gong, tai chi, reiki therapy, and massage. All have the same goal: to improve the balance and flow of energy. Traditional Chinese herbs are powerful tools that can benefit cancer patients. The same principles and underlying philosophy apply, but their use requires a greater degree of expertise than many Western physicians and healers can offer. In China herbal medicine is considered a specialty, much like internal medicine in the U.S. The clinical use of the herbal formulas is beyond the scope of this book. If you are interested in this approach to treatment, we urge you to consult with a care provider who has had specialized training in the field.

The following discussion focuses on acupuncture, qi gong and tai chi, which have been used widely in integrated cancer therapy programs.

Acupuncture

Acupuncture first gained wide recognition in the United States in 1971, when President Richard Nixon made a much-publicized tour of China. During that visit, a reporter for the *New York Times,* James Reston, had to undergo an emergency appendectomy. He was treated with acupuncture for postoperative pain. He wrote such a glowing report about the benefits that the American public became fascinated with this 5,000-year-old technique. Since then, interest has continued to grow and millions of Westerners have been treated with acupuncture for a range of complaints.

Acupuncture involves the use of extremely fine stainless-steel needles inserted into points along the meridians to direct the flow of energy. Practitioners have identified 365 major points and hundreds of minor points along the meridians where needles can be inserted.

There are many schools of acupuncture, each of which uses different techniques in choosing points for insertion. Some methods use only a few needles, some use many. Some focus on smaller meridian subsystems, such as relying mainly on points in the ear or on the hand. Whatever the system, the goal is to determine the form and location of energy blockage or imbalance and then remove the blockage to restore free movement of qi. We emphasize to our patients that the needles themselves are not doing any healing. Instead, the patients' bodies are enjoying the benefits that come from redirected energy.

From a scientific standpoint, stimulating these acupuncture points produces measurable biological effects. It increases levels of brain chemicals called endorphins, which act as the body's natural pain relievers. It produces favorable changes in blood chemistry and affects electrical stimulation of nerves.[3,4]

The acupuncture treatment for the cancer patient is designed to strengthen the immune system and strengthen the energy channels that are deficient or weak. The results that can be expected are that the patient has more stamina, less fatigue, and fewer of the side effects that result from conventional treatments, such as chemotherapy and radiation.

What is an acupuncture session like?
Practitioners each have their own way of treating patients. However, there are some general statements that can be made about almost all acupuncture therapy. Usually at the first visit the practitioner will ask you a series of questions. These will include questions about your main complaint but often will include seemingly unrelated questions about sleep, dreams, appetite, food cravings, digestion and elimination, emotions, moods, and fears.

The question-and-answer session will generally be followed by a brief exam. This may include an examination of the affected area as well as of the tongue and pulses. To the trained eye, the shape, color, and coating of the tongue reveal information about the internal state of the body, and the quality of the pulses (three in each wrist) gives information about the energy in the meridians and the organs.

From the information gleaned during the exam, the practitioner will determining if there is excess or deficient qi, where the areas of energy blockage are, the balance of yin and yang, and how best to address the problem. Once the imbalance is understood, the acupuncturist can correct it by selecting appropriate points. The goal is to restore balance without causing disturbances in other parts of the body.

During the session, you will lie on a table while the practitioner inserts the needles. Most patients find the process painless, but it can also be quite painful. Most people experience a momentary prick as the needle is inserted, followed by a sensation of tingling, pressure, warmth, or dull aching near the needle or along the meridian. Many patients find the process surprisingly relaxing—many even fall asleep during the treatment! A single session lasts anywhere from 20 to 60 minutes, after which all the needles are removed and discarded. When the session is over, some patients feel energized, while others feel sleepy and relaxed, depending on the points chosen by the acupuncturist.

How often you need treatment depends on the type and severity of the problem. As a general rule, patients go for sessions once every week or two, but it may be as often as three times a week or as seldom as once a month. Results will also vary. As is the case with Western medicine, deep-seated and complex problems will take longer to resolve, while milder and more acute problems are generally resolved more quickly.

Does acupuncture work?

Yes. According to an evaluation of acupuncture done by the National Institutes of Health, acupuncture can effectively relieve chronic pain, musculoskeletal injuries, and nausea from chemotherapy and anesthesia.[5] The World Health Organization confirmed that acupuncture offers these benefits and expanded the list to include dermatological complaints; asthma; digestive problems; mental and emotional problems, such as depression and PMS; reproductive problems, such as infertility and menstrual cramps; and infections such as bronchitis and hepatitis. In our personal experience, Chinese medicine has helped our patients to make some of the most remarkable improvements we have seen in our years of medical practice, especially in cases of long-standing pain.

Research has demonstrated that acupuncture and Chinese medicine as a whole are beneficial in certain aspects of cancer treatment.[6] For example, there are antiemetic medications available to prevent the vomiting associated with chemotherapy, but these drugs aren't as effective in alleviating the accompanying nausea. Studies have found that acupuncture, used alone or in conjunction with electrical stimulation, helps prevent nausea.[6–9] It's worth noting that several studies involved a placebo strategy in which needles were placed in "sham" acupuncture points. Patients in the placebo group did not experience the same benefits as patients who had needles placed in correct positions.

Acupuncture used as part of anesthesia for brain surgery was found to enhance the effectiveness of the anesthesia and to lead to smoother recovery with fewer complications.[10] Other researchers have reported that acupuncture prior to surgery reduces postoperative pain, nausea, and vomiting and the requirement for pain pills or morphine, and reduces pre- and postsurgical stress.[11,12]

Many patients who undergo radiation for head and neck cancer experience irreversible loss of salivary gland function. This results in dry mouth (xerostomia), a painful and annoying condition. Acupuncture has been shown to restore at least some level of salivation, even when medications fail.[13]

Other troublesome symptoms improved with acupuncture include hot flashes in prostate cancer patients, diarrhea and neuropathy from chemotherapy, and shortness of breath in advanced lung cancer patients.[6,14]

Several studies have found that acupuncture enhances immune function by increasing the number of white blood cells, T lymphocytes, natural killer cells, and cytokines such as interleukin-2. All these effects are valuable in the treatment of cancer.[11]

When done properly by trained personnel, acupuncture is extremely safe and side effects are rare. In fact, the NIH evaluation of acupuncture commented specifically on its safety record and the fact that the incidence of adverse effects was lower with acupuncture than with many Western drugs and medical procedures used to treat the same conditions.

Before you undergo treatment, however, be sure to verify that the acupuncturist has been adequately trained and uses sterile technique at all times to minimize the risk of infection. There are several questions to ask any practitioner before undergoing acupuncture treatment.

QUESTIONS TO ASK YOUR ACUPUNCTURE PRACTITIONER

Where did you go to school?
In general, acupuncturists have training equivalent to a master's degree. In some cases they may have a doctorate in Oriental medicine, which

represents even more extensive training. In all cases you want to go to someone who has been through an accredited program of training.

Do you have a license?
Acupuncturists in the United States have a national accrediting body, the National Commission for Certification of Acupuncture and Oriental Medicine (NCCAOM), which administers a national board exam and certification. If your state issues licenses, make sure the provider also has a state certificate. Even if your state does not license acupuncturists, be sure that the provider has a current certificate from NCCAOM.

What type of acupuncture do you do?
Understand whether your acupuncturist does Japanese, Korean, Chinese, or some other form of acupuncture. This is mainly important if you are looking for a particular type of treatment. Otherwise, the type of acupuncture is less important than the results.

Have you worked with cancer patients before?
Cancer is a complex illness, and experience in its treatment will help the acupuncturist to help you better.

What type of needles do you use?
You only want to go to someone who uses disposable, single-use needles. This eliminates the risk of infections such as hepatitis, which can come from improperly sterilized needles.

How will we evaluate progress?
Determine whether there is a measurable effect you can assess, such as levels of pain or nausea. Even for vaguer qualities, such as energy levels, try to rate yourself every day and see if the average level improves over time with acupuncture.

You should be able to evaluate results after 6 to 10 treatments. For a complex condition like cancer, it is not reasonable to expect a cure, but you should notice a reduction of symptoms such as nausea and perhaps an improvement of energy. Other symptoms such as nerve numbness or insomnia may also improve.

Are there other strategies we should try?

In addition to acupuncture, your practitioner may recommend tui na, Chinese massage, and may suggest an herbal formula or dietary changes designed to help your body move back toward a healthier balance.

Qi Gong

The term *qi gong* means "energy cultivation" and involves a series of internal exercises designed to stimulate the production and flow of energy. Training in qi gong teaches you how to regulate your own energy flow more consciously, reducing the need for external treatments such as acupuncture.

Qi gong consists of a series of movements and breathing exercises done repeatedly over time. Each exercise is designed to teach you how to breathe in a relaxed yet deliberate manner and to learn to coordinate the breath, mind, movement, energy, and intention to a single focus. There are over 80,000 different qi gong exercises. Some are very simple and others are more complex. There are even qi gong exercises you can do while lying in bed or while seated.

Qi gong has been practiced for 3,000 years in China and is taught to patients in many Chinese hospitals as part of their recovery program. To succeed with qi gong you must be persistent, because change happens slowly. But just as dripping water can eventually erode a mountainside, the daily use of qi gong can improve the flow of qi and the balance of yin and yang, leading to improved health and vitality.

It is best to learn qi gong from a teacher, but for those who have no teacher nearby there are books and videos available. One source of information is the Qi Gong Association of America (www.qi.org).

Tai Chi

Tai chi is a series of gentle flowing movement exercises derived from the martial arts. The goals of tai chi are to improve physical balance and to integrate inner and outer strength. Over time one learns to sense and regulate the flow of chi energy. Tai chi has sometimes been called a "moving meditation," because the concentration required often helps quiet the mind. The technique is valuable for those who would benefit from some form of relaxation or meditation exercise but find it difficult to sit still for the required time. Tai chi has also been shown to help improve heart and respiratory function and immune capacity and improve physical balance for those who may be at risk of falling. It helps patients regain both physical and inner strength.[15]

Tai chi is best learned from an experienced instructor. Most cities have several teachers who work through schools, colleges, and fitness centers. However, if there are no teachers in your area, it is possible to learn some of the basics from videos and books. For beginners, we recommend the videotape program *Tai Chi for Busy People* by Keith Jeffery (www.easytaichi.com).

Reiki Therapy

Reiki is a form of therapy that resembles the "laying on of hands," an ancient technique common to many spiritual traditions. The basic concept behind reiki, as in other forms of traditional Asian medicine, is that the body has an energy field that is central to health and proper functioning and that this energy travels in certain pathways that can become blocked or weakened.

In a typical reiki treatment, the patient, fully clothed, reclines comfortably on a massage table or sits in a chair. While standing in a sequence of standardized positions, the practitioner places his hands on the patient and transfers his energy, beginning at the crown of the head and moving toward the feet. The patient usually turns over once during the session. The practitioner's hands are held in each position, usually for as long as 5 minutes, to allow the transfer of energy and the healing process to take place. In each position, the hands are kept stationary. This is different from a typical massage, in which the hands move constantly. During the session, both the giver and receiver attempt to maintain an attitude of awareness, openness, and healing.

Although reiki practitioners believe that formal training is necessary to learn the proper methods of energy channeling and healing, individuals can still use some of the basic positions of reiki to relieve stress and to stimulate healing (see the "Healing Hands" box). Applying reiki to a

Healing Hands

Following is a general outline of a reiki session. As you'll see, the hands generally move from the top of the body down, but feel free to apply hands wherever there is pain or stress.

Position one: The hands are placed on the top of the head, with the wrists near the ears and the fingertips touching the crown of the head. Eyes should be closed. Hold for 5 minutes or more, until the mind feels clear and calm.

Position two: Cup the hands slightly and place the palms over the closed eyes, with the fingers resting on the forehead.

Position three: Place the hands on the sides of the head, with the thumbs behind the ears and the palms over the lower jaws, with the fingers covering the temples.

Position four: Place one hand on the back of the neck, at the base of the skull, and put the other hand just above it, on the back of the head and parallel to the first hand.

Position five: Wrap the hands around the front of the throat and rest them there gently with the heels of the hands touching in front.

Position six: Place each hand on top of a shoulder, close to the side of the neck, on top of the trapezius muscle.

Position seven: Form a T shape with the hands over the chest, with the left hand covering the heart and the right hand above it, covering the upper part of the chest.

Position eight: The hands are placed flat against the front of the body with the fingertips touching. Hold for 5 minutes or so, and repeat 4 or 5 times, moving down a hand width each time until the pelvic region is reached, which is covered with a V shape of the hands. Then, for the final position, repeat this technique on the back, beginning as close to the shoulders as the hands can reach and ending by forming a T shape with the hands at the base of the spine.

Reiki is
- a subtle and effective form of energy healing using the hands
- practiced in every country of the world
- being used in many settings, including hospitals and hospices, as well as in private practice and in self-care
- a complementary modality in any healing program

Reiki is not
- affiliated with any particular religion or religious practice
- new, but at least thousands of years old

loved one with cancer can be extremely gratifying for both the giver and receiver. The important thing is to focus on filling the mind and heart of both participants with peaceful, loving, caring, and healing thoughts and energy.

For more information on reiki and to find a practitioner in your area, contact:

International Association of Reiki Professionals
P.O. Box 481
Winchester, MA 01890
Phone: 781-729-3530
Fax: 781-721-7306
Web site: www.iarp.org

Part Three

Using Natural Medicine to

Cope with the Side Effects of

Chemotherapy, Radiation,

and Surgery

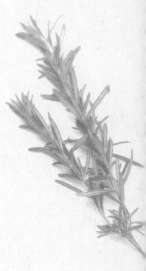

Chapter Eleven

Natural Strategies for Support Before and After Surgery

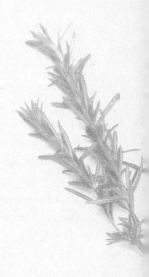

Surgery is the oldest medical treatment of cancer and is still the first approach used in treating many forms of cancer. Surgical removal often results in a cure, especially if the tumor is small—and localized, not having yet spread to neighboring tissues. Cancer surgery may involve a relatively minor procedure, such as removing a skin lesion. Or it can be extremely invasive, resulting in the removal of all or part of an organ, such as the lung, liver, or colon. In addition to removing tumors, surgery is often used as a means to control the spread of the tumor, relieve pain, or deal with other problems such as intestinal blockage or nerve damage.

If surgery alone is likely to cure the disease, it certainly makes complete sense to follow this course of action. Your physicians may also recommend using chemotherapy or radiation prior to surgery to shrink the tumor and reduce the likelihood of damage to nearby tissues.

Surgery does not produce the same type or degree of toxic side effects as chemotherapy or radiation, but operations carry a spectrum of risk. Although minor procedures are usually very safe, major surgery can cause serious, even life-threatening, complications, such as postsurgical infections and reactions to anesthetics.

Laser Surgery

Ordinary light, such as that from a lightbulb, contains many wavelengths and spreads in all directions. Laser light is very different; it uses one or more specific wavelengths and is focused in a narrow beam. Lasers can cut through steel or shape diamonds. They also can be used for very precise surgical work, such as repairing a damaged retina or cutting through delicate tissue.

Lasers were first used on skin tumors in 1961, and today one of the most common medical applications of lasers is in cancer treatment. Lasers are often used with endoscopes—tubes that allow physicians to see into certain areas of the body, such as the bladder. The light from some lasers can be transmitted through a flexible endoscope fitted with fiber optics. This allows physicians to see and work in parts of the body that could not otherwise be reached except by open surgery. Endoscopes allow surgeons to aim their laser beams very precisely. Lasers also can be used with low-power microscopes, giving the doctor a clear view of the site being treated. When used with a micromanipulator, laser systems can produce a cutting area as small as 200 microns in diameter—less than the width of a very fine thread.

Lasers are used to treat several kinds of cancer. They can remove precancerous polyps from the colon and can remove early cancers of the cervix, vagina, and vulva. Laser surgery for other cancers, such as breast cancer, is becoming more common. Among the advantages of this approach are shorter hospital stays and less risk of pain. A recent innovation is the contact laser, also known as a laser scalpel. To a surgeon, using this tool "feels" more like a performing a standard operation with a steel scalpel.

Lasers have several advantages over standard surgical tools:

- Lasers are more precise than scalpels. Tissue near an incision is protected, since there is little contact with skin or other tissue.
- The heat produced by lasers sterilizes the surgery site.
- Less operating time may be needed, because the precision of the laser allows for a smaller incision.
- Healing time is often shortened; since laser heat seals the blood vessels, there is less bleeding, swelling, and scarring.
- More procedures can be done on an outpatient basis.

Cryosurgery

Cryosurgery is a technique that uses extremely cold temperatures to freeze and destroy cancer cells. Most often, cryosurgery is used to treat cervical cancer and skin tumors, but recent technological advances have made it possible to use the method on tumors arising inside the body, such as in the prostate gland and the liver. Researchers also are studying its effectiveness as a treatment for some tumors of the bone, for brain and spinal tumors, and for tumors in the windpipe that may develop along with non-small-cell lung cancer. Some investigators use cryosurgery in combination with other treatments such as radiation, surgery, and hormone therapy. While initial results have been encouraging, more studies are needed to show the long-term effectiveness of this method.

Cryosurgery offers some advantages over conventional surgery. It's less invasive, involving only a small incision to allow insertion of the cryoprobe through the skin. Consequently, the risk of pain, bleeding, and other complications of surgery is minimized. Cryosurgery may be less expensive than other treatments and usually requires shorter hospital stays and recovery times. Because physicians can focus cryosurgical treatment on a limited area, they can avoid the destruction of nearby healthy tissue. The treatment can be safely repeated and can be used along with standard treatments such as conventional surgery, chemotherapy, and radiation. Furthermore, cryosurgery might offer an option for treating cancers that once were considered inoperable or that do not respond to standard treatments.

Use of cryosurgery for internal tumors is still in the experimental stage, so many insurance companies will refuse to pay for it. Another disadvantage is that sometimes it can be difficult for the surgeon to control how much tissue is frozen. If the probe goes too deep, healthy tissue adjacent to the tumor can be damaged. In prostate cancer, for example, this may result in damage to the urethra (the tube through which urine flows), resulting in difficulty urinating.

Music Therapy for a Quicker Recovery

The idea of music as a healing influence that could affect health and behavior is at least as old as the writings of Aristotle and Plato. Clinical studies have shown that music can ease pre-surgical anxiety as well as promote a quicker recovery.[1] Music has also been shown to alleviate pain when used in conjunction with anesthesia or pain medication, resulting in lesser amounts of these drugs being necessary.

Even during surgery, music appears to be of benefit, according to the results of a double-blind study to determine whether music or music in combination with therapeutic suggestions in the intra-operative period under general anesthesia could improve the recovery of hysterectomy patients.[2] In the study, 90 patients who underwent hysterectomy under general anesthesia were exposed to music, music in combination with therapeutic suggestion, or operating-room sounds. On the day of surgery, patients exposed to music in combination with therapeutic suggestions required less pain-relieving medications compared with the controls. Patients in the music group experienced more effective analgesia the first day after surgery and recovered earlier after the operation. At discharge from the hospital, patients in the music and music-combined-with-therapeutic-suggestion group were less fatigued compared with the controls. No differences were noted in nausea, vomiting, bowel function, well-being, or length of hospital stay between the groups.

Dietary Support for Surgery

Please follow the general guidelines given in Chapter 7, Battling Cancer Through Diet, prior to your surgery, along with any specific dietary instructions given by your physician.

Supplemental Support for Surgery

How aggressive should you be in using natural remedies as part of your surgical treatment? That depends on how extensive your operation will be. Someone undergoing a relatively minor operation, such as a woman who undergoes a simple lumpectomy requires only minimal support, while another who has a complete mastectomy or major abdominal surgery needs much more extensive and continued support.

High-quality nutrition is essential for promoting recovery from any surgery. Extensive surgery, in particular, imposes extreme demands. Your body will need to create new tissue and blood vessels, repair damaged tissue, and manufacture extra cells needed to heal the wound, fight infection, and control inflammation. If you are lacking any of the essential nutrients necessary for creating these cells and regulating these healing systems, your recovery will take longer and you're more likely to experience complications. Nutrients like protein, vitamins A and C, magnesium, copper, iron, and zinc are especially important in promoting wound repair and overall healing after a surgery.

Making sure that your body has plenty of reserves for healing prior to and after a surgery should become a primary goal to give yourself the best chance of success and a speedy recovery.

Important Warnings Before Surgery

It is essential that you notify your physicians and other caregivers about all the natural products you're using. Ask specifically if there are any supplements or herbal medicines you should avoid before or after the operation. In all cases, be sure to follow the guidelines and recommendations given to you by the surgeon and other health care staff.

Even something as simple as vitamin E can cause a problem during surgery. Specifically, vitamin E at doses above 200 IU per day may increase your risk of bleeding. You will need to stop using vitamin E supplements at least two weeks prior to surgery, or at least be sure your daily dose is less than 200 IU. Also, discontinue use of fish oils two weeks prior to the operation, because of their ability to prolong bleeding time. Here are some other natural products that you may be using that might increase the risk of bleeding during a surgery and when their use should be discontinued prior to a surgery:

- Garlic *(Allium sativum):* Discontinue at least seven days before surgery.
- Ginkgo *(Ginkgo biloba):* Discontinue at least 36 hours before surgery.
- Ginseng *(Panax ginseng, Panax quinquefolius):* Discontinue at least seven days before surgery.

In addition, it's wise to discontinue some herbs that may increase or interfere with the effects of anesthesia:

- Kava *(Piper methysticum):* Discontinue at least 24 hours before surgery.
- St. John's wort *(Hypericum perforatum):* Discontinue at least five days before surgery.
- Valerian *(Valeriana officinalis):* Discontinue at least five days before surgery.

These recommendations are based more on theoretical concerns than actual case reports or clinical trials. Still, discontinuing their use prior to surgery is a prudent precaution.

Modified Citrus Pectin (MCP)

One of the most important times to take MCP is when having any biopsy or surgery that could release tumor cells into circulation. It is well accepted that increased levels of tumor cells in circulation occur after the surgical removal of any primary tumor. Even relatively noninvasive procedures such as fine-needle biopsies of breast tumors can release free tumor cells into circulation. Having high levels of MCP in the bloodstream at these times can reduce the risk of the cancer being spread by the very procedures being done to treat it.

Like other fiber sources, MCP may interfere with the proper absorption of drugs. If you are taking any oral chemotherapy agents, you must time your dose of MCP carefully. Take it midway between doses of your chemotherapy medicine. For example, if you take a drug every eight hours, take MCP four hours after the last dose (four hours before the next one). This makes sure your body will get the full benefit out of both your cancer medication and the MCP.

Take either modified citrus pectin (MCP) at a dosage of 6 g dissolved by blending in water or juice twice daily. To ensure the best absorption, MCP should be taken on an empty stomach.

Probiotics Are Essential

If you are undergoing a major surgery, it is absolutely imperative that you take a probiotic before and after the surgery. Why? Just prior to and after a major surgery, you will be given antibiotics to reduce the likelihood of an infection. You will need to comply with this prescription, but we want to add another of our own—probiotics.

Probiotic supplements have shown good results in preventing and treating antibiotic-induced diarrhea.[3,4] Antibiotics often cause diarrhea by altering the type of bacteria in the colon or by promoting the overgrowth of *Candida albicans*. Antibiotic use can result in a severe form of diarrhea known as pseudomembranous enterocolitis. This condition is attributed to an overgrowth of a bacterium *(Clostridium difficele)*, resulting from the death of the bacteria that normally keep this Clostridium under control. Pseudomembranous enterocolitis can be quite serious and even deadly.

Reductions of friendly bacteria, the development of pseudomembranous enterocolitis, and/or infection with antibiotic-resistant bacteria may be prevented by administering probiotics products during antibiotic therapy, in particular, a specific strain—*Lactobacillus rhamnosus*.

Although it is commonly believed that acidophilus supplements are not effective if taken during antibiotic therapy, research actually supports the use of *L. rhamnosus* during antibiotic administration. A dosage of 10 to 20 billion organisms is required. Lactobacillus preparations do not appear to interfere with the effectiveness of antibiotics, but just to be as safe as possible, take the *L. rhamnosus* supplement as long as possible after taking the antibiotic.

If pseudomembranous enterocolitis does develop, then you will need to take *L. rhamnosus* and another probiotic product—*Saccharomyces boulardii*.[3,4] The effectiveness of this yeast in reducing recurrences of pseudomembranous enterocolitis has been proven in clinical trials and is even mentioned in many medical textbooks as an important adjunct to antibiotic therapy in the treatment of pseudomembranous enterocolitis. The dosage of *Saccharomyces boulardii* in this application is 3 billion live organisms daily.

Gotu Kola *(Centella asiatica)*

Gotu kola is an herbal product that promotes wound healing by stimulating the manufacture of structural proteins like collagen. Gotu kola extract has demonstrated impressive clinical results in promoting wound repair. The types of wounds healed include surgical wounds such as episiotomies and ear-nose-throat surgeries, skin ulcers due to arterial or venous insufficiency, traumatic injuries to the skin, gangrene, and skin grafts.[5]

It is very important to use gotu kola to prevent the formation of adhesions. Adhesions are large internal scars that can be quite problematic. For example, the formation of adhesions after an abdominal operation can lead to bowel obstruction—a potentially life-threatening scenario.

The majority of clinical studies have used an extract of gotu kola containing only molecules known as triterpenic acids at a dosage of 50 to 100 mg daily. This dry powdered extract is available in capsules and tablets at your local health food store. Gotu kola is also available in crude form (bulk or in capsules, tablets, or tea bags), tinctures, and fluid extracts, but since the concentration of triterpenes in gotu kola can vary between 1.1 and 8 percent, it is best to use extracts standardized for triterpenic acids. Here are the approximate dosages for other forms:

Crude dried plant leaves: 1 to 2 g twice daily
Tincture (1:5): 5 to 10 ml twice daily
Fluid extract (1:1): 1.0 to 2.0 ml twice daily

Proteolytic Enzymes

Proteolytic enzymes (see page 166) can help promote recovery after surgery, but they should not be used prior to surgery, as they may increase bleeding time. For best results, begin taking them no sooner than three days after surgery.

Several clinical studies have shown that, in addition to reducing inflammation and swelling, proteolytic enzymes can prevent the development of lymphedema.[6] Lymphedema refers to a buildup of lymphatic fluid that results in swelling. In lymphedema, the swelling can be so severe that it results in permanent loss of function of an arm or leg.

The lymphatic system collects fluid from body tissues, filters out harmful substances, and returns the fluid to the bloodstream. In a sense, the lymphatic system is a crucial part of your body's water-treatment facility. The lymph nodes are like little filtering stations. Sometimes lymph nodes are removed during surgery, especially following a mastectomy, creating a blockage in lymph flow and the development of lymphedema.

Edema can occur if the fluid contains too many large particles, such as fragments of bacteria or the debris from dead cells. This often happens when the system is working hard to manage a serious disease, such as infection or cancer. Like a sewage drain, the system can become clogged. The fluid then backs up, causing swelling. The most frequently affected lymph nodes are those in the pelvis and the legs and under the arms.

In many cases, the lymphedema after a surgery is quite mild and subsides in less than six months. But some people suffer from chronic lymphedema, which is constant or recurs frequently. This can happen if the lymph nodes are removed or if a tumor recurs or grows in an area where there are lymph nodes.

Patients at risk for lymphedema are those with

- Breast cancer if they have received radiation therapy or had lymph nodes removed. Radiation to the underarm area after the lymph nodes have been removed increases the occurrence of lymphedema.
- Melanoma of the arms or legs, especially if the patient has had lymph nodes removed from the underarm area and/or received radiation therapy.
- Prostate cancer treated by surgery or by radiation therapy to the whole pelvis.
- Cancer of the female reproductive tract that is advanced, treated with surgery to remove the lymph nodes, or treated with radiation therapy.
- Cancer that has spread to the lower abdomen, such as metastatic ovarian, testicular, colorectal, pancreatic, or liver cancer. The pressure from the growing tumor can destroy the lymphatic vessels and block lymphatic drainage.

Proteolytic enzymes can dramatically improve lymphedema, according to published clinical trials. The best results occur when enzymes are combined with complex decongestive therapy (CDT), a technique that includes massage, the use of special compression wraps or clothing, individualized exercises, weight loss, and skin care.

Chapter   Twelve

Natural Strategies for Support Before, During, and After Radiation

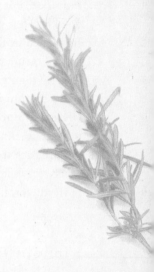

Radiation therapy is the use of radiation (x-rays, gamma rays, proton rays, and neutron rays) to kill cancer cells. Its main role is destroying or shrinking localized cancers (as opposed to cancers that have spread to distant parts of the body). About 60 percent of cancer patients get radiation at some point during their treatment. Sometimes radiation cures the disease, but if a cure is not possible, radiation can reduce tumor size to relieve pain or make surgery easier.

Certain types of cancers—such as Hodgkin's disease, some lymphomas, and prostate cancer—respond very well to radiation. In fact, sometimes radiation alone works best in these cancers. But for other cancers, radiation offers only partial benefit. For example, receiving radiation for advanced lung cancer increases your chances for living an additional five years by only 10 percent.

If radiation alone won't be enough to get the best results, you may need to have surgery, or chemotherapy, or both. Combining strategies often improves your odds of surviving. For example, radiation can shrink tumors, making them easier for the surgeon to remove. And if surgery doesn't "get it all," your doctors may use radiation to destroy or control the remaining cancer cells.

Of course, radiation kills normal cells about as effectively as it kills cancer cells. It's especially good at destroying cells that grow and divide quickly. That means cells in cancer tumors—but it also means normal cells, such as those of the skin, blood, immune system, and digestive tract. Fortunately, most normal cells are better at repairing radiation damage than are cancer cells.

To minimize damage to healthy cells, radiation treatments are usually given in small doses—"fractions"—over a course of time, usually five to seven weeks. That gives cells a chance to recover. Healthy cells usually bounce back more quickly than cancer cells. By the next dose, they hold up better while the weakened cancer cells suffer another blow. By the end of treatment, hopefully all of the cancer cells have been destroyed.

Kinds of Radiation Used to Treat Cancer

Photon Radiation

Early radiation therapy used high-energy, ionizing electromagnetic x-rays and gamma rays composed of particles of energy called photons. These particles have no mass and no electrical charge. Photon rays are part of the electromagnetic spectrum, as are ultraviolet, visible, and infrared light; radio waves; and microwaves. They are called ionizing because they act by knocking out small atomic particles called electrons. Damaging a cell's molecules in this way disrupts its function, especially its ability to divide and make new cells. While this method is effective, the risk of side effects, including destruction of healthy tissue, is high.

Particle Radiation

Many cancer treatment centers provide newer, more focused forms of radiation therapy that have advantages over photon radiation in some circumstances. One example is neutron therapy. Neutron rays are very high-energy rays composed of neutrons, which are particles that have mass but no electrical charge. These rays don't affect the tiny electrons. Instead, they go for bigger targets, destroying atoms in the cell's nucleus. In a sense, they wipe out the cell's headquarters rather than picking off a few soldiers guarding the front door. It's much harder for cells (whether cancerous or normal) to survive such an attack and to repair the damage.

Another advantage of neutron radiation is that, unlike conventional radiation, it can work even in the absence of oxygen. For that reason, neutrons can destroy cells hidden deep in the centers of large tumors. Neutron therapy is especially effective for the treatment of inoperable salivary gland tumors, bone cancers, and certain advanced cancers of the pancreas, bladder, prostate, and uterus.

Another new type of radiation therapy is proton radiation. Protons are particles that have mass and a positive electrical charge. Proton rays can be shaped to conform to the shape of the tumor more precisely than can x-rays or gamma rays. They thus allow delivery of higher radiation doses to tumors without increasing damage to the surrounding tissues. For these reasons, proton therapy is more effective than neutron therapy, requires fewer treatment sessions, and produces fewer side effects. The drawback is that proton radiation is not yet as widely available as the other methods.

Modes of Delivery

Traditionally, radiation therapy is delivered from a beam of radiation originating outside the body. This is called *external beam therapy*. Because the beam passes through the body before and after it gets to the tumor, it can injure tissue in its path.

To reduce such damage, physicians have developed new techniques that allow the radiation to emanate from inside the body. This method, called brachytherapy, involves the use of radioactive materials placed in small tubes, called seeds, that are implanted near the tumor (*brachy-* means "near"). Brachytherapy is especially useful in cases where surgery or radiation poses too great a risk of damage to tissues near the tumor, as is often the case in prostate cancer or cervical cancer. A newer form of brachytherapy, called high dose rate (HDR) brachytherapy, is more versatile than standard seed implantation and in many cases offers a more precise way to deliver this form of radiation.

Another method, known as radioimmunotherapy, is still in the experimental stage. This technique uses special protein molecules called antibodies. Attached to each antibody is a special radioactive molecule that emits gamma rays. Injected into the patient's bloodstream, the antibody carries its cargo through the body until it encounters a cancer cell. Then it attaches itself to a special receptor on the cell's surface. Once the antibody is docked, the gamma radiation is released directly at its target, spelling doom for the cancer cell. This new therapy is not widely available, but if it is of interest to you, please talk to your oncologist about it.

Practical Matters

Before radiation therapy begins, your doctors will carefully evaluate the size and location of the tumor and its surrounding tissue. Their goal is to design the treatment as carefully as possible to aim the right dose of radiation at the target while minimizing the risk of adverse effects. They'll probably use magnetic resonance imaging (MRI) or computed tomography (CT scans) to map out their strategy. Depending on the tumor's type, size, and location, the health care team will determine the total radiation dose, the number of sessions (fractions) needed, the interval between sessions, and whether to give each fraction from the same direction or from different directions.

In all cases, physicians will try to deliver only the dose needed, and only to the targeted area. To protect other parts of your body, they may construct a special shield. Newer techniques, such as 3-D conformal radiation and intensity-modulated radiotherapy (IMRT), can also reduce the amount of radiation that reaches healthy tissue. Your skin may be marked with ink or temporary tattoos to help achieve correct positioning for each treatment. In some cases, molds can be built to hold tissues in exactly the right place each time.

Toxicity and Side Effects

Because it kills normal cells along with the diseased ones, radiation therapy can be highly toxic. Newer, more targeted radiation treatments are less dangerous than some of the older techniques, but there are still risks of anemia, nausea, vomiting, diarrhea, hair loss, skin burn, and sterility. Which of these complications arises depends on the total volume of the area being treated, the dose of radiation, and the area of the body included in the field. For example, nausea occurs primarily if the abdomen is irradiated, whereas hair loss generally results from treatment of the head. The greater the total area being treated, the more likely it is that systemic effects such as anemia and fatigue will occur.

The side effects from radiation treatment occur in three different phases: early, intermediate, and late. The early side effects of radiation treatment occur while treatment is being given. Although these complications can be quite severe, they almost always completely resolve once the course of treatment is completed. Intermediate effects are those that appear weeks to months after the radiation treatment is completed. Late effects of radiation treatment, which are fairly rare, do not appear until many months or even years after therapy. These can include radiation necrosis (breakdown of a region of bone), pulmonary fibrosis (stiffening of lung tissue), secondary cancers, and scarring or hardening of tissues in the region exposed to radiation. Because these late effects are often extremely difficult to treat, the best strategy is to prevent them through the use of the natural therapies described later in this chapter.

Nausea and vomiting are more likely to occur when the dose is high or if treatment involves the abdomen or digestive tract. Sometimes nausea and vomiting occur after radiation to other regions, but in these cases the symptoms usually disappear within a few hours after treatment. Fatigue frequently starts after the second week of therapy and may continue until about two weeks after the therapy is finished. We recommend that patients limit their activities, cut back their work hours, take naps, and get extra sleep at night, but it is important to get some exercise in the form of tai chi, yoga, or stretching exercises to gently stimulate the circulation and the immune system.

Unlike chemotherapy, which is a systemic treatment designed to destroy cancer cells wherever they may be lurking in the body, radiation therapy is usually a local or regional therapy, affecting only the tumor and the immediately surrounding area. For this reason, many of the side effects are specific to the region of the body being treated. Typically there is some reddening of the skin, and the area may become irritated, dry, or sensitive. A skin reaction may progress to look like a sunburn.

Aloe Vera

The aloe plant has thick leaves that produce a slightly viscous, clear gel with many healing properties. The gel is 96 percent water; the rest is various polysaccharides (complex sugars), enzymes, minerals, and amino acids in solution.

The soothing and wound-healing effects of aloe vera have been chronicled since ancient times. Both Pliny (A.D. 23–79) and Dioscorides (first century A.D.) wrote of aloe's ability to treat wounds and heal infections of the skin. In 1935, physicians first successfully used the fresh juice to treat a patient suffering from facial burns due to x-rays.[1] The beneficial effects of aloe are now so well accepted that virtually every over-the-counter product for the topical treatment of burns, minor irritations, skin ulcers, and other skin disorders incorporates aloe into the formulation.

We recommend using pure, 100 percent aloe vera gel—the naturally occurring, undiluted material obtained directly from the leaves of the aloe plant. It is available at most drug stores and health food stores. If the skin has not been broken, the gel can be applied liberally to areas of inflammation and damage.

Treat the skin gently to avoid further irritation; bathe carefully using only warm water and mild soap. Avoid perfume and scented skin products and protect affected areas from the sun. We also recommend using aloe vera gel on areas of radiation burn (see box).

Dietary Support for Radiation Therapy

Please follow the guidelines give in Appendix B, Battling Cancer Through Diet. After the cancer is in remission, the guidelines provided in Chapter 2 can be followed. Several supplements deserve special mention:

Vitamin A and Beta-Carotene

Several studies have shown that vitamin A and its precursor, beta-carotene, offer significant benefits to people undergoing radiation therapy.[2-4] For example, these compounds reduce inflammation after radiation treatment. This allows physicians to administer higher, and hopefully more effective, doses. In a study of advanced squamous cell carcinoma of the mouth treated with radiation therapy, beta-carotene (75 mg daily) significantly reduced the incidence of severe oral inflammation.[4]

In addition to preventing some of the side effects of radiation therapy, vitamin A can also enhance the effectiveness of radiation therapy. Test tube studies have shown that vitamin A increases the sensitivity of cancer cells to radiation therapy.[5] In animal studies, the effect of local radiation was enhanced by supplemental vitamin A and beta-carotene given during treatment.[6] The animals receiving the antioxidant showed better tumor shrinkage and increased survival time. The results from these preliminary studies have been upheld in human studies.

We recommend taking an extra 75 mg of beta-carotene and 10,000 IU of vitamin A at least one week prior to radiation therapy. After this one-week usage, do not continue with these supplements at this dosage. You may supplement at a maintenance dosage of 15 mg of beta-carotene and 5000 IU of vitamin A if you so desire.

Vitamin C

Vitamin C therapy appears to be helpful during radiation therapy. In one human study, 50 cancer patients were given either vitamin C (5 daily doses of 1 g each) or placebo along with their radiation therapy.[7] More complete responses to radiation were noted in the vitamin C group at one month (87 to 55 percent) and four months (63 to 45 percent) after treatment. Side effects tended to be fewer in the subjects given the vitamin C as well.[8] We recommend a more modest intake of 500 to 1000 mg three times per day in light of our other antioxidant recommendations.

Vitamins C and E Prevent
Radiation-Induced Fibrosis

Vitamin E reduces the risk of radiation-induced fibrosis (excessive scar formation) and is extremely helpful if radiation-induced fibrosis or inflammation occurs.

In a study conducted at Loyola University Medical Center in Maywood, Illinois, vitamin E in combination with vitamin C was shown to be relieve chronic radiation proctitis, a common complication of pelvic radiation that causes pain and inflammation in the rectal area.[9] The study involved 20 patients who had received radiation treatment for prostate or gynecologic cancers and who had developed radiation proctitis involving one or more symptoms: rectal bleeding, rectal pain, diarrhea, or fecal urgency (overwhelming urges to have a bowel movement). They were given a combination of vitamin E (400 IU three times daily) and vitamin C (500 mg three times daily). Before and after treatment, they rated the frequency and severity of their symptoms on a questionnaire. They also described the impact of their symptoms on their lifestyle, on a scale from 0 (no effect on daily activity) to 4 (afraid to leave home).

Results showed that treatment significantly improved all of the symptoms except rectal pain. In some cases, the symptoms resolved completely. Of the 20 patients, 13 reported that their quality of life was significantly better—some even said their lives had returned to normal. A year later, the symptoms showed sustained improvement.

Vitamin E

Some studies on animals concluded that high doses of vitamin E can reduce the effectiveness of radiation.[10,11] But when you take a close look at the way that research was conducted, it's easy to question this finding. The mice in one such study were given doses of vitamin E that were 45 times higher than the maximum recommended daily dose for humans.[10] At those extreme levels, it's not surprising that there might have been adverse effects on the cells.

In contrast, in another study, giving vitamin E to animals before, during, and after radiation enhanced the killing power of the beam and reduced the ability of cancer cells to divide.[12] At the same time, the antioxidant protected normal cells from these effects. We recommend a dosage of 400 to 800 IU daily.

About Co-enzyme Q10 and Radiation

In 1998, a study was published warning that Co-enzyme Q10—abbreviated to CoQ10—reduced the effects of radiotherapy on small-cell lung cancer in mice.[13] While this animal study did indeed show a significant inhibition of radiation damage to cancer cells, the oral dosage required to produce this effect was 40 mg/kg, a dose roughly equivalent to 2800 mg in an adult human. Borderline inhibition was found at 20 mg/kg (approximately equal to a 1400-mg adult human dose), and no inhibitory effect on radiotherapy was noted at 10 mg/kg CoQ10, a dose roughly equivalent to 700 mg in an adult human. Based on this information, the normal human dosage range for CoQ10 of 50 to 300 mg a day would appear to have no adverse impact on concurrent radiotherapy.

Curcumin and Quercetin

Curcumin and quercetin protect healthy cells against the harmful effects of radiation without reducing its effectiveness. You won't need to take both curcumin and quercetin. Quercetin reduced skin damage from radiation in patients with head and neck cancers, so it is probably the best choice for this type of cancer.[14] For head and neck cancers, take

Table 12-1. When to Use Curcumin or Quercetin (with Radiation)

TYPE OF CANCER/TREATMENT	CURCUMIN	QUERCETIN
Brain		X
Breast	X	
Colon	X	
Leukemia		X
Liver	X	
Lung		X
Lymphoma		X
Ovarian		X
Prostate	X	
Skin	X	
Stomach	X	

quercetin (200 to 400 mg daily). For other cancers being treated by radiation, take curcumin (200 to 400 mg daily). Continue for at least one month after the last radiation treatment. After this period, choose either quercetin or curcumin based on the type of cancer.

Maitake MD-Fraction or PSK/PSP

These mushroom products are discussed more thoroughly in Chapter 8. Take either maitake MD-fraction, or PSK/PSP, at either 1 mg per 2.2 pounds per day for the maitake products or 3000 mg for the PSK/PSP products. Continue at this dosage until the cancer is in remission, then cut the dosage in half. In one study, PSK used with radiation therapy in non-small-cell lung cancer increased the five-year survival up to 39 percent in stages I and II disease and 22 percent in stage III disease, compared with 16 percent and 5 percent, respectively, in the groups that did not receive PSK.[15]

Melatonin

Melatonin is a hormone secreted by the pineal gland, a pea-sized gland at the base of the brain. It is available as a dietary supplement. Melatonin produces benefits for people undergoing radiation therapy, according to preliminary evidence. In one human study, the effect of radiotherapy plus 20 mg a day of melatonin was compared to that of radiotherapy alone in 30 patients with brain cancer (glioblastoma).[16] Patients with this form of brain cancer generally live only about six months after diagnosis. But at the end of one year, 6 of the 14 patients receiving melatonin were still living, compared with just one of the 16 undergoing radiotherapy alone. The researchers also noted fewer side effects from radiation therapy in patients taking melatonin.

We recommend 20 mg per day at bedtime one week prior to radiation, to be continued until the cancer is in remission.

Alkylglycerols

Alkylglycerols are compounds found in shark oil. In commercial alkylglycerols preparations, the high levels of vitamins A and D, along with other constituents found in shark liver oil, are removed. The effects of alkylglycerols in the treatment of radiation-induced leukopenia have been studied extensively. The major finding in most of these studies was that in radiation-treated cancer patients, alkylglycerols prevent the severe reduction in white blood cell counts and increase white blood cell production.[17,18]

Alkylglycerols also exert immune-enhancing effects and can also increase cancer survival rate. In one study of a series of 350 patients with cervical cancer treated with alkylglycerols and given radiation therapy, there was a greater survival rate for one year and five years compared with a matched control group who did not receive alkylglycerols.[18]

For protection from the damaging effects of radiation, we recommend a dosage of 1200 mg a day for at least one week before and after treatment. A dosage of 600 mg a day should be continued until normal white blood cell counts are achieved.

Chapter Thirteen

Natural Strategies for Support Before, During, and After Chemotherapy

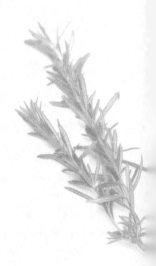

*C*hemotherapy is a broad term that means the use of one or more drugs in the treatment of cancer. For many people, the very thought of chemotherapy evokes horrific images of debilitating nausea, vomiting, diarrhea, and weakness. It's true that the benefits of chemotherapy come at a cost (see the list of side effects below). One of the problems with standard chemotherapy is that the drugs work by attacking cells that are actively dividing, whether they are cancerous or not. But certain normal cells—including those that line the intestines, bone marrow, and hair follicles—divide constantly, so they are more prone to damage by chemotherapy. Which side effects develop depends on many factors: the agents used, the combination of drugs, the dosage and timing of treatments, the patient's general health, and the history of prior chemotherapy.

Side Effects of Chemotherapy

Short-Term
  Anorexia
  Bladder inflammation
  Bone marrow suppression
  Confusion and short-term-memory impairment
  Diarrhea
  Fatigue
  Hair loss
  Infections
  Muscle pain
  Nausea
  Nerve irritation

Longer-Term
  Infertility
  Persistent bone marrow suppression
  Persistent fatigue
  Secondary cancers

Good News

The good news is that there are natural measures to reduce the toxicity of chemotherapy. There have also been advances in treatment that have made most chemotherapy regimens less toxic and more tolerable than in the past.

Complementary natural medicines can help in three ways: by acting directly against cancer cells, by protecting and supporting normal cell function, and by reducing the risk of adverse effects of therapy. When selected carefully and used judiciously, natural medicine has been found to improve your chances for achieving the best possible outcome.

As detailed in Chapter 7, Battling Cancer Through Diet, the importance of high-quality nutrition in the battle against cancer cannot be overstated. Cancer patients who have higher nutritional status are not only more likely to fight off infections and recover from their illness but are also better able to tolerate chemotherapy and its side effects. The following dietary suggestions are especially important for anyone undergoing chemotherapy, especially the chemotherapy-treated patient suffering from anorexia (loss of appetite) or cachexia (severe muscle wasting).

Key Dietary Recommendations for Chemotherapy Support

- Drink a high-protein smoothie once or twice daily (see page 153 for more information and pages 320–332 for delicious recipes). Smoothies can take the place of breakfast and can also be used as between-meal snacks.
- Stay well hydrated and drink 18 to 24 ounces of fresh vegetable juice daily, which can be taken with food—or better yet, take a midmorning juice break.
- It may be necessary to eat small frequent meals (every 1 to 2 hours) rather than larger meals less often.
- Use extra seasonings, spices, and flavorings to improve food's taste appeal. A higher sensitivity to the taste of food may cause them to taste flavorless or boring.
- Avoid flavorings that are very sweet or very bitter.
- Eat soft, moist foods like smoothies, bananas, brown rice, yams, and so on, and avoid hard, dry foods like cereals, crackers, and hard candies.
- Take small bites and chew completely.

Antioxidants and Chemotherapy

One of the most controversial natural measures to support chemotherapy is the recommendation to use antioxidant nutrients during the active phase of the treatment. This issue was briefly discussed in Chapter 7, Battling Cancer Through Diet. While there is little concern with using antioxidant nutrients after the completion of a course of chemotherapy or radiation treatment, many oncologists fear that antioxidant nutrients may interfere with the effectiveness of conventional therapies. Is this fear valid? According to many experts, the answer is no. We prefer to simply say, since you can always find exceptions, that it depends upon the nature of the treatment and the antioxidant in question. The biggest issue is not whether to use an antioxidant, but rather which antioxidant offers the greatest benefit and what dosage should be used.

Deciding to recommend any treatment or supplement for any condition is a balancing act of risk versus benefit. While there are many questions that beg to be answered in well-designed clinical studies, we believe that appropriate antioxidant support has virtually no risk, yet can produce significant benefits, as the majority of human studies have shown that patients treated with antioxidants during chemotherapy and/or radiation have been noted to tolerate standard treatment better, have a better quality of life, and, most important, live longer than patients receiving no supplements.

The issue of combining antioxidant therapy with conventional cancer therapy is being championed by many experts, including Kedar Prasad and his colleagues at the Center for Vitamins and Cancer Research at the University of Colorado Health Science Center's Department of Radiology in Denver. Dr. Prasad has stated that the concerns over the use of high-dosage antioxidants during chemotherapy and radiation "are not valid."[1] Dr. Prasad feels that "high doses of multiple antioxidant vitamins, together with diet modification and lifestyle changes, may improve the efficacy of standard and experimental cancer therapies by reducing their toxicity on normal cells and by enhancing their growth-inhibitory effects on cancer cells."[1] We agree with him wholeheartedly.

How can antioxidants protect healthy cells and not cancer cells? The answer to this question is attributed to the fact that cancer cells actually increase the intracellular level of antioxidants beyond normal levels, resulting in increased expression of growth-inhibitory genes, reduced expression of growth factors, and increased cellular suicide (apoptosis). The initial protection offered by the antioxidants in cancer cells to chemotherapy and radiation becomes irrelevant to the mechanism of action of the chemotherapy drug or radiation. Antioxidant supplementation at the dosages we recommend offers about as much protection to the cancer cell as a bulletproof jacket would during a nuclear attack. In contrast, normal cells are able to utilize the antioxidant to protect against the toxicity and damage caused by standard cancer treatments.

Chemotherapy Supplementation Program

There are so many natural products that offer benefit in supporting the chemotherapy patient that it can be overwhelming. In order to provide you with the best possible support, we have supplied a basic supplementation program for chemotherapy followed by some specific recommendations based on the type of chemotherapy agent being used. (See Appendix E, page 338.)

The Importance of Fish Oil Supplements

Again, we cannot stress enough the importance of utilizing fish oil supplements rich in the omega-3 fatty acids EPA and DHA in cancer patients. Fish oil supplements boost immune function and prevent cachexia—the severe wasting syndrome in cancer.[2–5] Fish oil supplementation benefits anyone taking chemotherapy, especially anyone receiving the drug doxorubicin. Not only has it increased survival time in humans and animals taking the drug, but there is considerable evidence in test tube studies that fish oils (especially DHA) increase the effectiveness of the drug.[4–7] Use fish oil supplements at a daily dosage of 700 to 1200 mg of EPA and 400 to 700 mg of DHA.

Maitake MD-Fraction and PSK/PSP

The benefits of these natural immune enhancers derived from mushrooms were discussed in Chapter 8, The Super Eight: Fighting Cancer Through Key Natural Products. It is very important to choose one of these two products. Either can reduce the side effects of conventional chemotherapy and radiation while at the same time enhance the effectiveness of these treatments. For example, here are some of the results from studies with PSK:

- A randomized study of 253 patients with surgically treated stomach cancer showed that adding PSK to standard chemotherapy

(5-FU) significantly increased the five-year disease-free survival rate from 59 to 71 percent.[8]

- Two randomized studies showed statistically significant increases in survival when PSK was added to standard chemotherapy after complete surgical removal of primary tumors.[9,10] In one of the trials, survival time more than doubled.[10]

- PSK used with radiation therapy in non-small-cell lung cancer increased the five-year survival rate by 39 percent in stages I and II disease and by 22 percent in stage III disease, compared with 16 percent and 5 percent, respectively, in the groups that did not receive PSK.[11]

- PSK significantly increased the survival rate in women with breast cancer undergoing surgery and chemotherapy, compared with the control group receiving only conventional treatment.[12] The women receiving PSK also showed no significant drop in their peripheral white blood cell and platelet counts.

The dosage for maitake MD-fraction is 1 mg per every two pounds of body weight, while the dosage for PSK or PSP is 3000 mg a day. Either should be taken on an empty stomach. Continue at this dosage until the cancer is in remission, then cut the dosage in half.

Curcumin or Quercetin?

Curcumin and quercetin share many common features (both are discussed in Chapter 8, The Super Eight: Fighting Cancer Through Key Natural Products). The choice of which to use depends on the type of cancer or the chemotherapy agent.

Both curcumin and quercetin protect healthy cells against the harmful effects of radiation and chemotherapy agents without reducing the effectiveness of these therapies against cancer cells. In particular, curcumin has been shown to enhance the action of the chemotherapy drug cisplatin, while quercetin increases the therapeutic efficacy of busulphan, Adriamycin (doxorubicin), cyclophosphamide, gemcitabine, topotecan, and cisplatin.[13-20]

Table 13-1. When to Use Curcumin or Quercetin (with Chemotherapy)

TYPE OF CANCER/TREATMENT	CURCUMIN	QUERCETIN
Brain		X
Breast	X	
Colon*	X	
Leukemia		X
Liver	X	
Lung		X
Lymphoma		X
Ovarian		X
Prostate	X	
Skin	X	
Stomach	X	
Radiation Therapy		
Head and neck cancers		X
Others	X	
Type of Chemotherapy		
Alkylating agents and platinum compounds	X	
Antimetabolites		X
Antitumor antibiotics		X*
Microtubule and chromatin inhibitors		X

*Note: Do not use quercetin in colon cancer if being treated by antitumor antibiotics like doxorubicin (rarely used in colon cancer). Curcumin is the better choice.

Melatonin

Melatonin is a hormone secreted by the pineal gland, a pea-sized gland at the base of the brain. Melatonin is a popular dietary supplement for the treatment of jet lag and insomnia. But tantalizing new evidence suggests that melatonin may have some benefit as an adjunct to cancer therapy. It has been shown to inhibit several types of cancers in test tube and animal studies and appears to work by increasing the expression of the p53 gene (see page 20), which acts to reduce cell proliferation by literally signaling cellular suicide (apoptosis).

Melatonin may help regulate some of the immune system's signaling proteins, including interleukins and gamma-interferon, which work by increasing the ability of white blood cells to identify and destroy tumor cells. Evidence also suggests that melatonin reduces the toxicity and/or enhances the effectiveness of other chemotherapy agents. Melatonin should not be used in acute leukemias, children, or people taking antidepressant drugs, however.

In studies involving patients with metastatic solid tumors, melatonin has been shown to enhance the anticancer effects of certain chemotherapy drugs, including cisplatin, etoposide, interleukin-2, interferon, tamoxifen, and lupron, as well as radiation.[21–28] It also may reduce cachexia.[29] Studies have shown that patients taking melatonin (20 mg a day) had significantly less weight loss (3 kg vs. 16 kg) and a lower chance of disease progression (53 percent vs. 90 percent) compared with those treated with supportive care alone.

A randomized trial in patients with advanced non-small-cell lung cancer investigated the effects of adding melatonin (20 mg a day) to a regimen of cancer drugs (cisplatin and etoposide). In this study, 15 of 24 patients who received the melatonin were still alive after one year, compared with 7 of the 36 patients who received chemotherapy alone. There was some evidence that tumors in the melatonin group responded better to treatment, but the difference was not statistically significant. The melatonin group also had less nerve damage, cachexia, and bone marrow suppression.[22]

In another study, 63 patients with non-small-cell lung cancer that was not responding to cisplatin therapy were randomized to receive either 10 mg a day of melatonin or supportive care alone. Patients receiving melatonin lived longer on average (6 months vs. 3 months) and were more likely to survive for one year (8 of 31 survived vs. 2 of 32).[23]

Treatment with melatonin (20 mg a day) was also associated with greater one-year survival than supportive care alone in patients with brain metastases.[24] Other studies have noted that melatonin increased survival in malignant melanoma and in patients with metastatic disease.[25] A European study of 250 stage IV (advanced metastatic) cancer patients found that patients given 20 mg of melatonin daily along with standard chemotherapy had double the response rate and double the one-year survival rate of those given chemotherapy alone.[27]

Melatonin also has benefits for people undergoing radiation therapy, according to preliminary evidence. In one human study, the effect of radiotherapy plus 20 mg a day of melatonin was compared with that of radiotherapy alone in 30 patients with brain cancer (glioblastoma).[28]

Patients with this form of brain cancer generally live only about 6 months after diagnosis. But at the end of one year, 6 of the 14 patients receiving melatonin were still living, compared with just one of the 16 undergoing radiotherapy alone. The researchers also noted fewer side effects from radiation therapy in patients taking melatonin.

Proteolytic Enzymes in Herpes Zoster (Shingles): A Common Side Effect of Chemotherapy

Because of the immune-suppressing effects of chemotherapy, a common side effect is shingles—a painful rash of blisters that is due to the same herpes virus that causes chicken pox. After someone recovers from chicken pox, the virus remains quiet, or dormant, in nerves. The infection can reactivate for various reasons later in life.

Shingles symptoms are usually limited to a small area of the body. This area is usually a small strip of skin on one side of the chest or abdomen. In some cases, the face can be involved, and this may cause an eye infection. The first symptoms are usually related to sensation. People may experience pain, numbness, tingling, or itching. Pain usually occurs at some point, and can be quite severe. This is usually followed by the development of groups of blisters. The areas around the blisters are often quite painful. The pain can be severe and last for weeks. If the immune system is severely compromised, the infection can be very serious, causing infection in the liver, lungs, and brain.

Orally administered pancreatic enzyme preparations have been used in Germany in the treatment of shingles for over 30 years. Even in Germany, however, the standard treatment is now oral acyclovir. The positive results obtained in earlier studies with proteolytic enzymes led researchers to design a study to determine the effectiveness of enzyme therapy versus acyclovir (Zovirax)—a popular drug used to treat shingles and other herpes virus infections.[30]

The study design was a double-blind, controlled, multicenter trial of

90 immunocompetent patients with herpes zoster. Patients were randomly assigned to receive either acyclovir (800 mg) or an enzyme preparation (120 mg trypsin, 40 mg chymotrypsin, and 320 mg papain) five times a day for a treatment period of 7 days. The parameters of pain and skin lesions were measured over 14 to 21 days. Results indicated no statistically significant difference in either parameter between the two groups, indicating that the enzyme preparation is as effective as acyclovir. The proposed mechanism of action for the enzyme preparation was stimulation of the breakdown of immune complexes, as well as enhancement of immune function.

Hand-Foot Syndrome

Hand-foot syndrome (also known as palmar-plantar erythrodysthesia) is an adverse reaction to chemotherapy characterized by reddening of the skin. Doxorubicin, cytarabine, docetaxel, and fluorouracil are the most frequently implicated agents. Although, as the name implies, it usually affects the hands and feet, it can also affect any area that is subjected to heat or pressure. The redness is often accompanied by blistering, pain, and swelling. Eventually, the affected skin peels off, as healthy skin underneath regrows. There is rarely any permanent scarring unless a secondary infection occurs.

Hand-foot syndrome usually appears after two or three cycles of chemotherapy, but it can occur sooner or later. It is graded according to severity:

Grade 1: Mild redness or peeling, not severe enough to interfere with usual activity.

Grade 2: Symptoms have a mild impact on daily activity.

Grade 3: Symptoms severe enough to interfere with walking and normal wearing of clothes.

Grade 4: Severe symptoms involving infections or the need for hospitalization.

It is important to recognize hand-foot syndrome early. Report any symptoms of tingling, numbness, or redness to your oncologist. Avoid any unusual trauma to the hands and feet, as well as to other pressure areas, such as the elbows and knees.

To minimize absorption of the drug into the skin, limit skin exposure to external heat for one day prior to each chemotherapy infusion and three to five days afterward. For example, avoid hot baths, saunas, and heated whirlpools. Don't wear any tight clothing that causes pressure on the skin. Reduce sun exposure and be sure to wear sunblock with a sun protection factor (SPF) of at least 15 whenever going outdoors.

To relieve symptoms of hand-foot syndrome, take cool baths or showers. Take vitamin B_6 at dosages of 50 mg twice daily and use aloe vera gel topically to speed healing. In severe cases, it might be necessary for your physicians to change the dosage or timing of chemotherapy to allow more recovery time.

Types of Chemotherapy

The hundreds of different chemotherapy agents available today can be divided into seven main categories:

- Alkylating agents and platinum compounds
- Antimetabolites
- Antitumor antibiotics
- Biological response modifiers
- Hormones and hormone inhibitors
- Microtubule inhibitors and chromatin function inhibitors
- New-breed agents

How a chemotherapy drug is administered—by mouth or intravenously or through some other means—depends on many factors. Some drugs can't be absorbed through the digestive system, or they may cause unacceptably severe side effects if taken orally. Another way to take cancer drugs involves use of a small catheter that's threaded through the arteries to reach the blood vessels feeding the tumor. The drug is delivered right to the cancer rather than having to circulate throughout the entire body. That means smaller doses can be given, with a lower risk of side effects. One

Table 13-2. Chemotherapy Agents

CLASS (SUBCLASS)	COMMON NAME	TRADE NAME
Alkylating agents and platinum compounds	altretamine	Hexalen
	BCNU	Carmustine
	busulfan	Myleran
	chlorambucil	Leukeran
	cyclophosphamide	Cytoxan, Endoxan, Neosar
	fotemustine	Muphoran
	iphosphamide	Ifex
	lomustine	CCNU
	melphalan	Alkeran, L-PAM
	nitrogen mustard (mechlorethamine)	Mustargen
	pipobroman	Vercyte
	procarbazine	Matulane, MIH
	streptozocin, streptozotocin	Zanosar
	temozolomide	Temodar
	thiotepa	Thioplex
	triethylenemelamine	TEM
Platinum-containing compounds	carboplatin	Paraplatin
	cisplatin	Platinol, Platinol-AQ
Antitumor antibiotics	actinomycin D	Cosmegen
	bleomycin sulfate	Blenoxane
	daunomycin daunorubicin,	Cerubidine
	doxorubicin	Adriamycin, Doxil
	epirubicin	Ellence
	idarubicin	Idamycin
	mitomycin, mitomycin-C	Mutamycin
	mitramycin	Mithracin
Antimetabolites	asparaginase	Elspar
	chlorodeoxyadenosine	Leustatin
	cytosine arabinoside	Ara-C, Cytosar-U
	deoxycoformycin, pentostatin	Nipent
	floxuridine	5-FUDR

Table 13-2. Chemotherapy Agents *(Continued)*

CLASS (SUBCLASS)	COMMON NAME	TRADE NAME
Antimetabolites *(cont.)*	fludarabine phosphate	Fludara
	fluorouracil	5-FU
	gemcitabine	Gemzar
	hydroxyurea	Hydrea
	mercaptopurine	6-MP
	methotrexate	Folex, MTX
	thioguanine	6-TG
Biological response modifiers	alpha interferon	Intron A, Roferon-A
	bacillus Calmette-Guerin	BCG, TheraCys, TICE
	erythropoietin	EPO, Epogen, Pocrit
	G-CSF	Neupogen
	GM-CSF	Leukine, Prokine
	interleukin-2 (IL - 2)	Aldesleukin, Proleukin
Hormones		
Corticosteroids	betamethasone sodium phosphate	Adbeon, Celestone phosphate
	cortisone acetate	Cortisone, Cortone Acetate
	dexamethasone	Decadron
	dexamethasone acetate	Dalalone D.P.
	hydrocortisone	Hydrocortone
	prednisolone	Prelone
	prednisolone tebutate	Hydeltra-T.B.A.
Anticorticosteroid	aminoglutethimide	Cytadren
Estrogens	chlorotrianisene	Tace
	diethylstilbestrol	DES
	estradiol	Alora, Climara, Esclim, Estrace, Estraderm, Estradiol, Fempatch, Gynodiol, Vivelle
	estradiol valerate	Delestrogen, Dioval, EstroSpan, Valergen
	estrogens, conjugated, equine	Premarin
	estrogens, conjugated, synthetic A	Cenestin
	estrogens, esterified	Estratab, Menest

Table 13-2. Chemotherapy Agents *(Continued)*

CLASS (SUBCLASS)	COMMON NAME	TRADE NAME
Estrogens (cont.)	estropipate	Ogen, Ortho-Est
	ethinyl estradiol	Estinyl
Estrogen/Progesterone combinations	estrogens, conjugated/ Medroxyprogesterone acetate	Premphase, Prempro
Progestins	medroxyprogesterone acetate	Amen, Curretab, Cycrin, Depo-Provera, Prodoxy-10, Provera
	progesterone	Crinone, Progestasert, Prometrium
Antiestrogens	anastrozole	Arimidex
	letrozole	Femara
	raloxifene	Evista
	tamoxifen	Nolvadex
Progestin/Antiestrogen	megestrol acetate	Megace
Antiprogestin	mifepristone	Mifeprex
Testosterones	fluoxymesterone	Halotestin
	testosterone	Adroderm, Testoderm, Testopel, Testro
	testosterone cypionate	Andro-Cyp, Depotest, Virilon-Im
	testosterone enanthate	Adro LA, Delatestryl, Everone, Testro LA
Antitestosterones	bicalutamide	Casodex
	flutamide	Eulexin
	goserelin	Zoladex
	ketoconazole	Nizoral
	leuprolide	Lupron
	nilutamide	Anandron, Nilandron
Microtubule inhibitors	docetaxel	Taxotere
	paclitaxel	Taxol
	rinorelbine	Navelbine
	vinblastine sulfate	Velban
	vincristine sulfate	Oncovin
Chromatin function inhibitors	etoposide	Vespid, VP-16
	irinotecan	Camptosar

Table 13-2. Chemotherapy Agents *(Continued)*

CLASS (SUBCLASS)	COMMON NAME	TRADE NAME
Chromatin function inhibitors *(cont.)*	teniposide	Vumon
	topotecan	Hycamtin
New-breed agents	rituximab	Rituxan
	STI571	Gleevec
	trastuzumab	Herceptin

promising technique involves binding chemotherapy drugs to antibodies, which attach themselves to cancer cells and deliver their drug payload directly to the tumor while sparing healthy cells from destruction.

How often you take chemotherapy drugs is also a complex decision. Typically a drug protocol involves cycles: You take the drug for a period of time (often three or four weeks), followed by a drug "holiday." Then the cycle starts again. A new strategy, "fractionated chemotherapy," involves smaller doses taken more frequently. This method appears to be equally effective, and usually people experience fewer and milder side effects. A new science, chronotherapy, is exploring the optimum strategy for timing the administration of cancer drugs.

Alkylating Agents and Platinum Compounds

Alkylating agents and platinum compounds cause damage to cells by directly damaging DNA. The various alkylating agents and platinum-based drugs differ in their patterns of antitumor activity, sites of activity, and side-effect profiles. These highly reactive chemicals are very toxic to cancer cells, but they also damage normal cells. They are especially toxic to rapidly proliferating normal cells, such as bone marrow and the cells that line the gastrointestinal tract. Cyclophosphamide, the most widely prescribed alkylating agent, is used to treat Hodgkin's disease and other lymphomas, acute lymphocytic leukemia, and a variety of solid tumors.

Platinum compounds work in a slightly different way from alkylating agents, but the result is the same: damage to DNA. These agents are most often used in the treatment of testicular cancer (in combination with bleomycin and vinblastine), bladder cancer, head and neck cancer (with bleomycin and fluorouracil), ovarian cancer (with cyclophosphamide or doxorubicin), and lung cancer (with etoposide or Taxol). Cisplatin causes severe side effects, and its use today is limited to a few specific types of cancer or as an alternative if cancer recurs after other forms of treatment have been tried. A newer platinum compound, carboplatin, is becoming more widely used because it has a more favorable side-effects profile.

TOXICITY AND SIDE EFFECTS | The biggest problem with alkylating agents is bone marrow suppression. The bone marrow is responsible for manufacturing white and red blood cells and platelets. When the marrow is suppressed, you may experience low white cell counts and anemia. Signs and symptoms include fatigue, greater susceptibility to infections, especially yeast infections (candidiasis, also known as thrush), shingles, and slow healing. Your physicians will want to monitor your blood cell and platelet counts carefully during therapy with these drugs.

Platinum compounds pose many of the same risks. Besides suppression of bone marrow function, the biggest concern about use of cisplatin is toxicity to the kidneys. Other complications include severe nausea and vomiting (in virtually all patients), damage to the ear drums (ototoxicity) leading to hearing loss, heart damage, hair loss, allergic reactions, and peripheral nerve damage (feelings of pins and needles or loss of feeling or pain in the hands or feet). Some patients experience changes in their sense of taste or color perception. Carboplatin is less toxic to nerves and kidneys and causes less nausea and vomiting, although it is more likely to suppress bone marrow. Some patients develop allergic (rashlike) reactions.

WHAT TO DO IF YOU TAKE ALKYLATING AGENTS | For natural support when you are taking alkylating agents, as well as dealing with bone marrow suppression, we recommend utilizing the basic guidelines on diet given on page 238, as well as those described in Chapter 7, Battling Cancer Through Diet, and the chemotherapy supplement program listed in Appendix E on page 338. We also recommend the use of hydrotherapy at home, acupuncture, and Polyerga (a special spleen extract from hogs; for more information, see page 181). In one double-blind, placebo-controlled study, Polyerga was shown to work in patients with head and neck cancers who were receiving 5-FU and cisplatin.[31] These drugs typically cause a decline in the number of white blood cells called lymphocytes, but use of Polyerga stabilized lymphocyte levels. In

> ## Warning
>
> The anemia that develops as an adverse event of cancer chemotherapy is rarely due to low levels of iron. Unless blood tests such as serum ferritin show that you have an iron deficiency, do not take supplemental iron. Too much iron in the blood can promote tumor growth and worsen the side effects of chemotherapy. Consult your physician before taking an iron supplement for anemia.

contrast, the placebo group did experience a drop in lymphocyte counts. The Polyerga group also reported less fatigue and higher energy levels than the placebo group, and there was no weight loss. In addition to the goal of boosting white blood cell counts, preventing weight loss is a major goal in the support of cancer patients, since weight loss reduces the tolerance to anticancer drugs, alters the functioning of the immune system, and can be a cause of death. For people of up to 140 pounds body weight, take one Polyerga tablet three times a day. For every additional 40 pounds body weight, add an additional tablet (e.g., a 220-pound person would take 5 tablets daily in divided dosages). For best results, take Polyerga on an empty stomach before meals. Also, do not take Polyerga at the same time you take digestive enzymes such as pancreatin, bromelain, or papain.

Keep in mind that chemotherapy will almost always cause some drop in blood counts. The goal is to prevent such a severe drop that complications ensue. If the natural methods are not adequate, it's reassuring to know that modern medicine can offer some very effective treatments to help with low blood counts. These are bioengineered versions of growth factors normally made in the body. Erythropoeitin (EPO) stimulates the growth of red blood cells, and Neupogen stimulates the growth of white blood cells. These compounds have some drawbacks. They must be injected daily for up to five days; many people dislike having to administer injections to themselves. The other disadvantage is cost. A series of injections can cost thousands of dollars.

WHAT TO DO IF YOU TAKE PLATINUM COMPOUNDS | For protection when taking cisplatin or carboplatin, follow the basic dietary program given in Chapter 7 as well as the chemotherapy supplement program given above. We especially recommend being sure to get appropriate levels of vitamin C (500 mg three times daily), vitamin E (400 to 800 IU daily), selenium (100 to 400 mcg daily), and melatonin (20 mg daily at bedtime) to enhance the effects of cisplatin and reduce its toxicity.

Selenium supplementation alone has been shown to be of value, but as we have stated repeatedly, when using antioxidants be sure they are used along with other antioxidants. In a study of patients given cisplatin alone or cisplatin plus selenium, white blood cell counts were significantly higher and fewer transfusions were needed during the cycles in which selenium was used.[32] The same study found that blood markers that indicated kidney damage were lower in the selenium group. Animal studies have concluded that administering selenium with cisplatin allows larger doses to be used, resulting in better therapeutic efficacy with less toxicity.[33]

We also recommend increasing the consumption of soy foods. The soy isoflavonoid genistein increases the uptake of cisplatin into cancer cells. In one study, genistein was able to reestablish the effectiveness of cisplatin in ovarian cancer cells that had developed resistance to the drug.[34]

CAUTIONS WHEN USING PLATINUM-BASED DRUGS | Do not take N-acetylcysteine (NAC), a derivative of the naturally occurring amino acid cysteine. Some people use NAC as a nutritional supplement to boost glutathione levels. However, two laboratory studies have shown that NAC inhibits the antitumor activity of cisplatin.[35,36] In fact, we recommend that you avoid NAC during active treatment with *any* chemotherapy agent. After your treatment is complete, NAC may be of benefit—for example, by helping reverse kidney damage.

Also, avoid dosages of vitamin B_6 over 200 mg a day. At higher levels, B_6 may interfere with platinum-containing compounds.[37]

Antitumor Antibiotics

The antibiotics you take to treat an infection are designed to attack and destroy bacteria, the one-celled creatures that make you sick. In cancer treatment, certain drugs can also be used to attack cancer cells. These drugs, known as antitumor antibiotics, work by binding directly to DNA components in the nucleus, thus interfering with DNA synthesis

A Special Licorice Extract Helps Mouth Ulcers

A special extract of licorice root can be extremely helpful in healing mouth ulcers that are often experienced by people on chemotherapy. The extract is known as DGL. That's the abbreviation for de-glycyrrhizinated licorice, but we like to think it stands for "darn good licorice." DGL is produced by removing glycyrrhetinic acid from concentrated licorice. This compound can result in elevations in blood pressure because of sodium and water retention. Yes, eating too much licorice candy, if it contains real licorice extract, can raise blood pressure. Because the glycyrrhetinic acid has been removed, DGL does not raise blood pressure.

In addition to having shown clinical benefit in healing mouth ulcers, DGL is also extremely useful in treating peptic ulcers (gastric or duodenal ulcers).[38] In fact, in several head-to-head studies, DGL has been shown to be more effective than Tagamet, Zantac, or antacids in both short-term treatment and maintenance therapy of peptic ulcers.[39,40] Rather than inhibit the release of acid, DGL stimulates the normal defense mechanisms that prevent ulcer formation, whether in the mouth, stomach, or intestines. It improves both the quality and quantity of the protective substances that line the intestinal tract, increases the life span of the intestinal cell, and improves blood supply to the intestinal lining. There is also some evidence that it inhibits growth of *H. pylori,* the bacterium that is linked to peptic ulcer disease and stomach cancer.

The standard dosage for DGL is one or two chewable tablets containing 400 mg DGL taken between meals or 20 minutes before meals. You won't get good results if you take DGL after meals. For DGL to be effective, it must mix with saliva. Taking DGL in capsules doesn't work: In order for it to be effective, it must mix with saliva. If your mouth is too sore to chew the tablets, let them dissolve in your mouth, or you can crush them and dissolve them in water.

or with cell processes that are controlled by DNA signals. The drugs are used to treat a wide variety of cancers, including cancers of the breast, lung, and stomach; lymphomas; certain leukemias; myelomas; and sarcomas. The trouble is, these antitumor antibiotics are not very specific in their action—that is, they attack normal cells as well and so can produce serious side effects.

TOXICITY AND SIDE EFFECTS | The most serious of the toxicity problems with antitumor antibiotics is bone marrow suppression, leading to reductions in white blood cell levels. They can also cause damage to the heart muscle, which can be life-threatening. Bleomycin (Blenoxane) does not depress bone marrow function and is less likely to affect liver, kidney, and central nervous system function. But bleomycin is still quite toxic, especially to the lungs, and also to skin, hair, and mucous membranes.

Another concern is the risk of secondary cancers. Studies vary, but generally the risk for developing acute myelogenous leukemia ranges from 1 to 5 percent after five years. This form of leukemia is extremely dangerous, with a very poor prognosis.

Side effects such as nausea and vomiting, fatigue, malaise, mouth ulcers, gastrointestinal ulcers, and acne-like eruptions of the skin are common. Nausea, vomiting, and malaise begin several hours after treatment and last for as long as a day or two. Fortunately, it appears that several natural compounds can reduce the likelihood of this complication without interfering with the drug's efficacy.

WHAT TO DO IF YOU TAKE ANTITUMOR ANTIBIOTICS | To reduce the toxicity of these drugs, we recommend utilizing the basic guidelines on diet given on page 238, as well as those described in Chapter 7, Battling Cancer Through Diet, and the basic chemotherapy supplement program given in Appendix E on page 338. We also recommend using co-enzyme Q10 (CoQ10)—100 mg twice daily. The role of CoQ10 in the heart is similar to the role of a spark plug in a car engine. Just as the car cannot function without that initial spark, the heart cannot function without CoQ10. Over 20 double-blind studies have shown that CoQ10 supplementation improves heart function by increasing energy production in the heart muscle and by acting as an antioxidant. Doxorubicin depletes the heart of CoQ10, leaving it extremely susceptible to damage.

A number of studies have shown that CoQ10 prevents the cardiac toxicity associated with antitumor antibiotics like doxorubicin. A small study in humans showed CoQ10 administration at 1 mg per kg (2.2 pounds) body weight led to 20 percent or greater reduction in heart damage compared with patients who took doxorubicin alone.[41] Diarrhea and mouth ulcer formation were also significantly reduced. In a study of 20 leukemia patients undergoing treatment with daunorubicin (a drug similar to doxorubicin), taking 100 mg of CoQ10 twice daily significantly reduced adverse cardiac events as measured by echocardiography.[42] A study in mice also suggested that CoQ10 might enhance the antitumor activity of doxorubicin.[43] CoQ10 has demonstrated other anticancer effects, including some positive results in preliminary human studies.[44,45]

Another useful strategy is to take melatonin. In one study, melatonin (20 mg a day at bedtime) normalized platelet counts in 9 of 12 breast cancer patients who developed thrombocytopenia (reduced platelet counts) during treatment with epirubicin.[46] In 5 of the patients, the tumors regressed in size. Melatonin has also been shown to increase the tumor-killing action of doxorubicin while simultaneously reducing undesirable toxic side effects.[21]

Vitamin E may also reduce the toxicity of doxorubicin and may enhance the drug's anticancer effects. A study showed that giving mice vitamin E before administering the drug at lethal dosages reduced the death rate from 85 percent to 10 percent.[47] This dose of vitamin E did not alter the suppression of tumor cell DNA synthesis by doxorubicin, however. The mice who got vitamin E lived longer on average than those treated with doxorubicin alone. The authors theorized that the vitamin E prevented heart damage by blocking oxidation of lipid molecules without impairing the drug's antitumor effects. In an animal study, vitamin C also has been shown to reduce the toxicity of doxorubicin without diminishing its effectiveness.[48]

While quercetin has shown an ability to increase the concentration of doxorubicin in human breast cancer cells, it reduced concentrations in a colon cancer cell line.[49,50] Therefore, use it if you have breast cancer, but do not use quercetin with doxorubicin if you have colon cancer; use curcumin instead. Curcumin has shown good inhibition of colon cancer in experimental studies and has also been shown to protect the heart and the kidneys from doxorubicin toxicity.[51-53]

Studies in mice have shown that green tea increased doxorubicin concentrations in two types of tumors but not in normal tissue. The antitumor activity of the drug was enhanced 2.5 times in mice fed green tea.[54] Another report confirmed these results, showing that the tumor inhibition of doxorubicin increased from negligible to 62 percent.[55] This report suggested that the activity of green tea was due to an amino acid, theanine, rather than its flavonoid content. This association was solidified in several other studies,[56,57] indicating that regular green tea consumption or the use of green tea extracts that contain theanine is preferable to polyphenol extracts in this application. The protocol for supplements to take to support antitumor antibiotic therapy appears on page 339.

Antimetabolites

Antimetabolites are compounds that interfere with the production of genetic material or another key aspect of cellular reproduction. There are three main categories of antimetabolites, each with different activity:

- Antifolates, such as methotrexate (Folex, Mexate); these block folic acid, an essential component of enzymes that help manufacture DNA and RNA.
- Purine analogs, such as mercaptopurine (6-MP, Purinethol) and thioguanine (6-TG); these block cellular growth and reproduction by interfering with the purine compounds xanthine and guanine, respectively, which are necessary for the manufacture of DNA and RNA.
- Pyramidine analogs, such as 5-fluorouracil (5-FU, Adrucil) and fluorodeoxyuridine (FdUrd) (FUDR); these inhibit the manufacture of pyramidines, the other building blocks of DNA and RNA.

Antimetabolites, alone and in combination with other chemotherapy agents, are used in the treatment of many types of cancer, including cancers of the breast, lungs, liver, gastrointestinal tract, bone, ovaries, and pancreas, as well as certain leukemias and lymphomas.

TOXICITY AND SIDE EFFECTS | The toxicity of antimetabolites is somewhat less severe than other classes of chemotherapy agents. The most common side effects are bone marrow suppression (except floxu-ridine and asparaginase), mouth sores, hair loss, loss of appetite, nausea, and diarrhea. In fact, the presence of these side effects is often used as gauge that a sufficient dose has been given.

WHAT TO DO IF YOU TAKE ANTIMETABOLITES | These drugs can produce the same side effects as other chemotherapy drugs but usually in less severe forms. Follow the basic dietary program on page 238, as well as those described in Chapter 7, Battling Cancer Through Diet, and the chemotherapy supplement program given in Appendix E on page 338. There are some additional cautions worth noting:

The antimetabolite drug methotrexate (MTX) works by inhibiting the transformation of folic acid into compounds necessary for the repli-cation of DNA. For this reason, patients should avoid taking large doses of folic acid while being treated with MTX. But folic acid is still an im-portant nutrient for support of normal cell function. To err on the side of caution, we advise using no more than 800 mcg of folic acid daily during treatment with MTX. Between courses of MTX therapy, it is safe to take larger doses of folic acid if prescribed by your physician.

It is very important for people on MTX therapy to take whey pro-tein. One of the key amino acids in whey protein, glutamine, increases the intratumor levels of MTX in human and rat studies, thereby in-creasing its cancer-killing effect.[58] Within 24 hours, the rats who were given glutamine had a higher rate of tumor destruction. This result was due to the effect that glutamine exerts in decreasing the intratumor lev-els of glutathione, making tumors more susceptible to the MTX. For more information on this action of glutamine, see page 154. Again, we prefer whey protein over glutamine. Two servings of a whey-protein smoothie, each providing 20 to 30 g of whey protein, are recommended.

Be aware that some common medications can interact with MTX. For example, aspirin and other anti-inflammatory agents can reduce the elimination of MTX through the kidneys, which thus increases blood levels and may lead to higher risk of toxicity. Penicillin can also produce a similar effect and should be avoided during treatment. Be sure all your physicians are aware of what drugs you're taking to reduce the risk of such interactions.

Biological Response Modifiers

Biological response modifiers are compounds that affect the way the body's immune system reacts to cancer. Examples include interferons and interleukins, which work directly by slowing down cancer cell reproduction. They also act indirectly by signaling white blood cells to attack infecting organisms and cancer cells. The agent BCG works indirectly to enhance immune function. BCG is a live bacterial strain that is injected directly into tumors (usually of the bladder). White blood cells rush to the area of injection to kill the bacteria, and in their heightened state these immune cells kill the cancer cells as well.

Among the newest biological response modifiers are various growth factors. These work by overcoming the suppression of bone marrow that results from some forms of cancer treatment, thereby stimulating the bone marrow to manufacture blood cells. Erythropoietin is used to replenish red blood cells, while granulocyte-macrophage colony stimulating factor (GM-CSF, sold as Leukine or Prokine) and granulocyte colony stimulating factor (G-CSF, sold as Neupogen) are used to replenish white blood cells. Positive benefits include decreasing the frequency of infections and shortening the stay in the hospital.

The use of biological response modifiers in cancer therapy is gaining acceptance, but treatment with these agents can be very expensive.

TOXICITY AND SIDE EFFECTS | The toxicity of biological response modifiers, especially the bone marrow stimulators, is generally low compared with other chemotherapy agents. But they can still produce significant side effects, including flu-like symptoms (fever, chills, muscle aches, headache, fatigue, and joint pain).

WHAT TO DO IF YOU TAKE BIOLOGICAL RESPONSE MODIFIERS | As with all forms of chemotherapy, follow the basic dietary program on page 238, as well as those described in Chapter 7, Battling Cancer Through Diet, as well as the basic chemotherapy supplementation program given in Appendix E on page 338. Patients who are taking interleukin-2 (IL-2) should supplement with melatonin. One study found that melatonin (40 mg a day) increased the effect of IL-2 against a variety of solid cancers.[27] Another found that the combination of melatonin (40 mg a day) and IL-2 was a more effective treatment than cisplatin and etoposide in non-small-cell lung cancer.[24]

Hormones and Antihormones

Hormones are chemicals your body produces to signal other organs to function. Some cancer tumors respond to the presence of hormones, so treatment with hormonal agents can alter tumor activity. Antihormones block the effect of the corresponding natural hormone on the cancer cells. For example, antiestrogens are used against estrogen-dependent breast cancers, while antitestosterones are used against testosterone-dependent prostate cancers. Another type of hormone, the corticosteroids, are used primarily to suppress white blood cell growth in certain leukemias and lymphomas. The most commonly used corticosteroid is prednisone.

One of the more controversial antihormones is tamoxifen, which can prevent breast cancer in high-risk individuals and can reduce the risk of recurrence in women who have already had the disease. Tamoxifen has been used for more than 20 years. Here's how it works:

The surfaces of certain tumor cells have unique molecules, called receptors, that bind with molecules of estrogen. When that connection is made, it generates signals that tell the cancer cell to divide and thus causes the tumor to grow. Such cancers are described as estrogen-responsive tumors. Like estrogen, tamoxifen also binds with the estrogen receptor, but unlike the hormone, it does not trigger growth signals. When tamoxifen occupies the "parking space," estrogen can't bind to the receptor. Thus the cancer cells grow more slowly, or they stop growing altogether. Studies indicate that tamoxifen lowers cancer risk by about half. That is, a woman who has a 50 percent chance of breast cancer recurrence without the drug might have only a 25 percent chance if treated with tamoxifen.

In women who have not yet gone through menopause, most of their estrogen is produced by the ovaries. After menopause (or following surgical removal of the ovaries), estrogen levels fall, but some estrogen is still produced by other metabolic systems, such as the aromatase enzyme system, which converts other hormones into estrogen. There are antiestrogen drugs available, such as Arimidex and Femara, that inhibit the aromatase system. They can be used alone or in combination with tamoxifen to reduce estrogen activity in cancer calls. Recent studies suggest that aromatase inhibitors may be as effective as tamoxifen and have fewer side effects,[59] but these drugs do not yet have the long-term track record of tamoxifen.

Like breast cancer in women, prostate cancer in men is a hormone-responsive cancer. The hormone involved here is testosterone. Prostate cancer cells bind with testosterone, which triggers cell activity and growth. Drugs are available that affect testosterone production or metabolism. Leuprolide (Lupron) and goserelin (Zoladex) both work by blocking signals from the pituitary gland that tell the testicles to make testosterone. Drugs such as bicalutamide (Casodex) and flutamide (Eulexin) act the way tamoxifen does: They block the hormone receptors on the surface of prostate cancer cells.

One drawback of treatment with antitestosterone agents is that prostate cancer cells may become resistant to hormone blockade—they figure out how to grow and divide without depending on signals from testosterone. If that happens, the disease can become much more difficult to treat. As a countermeasure, physicians may recommend intermittent hormone blockade. In this approach, the patient takes antihormones until the cancer appears well controlled, then stops treatment until the PSA levels rise. (PSA, or prostate specific antigen, is a protein released by prostate tumors that can be measured to evaluate the extent of the disease; see page 22 for more information.)

Another approach is known as triple hormone blockade. In this strategy, the patient takes a combination of Lupron, Casodex, and Proscar to inhibit the three major ways testosterone can affect the prostate. After about 13 months, most patients are able to discontinue treatment, taking only Proscar as maintenance therapy. This approach avoids the side effects of radiation and surgery and also minimizes the side effects of hormone blockade, because the treatment period is relatively brief. An analysis of 110 patients treated with this protocol and followed for as long as 10 years found that all patients were off therapy and that none had to be re-treated.[60]

TOXICITY AND SIDE EFFECTS | Hormonal agents are generally well tolerated and usually do not produce severe toxicity. Side effects tend to be more annoying than debilitating.

ANTIESTROGEN AGENTS | Common side effects include nausea, vomiting, indigestion, and hot flashes. Some patients may experience mild bone marrow suppression. These complications tend to appear in the first few weeks of therapy and disappear fairly soon (although some women experience hot flashes for as long as they take tamoxifen).

Less common adverse reactions include depression, tiredness, dizziness, bone pain, and reduced sex drive. Rare side effects include:

Allergic reactions, such as skin rashes
Temporary thinning of the hair
Headaches (including changes in patterns of migraines)
Flaking fingernails (usually occurring only after years of treatment)
Thrombosis (blood clots)
Visual problems (blurred or reduced vision)
Endometrial hyperplasia and cancer

Women taking tamoxifen who have not yet reached menopause may notice changes in their monthly periods. Menstrual flow may become irregular or lighter; sometimes it stops altogether. Some women report vaginal discharge or itching in the vulva.

Thrombosis is particularly serious, since blood clots can block blood vessels and cause severe injury or death. Several of our patients have developed deep-vein thromboses after starting tamoxifen therapy. Symptoms of thrombosis include pain, warmth, and swelling or tenderness

Warning

Women who are taking the anticancer drug tamoxifen also should avoid soy. Tamoxifen works by attaching to estrogen receptors in cancer cells. By doing so, it blocks "real" estrogen or estrogen-like compounds from attaching and thus keeps them from stimulating tumor cell growth. But test tube studies have found that genistein and tamoxifen compete to bind with the estrogen receptors.[26] Usually genistein wins the race, thus negating the desired effects of tamoxifen. For this reason and others, it's prudent for women with estrogen-sensitive breast cancer to avoid and consume no more than four servings of soy foods weekly.

especially in the chest, arm, or leg. Report any such problems to your physician immediately.

ANTITESTOSTERONE AGENTS | Many men taking these drugs develop a greater sympathy for what women experience during menopause, because they too experience hot flashes. These agents frequently cause impotence, anemia, and a decrease in sexual drive. They can also cause muscle wasting and bone loss.

Oral corticosteroids: The side effects of oral corticosteroids depend on dosage levels and length of time on the medication. The longer you take them, the greater the risk of side effects. The number and severity of side effects is a matter of dosage and length of treatment. At lower dosages (less than 10 mg a day), the most common side effects are increased appetite, weight gain, retention of salt and water, and increased susceptibility to infection. These side effects are expected to develop in most people taking corticosteroids.

Long-term use of corticosteroids at higher doses can cause depression and other mental or emotional disturbances in more than half of patients; high blood pressure; diabetes; peptic ulcers; acne; excessive facial hair in women; insomnia; muscle cramps and weakness; thinning and weakening of the skin; osteoporosis; and susceptibility to the formation of blood clots.

WHAT TO DO IF YOU TAKE HORMONES OR ANTIHORMONES |

Breast cancer: Women with breast cancer should follow all the recommendations given in Chapter 4, Special Steps for Preventing Lung, Breast, Prostate, and Colon Cancers, as well as the chemotherapy supplement program given on page 338, including taking lycopene, calcium D-glucarate, indole-3-carbinol, and ground flaxseed.

For women taking tamoxifen, we recommend adding melatonin to the regimen. One study examined the combination of tamoxifen plus melatonin (20 mg a day) in the treatment of metastatic breast cancer that had progressed under treatment with tamoxifen alone.[61] Four of the 14 patients had a partial response to this combination: Progression of their disease was delayed by an average of eight months compared with tamoxifen treatment alone. Treatment was well tolerated, and relief of anxiety or depression was also noted by many patients.

There are a number of ways to help reduce or control hot flashes and sweats. Some women find it helpful to avoid or cut down on tea, coffee, nicotine, and alcohol. Interestingly, while black cohosh seems to work in most women, a recent double-blind trial in breast cancer patients found that it did not seem to work.[62]

Tamoxifen also causes severe elevation in blood triglycerides and possibly cholesterol levels as well. Elevation in these blood fats is associated with an increased risk for heart disease. Fortunately, vitamins C and E can help. In one study, supplementation of vitamin C (500 mg daily) and vitamin E (400 mg daily) for 90 days along with tamoxifen (10 mg twice a day) reduced total cholesterol, low-density lipoprotein (LDL) cholesterol, and triglyceride levels while significantly increasing the protective high-density lipoprotein (HDL) cholesterol level. The authors of the study concluded that "these results suggested that tamoxifen treatment is the most effective during co-administration of vitamin C and vitamin E."[63]

Prostate cancer: Men with prostate cancer should follow all the recommendations given in Chapter 4, Special Steps for Preventing Lung, Breast, Prostate, and Colon Cancers, as well as the basic chemotherapy supplement program given in Appendix E (see page 338), including taking lycopene, calcium D-glucarate, indole-3-carbinol, and ground flaxseed. Men taking antihormonal drugs should take extra calcium and should focus on weight-bearing and resistance exercise to prevent osteoporosis.

Usually prostate cancer is a slow-growing disease that can be monitored quite easily. That means it's sometimes possible to defer conventional therapy (one term for this strategy is *watchful waiting*) and try alternative treatments first. If you want to follow this approach, discuss your options with your physicians. Set up a plan for monitoring your condition on a regular basis. In general, we recommend having a PSA test and perhaps a testosterone level test once a month. We also recommend periodic imaging studies, including bone scans, CT scan, or transrectal ultrasound, depending on the stage of your cancer. If the disease appears to be progressing, you and your caregivers can decide on more aggressive strategies.

Microtubule Inhibitor and Chromatin Function Inhibitors

Many of the drugs in this category are derived from plants, including the periwinkle plant (source of the vinca alkaloids vincristine and vin-

PC-SPES

PC-SPES is a combination of eight herbs that many men use for treatment or prevention of prostate cancer. (PC stands for "prostate cancer," and SPES comes from the Latin word for "hope.") The product was developed by Sophie Chen, a Chinese-born scientist educated in the United States, as a remedy to help a friend with prostate cancer.

Following are the reported ingredients of PC-SPES:

- *Isatis indigotica* contains the component indirubin, which is reported to have anticancer activity and has been used in China in the treatment of leukemias.
- Licorice *(Glycyrrhiza glabra* and *Glycyrrhiza uralensis)* contains triterpenoids and flavonoids that might have anticancer effects.
- Ginseng *(Panax ginseng)* contains immune-enhancing and anti-cancer compounds known as ginsenosides.
- Reishi mushroom *(Ganoderma lucidum)* contains polysaccharide molecules (glycans) that have shown significant antitumor effects in test tube studies.
- Skullcap *(Scutellaria baicalensis)* contains baicalein, a flavonoid that has shown anticancer properties.
- Chrysanthemum *(Dendranthema morefolium)* is a less well-known Chinese herb with unspecified biologic effects.
- *Rabdosia rucescens* is thought to contain an antihormonal compound that has multiple antitumor effects.
- Saw palmetto *(Serenoa repens)* has been shown to inhibit the conversion of testosterone to its more potent form, dihydrotestosterone. Used primarily as a remedy for benign prostatic hyperplasia (BPH, a noncancerous condition causing prostate enlargement), saw palmetto has been shown to be as effective as conventional drugs in the treatment of mild to moderate cases.[64]

In user surveys, PC-SPES has been found to help about 70 percent of more than 1,700 men with prostate cancer.[65] A study conducted at the University of California at San Francisco found that most prostate cancer patients who have never been treated with hormones will have a significant response to PC-SPES.[66] In the study, of the 70 participating subjects, 100 percent had a decline in their PSA, and 56 percent achieved an undetectable PSA. This effect appears to result primarily from the antihormonal effects of the drug, since more than 80 percent of men taking PC-SPES showed a dramatic decline in their testosterone levels. In some cases the drop was equivalent to castration.

PC-SPES may also have effects against prostate cancer tumors that are not hormone-sensitive. Approximately 60 percent of such patients had significant declines in their PSA. Some of the patients also showed improvements on bone scans and other measures of disease.[67,68]

PC-SPES can cause side effects. When testosterone levels fall to a certain point, most men develop breast tenderness or breast enlargement, the same side effects seen following treatment with Lupron or DES (diethylsilbesterol). Other side effects include:

- Decreased libido (sexual desire)
- Decreased ability to achieve and maintain erections
- Frequent loose bowel movements or diarrhea (usually mild) in about a third of patients
- Leg cramps or muscle cramps in about a third of patients
- Change in urine flow (increase or decrease)
- Fatigue
- Allergic reactions
- Blood clots in legs or lungs (rare)

Our Take on PC-SPES

Even though PC-SPES is a "natural" product, its effects—that is, reduction in testosterone levels and activity—are not. It is an expensive herbal mixture whose active ingredients and mechanism of action are not well defined. We are especially puzzled by reports of dramatic reductions in testosterone levels. Such effects are much larger than are typically seen with most herbal medicines. And PC-SPES is not without side effects.

There have been reports from at least two independent laboratories that DES was found in at least two lots of PC-SPES. In February 2002, the FDA issued a warning on PC-SPES, citing that it contained another drug—warfarin (Coumadin), the powerful blood thinner. This report led to a total recall of the product by BotanicLab, the manufacturer. Until these contamination issues of PC-SPES are cleared up, we would recommend avoiding it. Keep an eye on the PSA Rising Web site (www.psa-rising.com) for up-to-date information on PC-SPES.

blastine), the Pacific yew tree (paclitaxel), and the May apple (podophyllin derivatives such as etoposide and teniposide). Some of these cellular poisons work by interfering with cellular structures known as microtubules. Microtubules are proteins that control the cell's shape and movement. The major component of microtubules is a protein called tubulin. This molecule contains two subunits, known simply as alpha and beta. Microtubule inhibitors like Taxol and the vinca alkaloids work by disrupting the balance between the alpha and beta units. As a result, they interfere with the physical actions of the cancer cell and disrupt its ability to function and reproduce.

Chromatin inhibitors like etoposide, teniposide, and irinotecan disrupt DNA (chromosome) dynamics. For DNA to carry out a function, part of the long, tightly wound molecule must untwist, change position, and split apart temporarily. That activity is controlled by enzymes known as topoisomerases, which break DNA strands apart and then reseal them. Chromatin inhibitors act by blocking these enzymes. Without those enzymes, the DNA can't do its job—and thus the cancer cell can't reproduce.

Paclitaxel and docetaxel are frequently used to treat ovarian cancer, breast cancer, carcinoma of the lung, and head and neck carcinoma. The response rate in these cancers is fairly high. Vincristine, usually in combination with prednisone, is used to induce remission in childhood acute leukemias; complete remissions occur in about 80 to 90 percent of cases. Vincristine is also used for the treatment of Hodgkin's and non-Hodgkin's lymphoma. Combined with bleomycin and cisplatin, vinblastine is very effective in the treatment of metastatic testicular cancer. The newest of the vinca alkaloids, vindesine shows significant activity in the treatment of acute leukemia, blast crisis of chronic myelogenous leukemia, and Hodgkin's and non-Hodgkin's lymphomas.

Etoposide, often combined with bleomycin and cisplatin, is active against a variety of tumor types, especially resistant testicular tumors. Etoposide plays an important role in the treatment of small-cell lung carcinomas, usually combined with cisplatin. Teniposide appears to be effective for the treatment of acute lymphoblastic leukemia and childhood neuroblastomas, as well as brain tumors in adults. Irinotecan appears to be one of the most active compounds available for the treatment of non-small-cell lung cancer.

TOXICITY AND SIDE EFFECTS | The principal dose-limiting toxicity of these drugs, with the exception of vincristine, is severe bone marrow suppression. Nausea and diarrhea are common but usually are not severe. Mouth sores can be severe at higher doses. Other toxic effects include fever, chills, skin rash, and allergic reactions. Vincristine can cause peripheral nerve damage as well as damage to the nerves that control internal organs. As a result, some patients experience abdominal pain, constipation, urinary retention, and orthostatic hypotension (low blood pressure upon standing). Taxol also causes muscle aches and some reversible neurotoxicities, most often numbness and feelings of pins and needles (paresthesias) in the hands and feet.

WHAT TO DO IF YOU TAKE MICROTUBULE INHIBITORS AND CHROMATIN FUNCTION INHIBITORS | As is the case with all forms of chemotherapy, follow the basic dietary program given above on page 228, as well as those described in Chapter 7, Battling Cancer Through Diet, as well as the basic chemotherapy supplementation program given in Appendix E on page 338. These drugs produce the same sort of side effects as other chemotherapy drugs. The principal dose-limiting toxicity of these drugs (except vincristine) is severe bone marrow suppression. People taking these agents drugs should also take Polyerga (see page 181) and be sure to have at least 40 to 60 mg of whey protein or 3 to 10 g of glutamine daily.

New-Breed Chemotherapy Agents

There are several promising chemotherapy drugs that we call new-breed chemotherapy agents. These drugs have great potential. They are highly selective in their actions, thus doing a better job of targeting cancer cells and leaving normal cells alone. For example, monoclonal antibodies are being developed that recognize specific molecules (called antigens) that appear on only cancer cells. Once attached to the cell, the antibody can inhibit its growth or can act as a "red flag," signaling the immune system to come and destroy the cell. Antibodies are being designed to deliver antitumor drugs, toxins, or radioactive material directly to cancer cells, thus avoiding damage to healthy cells. (You can recognize many of these drugs because their chemical names end with -*mab*, short for "monoclonal antibody.")

Other new "molecularly targeted" drugs are being developed that bind to specific genetic defects found only in cancer cells.

If you are on one of these new-breed chemotherapy agents, we still believe that it is important to follow the basic dietary program given in Chapter 7, as well as the basic general supplementation program given above.

GLEEVEC | Gleevec (STI571), used in the treatment of chronic myeloid leukemia (CML), is heralded as the first approved "molecularly targeted" drug. Gleevec treats CML by targeting a specific genetic defect found in cells of patients with this type of cancer. It blocks receptors of a certain enzyme (tyrosine kinase) that leukemic cells depend on to fuel their growth. Because Gleevec's action is so specific, it does not harm normal cells.

The results with Gleevec in CML have been nothing short of miraculous. In April 2001, Brian Druker and colleagues reported the results of a study on Gleevec in the *New England Journal of Medicine*. Their data showed that Gleevec restored normal blood counts in 53 out of 54 chemotherapy-resistant CML patients, a response rate rarely seen in cancer with a single agent. Fifty-one of these patients were still doing well after a year on the medicine, and most reported few side effects.[69,70]

While Gleevec is currently approved only for treating CML, studies have shown that it may have potential for the treatment of other cancers that express the specific receptors for tyrosine kinase, including gastrointestinal stromal tumor and small-cell lung cancer. Gleevec's success gives us hope that, in the future, more drugs can be designed to exploit the weaknesses of all types of cancer.

HERCEPTIN | Herceptin (trastuzumab) is a monoclonal antibody developed to specifically seek out a specific antigen known as HER2 receptors that lies on the surface of some cancer cells. About 30 percent of women with breast cancer have multiple copies of a gene, known as HER2, in a single cell. This gene is responsible for producing a protein, HER2 growth factor cell-surface receptor, which plays a role in cell growth and division. Multiple copies of the HER2 gene in a single cell lead to overproduction of the HER2 protein. This causes the cells to grow and divide at an abnormally fast rate. The result: cancer. Breast cancer resulting from HER2 overexpression tends to be very aggressive and resistant to treatment.

In individuals who overexpress the HER2 protein, Herceptin binds to the cell and helps shrink the tumor. Patients are given Herceptin intravenously once a week. Herceptin causes fewer side effects than traditional chemotherapy. The most common adverse reaction to the treatment—chills and fever—is usually a response to infusion of the drug and is generally not severe. Herceptin can also cause damage to the heart, however; if so, treatment is discontinued.

RITUXAN | More than 90 percent of people with B-cell type non-Hodgkin's lymphoma (NHL) have cancerous white blood cells (B-lymphocytes) that express a certain antigen known as CD-20. Rituxan (rituximab) is a monoclonal antibody that binds to CD-20 and destroys the cell. The drug has generated a lot of excitement because of its new way of attacking cancer cells, but it is not cure-all; according to clinical trials, it has a response rate of about 40 to 60 percent. Nor is it free of side effects, but the toxicities from treatment are usually mild and include fevers, chills, nausea, rash, and hives. In some cases, severe, even life-threatening, respiratory events have occurred.

Dealing with Hair Loss

For many patients, hair loss is one of the most devastating complications of chemotherapy. Hair loss occurs because treatment with drugs or radiation can kill the cells in the hair follicles. That's because these cells share a trait in common with cancer cells: They reproduce quickly. When the follicles die, the hairs they support fall out.

Some patients experience hair loss and others do not, even when they're taking the same drugs. And not all cancer drugs cause hair loss. Some treatments cause loss of hair from the scalp only, while others cause loss from the scalp and elsewhere on the body. Radiation therapy administered to the head often causes scalp hair loss; in these cases, depending on the radiation dose, the hair may not regrow naturally.

If hair loss does occur, it usually begins within 2 weeks of the start of therapy and gets worse 1 to 2 months after the start of therapy. In many cases, hair regrowth begins even before therapy is completed. Sometimes the hair that regrows is different in body or texture. In many cases, the next "batch" that grows in is more like the original hair.

Here are some tips for dealing with hair loss:

- Before hair loss begins, be gentle when brushing and shampooing your hair. Hair loss can be reduced somewhat by avoiding too much brushing or pulling of the hair and by avoiding heat from electric rollers, hair dryers, and curling irons.
- Before treatment begins or at the very start of treatment, buy a wig or toupee. Doing this before hair loss sets in makes it easier for the wig shop to match your hair color and texture.
- Be sure to get a prescription from your doctor for the wig, because it is often covered by insurance. Ask your health care team for referrals to wig shops in your area that specialize in dealing with cancer patients.
- Some women who have long hair go to a salon for a stylish short cut and then have a beautiful wig made from their own hair.
- If you buy a wig, try on many different ones until you find one that you really like.
- Consider buying two wigs, one for every day and one for special occasions.
- Use a sunscreen, sunblock, or hat to protect your scalp from the sun.
- Wear a hat or scarf outdoors in cold weather to prevent loss of body heat.

New hair growth after chemotherapy or radiation is influenced by age and a wide variety of nutritional and hormonal factors. It is harder for both men and women over the age of 55 years to quickly recover from chemotherapy-induced hair loss. By age 40 or so, the rate of hair growth slows down, and as we continue to age, new hair growth just runs out of steam. New hairs are not replaced as quickly as old ones are lost. Nevertheless, there are things that can be done regardless of age.

In our experience, besides age there are three common causes of failure to recover quickly from chemotherapy-induced hair loss (especially in women): (1) other drugs, (2) nutritional deficiencies, and (3) hypothyroidism.

Drug-Induced Hair Loss

There is a long list of drugs that can cause hair loss. Although all the drugs listed in Table 13-3 are capable of causing hair loss, it should not be interpreted that simply because a person is complaining of hair loss and is taking one of these drugs that the drug is the single cause of the hair loss. Of course, for some drugs, most notably chemotherapy agents such as fluorouracil, they are obviously the cause, because they are such powerful inhibitors of hair growth. When medically appropriate, natural alternatives to suspected culprits of hair loss should be employed.

Table 13-3. Classes of Drugs That Can Cause Hair Loss[71]

CLASS	EXAMPLES
Antibiotics	Gentamyacin, chloramphenicol
Anticoagulants	Coumadin, heparin
Antidepressants	Prozac, desipramine, lithium
Antiepileptics	Valproic acid, Dilantin
Cardiovascular drugs	ACE inhibitors, beta-blockers
Chemotherapy drugs	Adriamycin, vincristine, etoposide
Endocrine drugs	Bromocriptine, clomid, danazol
Gout medications	Colchicine, allopurinol
Lipid-lowering drugs	Gemfibrizol, fenofibrate
Nonsteroidal anti-inflammatory drugs (NSAIDs)	Ibuprofen, indomethacin, naproxen
Ulcer medications	Tagamet, Zantac

Nutritional Deficiencies

A deficiency of any of a number of nutrients can lead to significant hair loss. Deficiencies of zinc, vitamin A, essential fatty acids, and iron are the most common. Typically, in our experience in women with either noticeable hair loss or failure to regrow lost hair after chemotherapy, they will be suffering from apparent deficiencies of all these nutrients, but especially iron. For evaluating iron status, we recommend that you ask your doctor to perform a simple blood test called serum ferritin. When evaluating serum ferritin levels, please be aware that many reference laboratories report low ferritin levels, e.g., 10 to 30 mcg per liter, within the normal range. If the serum ferritin is less than 30 mcg per liter, iron supplementation is indicated at a dosage of 30 mg twice a day between meals (if this recommendation results in abdominal discomfort, take 30 mg with meals three times a day). When serum ferritin levels get below this, hair growth and regeneration are impaired, as the body seeks to conserve the iron.

Hypothyroidism

It is a well-known fact that hair loss is one of the cardinal signs of hypothyroidism. It is estimated that between 1 and 4 percent of the adult population have moderate to severe hypothyroidism, and another 10 to 12 percent have mild hypothyroidism.

Signs and symptoms of hypothyroidism
Hair loss
Dry, rough skin
Course, dry, and brittle hair
Thin and brittle nails
Depression
Weight gain
Sensitivity to cold weather
Cold hands or feet
Elevated cholesterol and triglyceride levels
Menstrual abnormalities in women
Muscle weakness and joint stiffness

Shortness of breath
Constipation
Low basal body temperature

We make the diagnosis of hypothyroidism by looking at signs and symptoms along with laboratory data. The diagnosis is straightforward when blood measurements of thyroid hormones are clearly abnormal. In milder cases of hypothyroidism, the diagnosis is not as clear. An elevation in thyroid stimulating hormone (TSH) with a normal thyroxine (T_4) level is generally considered "subclinical," but the accepted normal range for TSH is extremely broad—0.35 to 5.50 μIU per milliliter. We tend to begin thyroid hormone-replacement therapy in patients with TSH values greater than 2.5 μIU per milliliter, especially if they are demonstrating clinical signs of hypothyroidism. If you have signs or symptoms of hypothyroidism, talk to your doctor, as it may require prescription thyroid medication.

Final Comment

Because many cancers can increase the likelihood of forming life-threatening blood clots, many cancer patients are placed on the anticoagulant drug coumadin (Warfarin). For coumadin to be effective, certain safeguards must be followed. For example, your specific dose of coumadin will be determined according to results of a blood test known as the international normalized ratio (INR).

Your doctor will also counsel you about certain dietary strategies to follow while taking coumadin. You should know, for example, that coumadin works by interfering with vitamin K's role in promoting blood clots. Since green leafy vegetables and green teas contain high levels of vitamin K, you should avoid increasing your intake of these foods while taking coumadin. You can eat at the same levels you're accustomed to—just don't increase your consumption. Your physician will monitor your blood using the INR test to be sure the coumadin is working and to change your dose (up or down) as needed. The key is consistency: Eat approximately the same-size servings of green leafy vegetables every day.

You may need to adjust your use of other natural remedies if you take coumadin. Here are some guidelines:

- Co-enzyme Q10 and St. John's wort *(Hypericum perforatum)* may reduce coumadin's efficacy, while proteolytic enzymes and several herbs, including panax ginseng, devil's claw *(Harpagophytum procumbens),* and dong quai *(Angelica sinensis),* can increase its effects. It's likely that you can continue using these products, but don't change the dosage from what your body is accustomed to. INR values must be monitored appropriately.
- Garlic *(Allium sativum)* and ginkgo *(Ginkgo biloba)* extracts may reduce the ability of platelets to stick together, increasing the likelihood of bleeding, but neither appears to interact directly with coumadin. We generally tell patients taking coumadin to avoid these products at higher dosages (more than the equivalent of one clove of garlic a day for garlic or more than 120 mg a day of ginkgo extract) but not to worry if they are just on the typical support dose.
- Iron, magnesium, and zinc can bind with coumadin, potentially decreasing its absorption and activity. Take coumadin and iron/magnesium/zinc–containing products at least 2 hours apart.

Appendixes

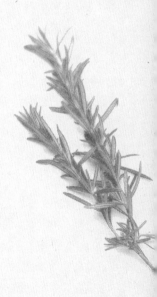

Daily Plan for Preventing Cancer

Constructing your own personal daily plan for preventing cancer involves strategies for strengthening the "four cornerstones of good health." You can liken these cornerstones to the four legs on a chair or table. If you want that chair or table to remain upright when stress is placed on it, the four legs must be intact and strong. Likewise, if you want to have good or, better yet, ideal health, including preventing cancer, it is essential that the following four areas be strong:

- A positive mental attitude
- A healthy lifestyle
- A health-promoting diet
- Supplementary measures

Develop a daily routine that is consistent with supporting and strengthening these four cornerstones of good health.

Here is a sample daily routine based on a 9-to-5 workday.

6:30 A.M.—Wake up
6:40 to 7:30—Exercise (including stretching, warm-up, training in target heart range for 20 to 30 minutes, and a 5-minute cool-down)
7:30 to 9:00—Personal time for shower, breakfast, catching up on the news, getting ready for the day, and commuting to work
10:30 to 10:45—Healthy break
12:30 to 1:30 P.M.—Lunch break
3:00 to 3:15—Healthy break

5:45 to 6:00—Quiet time filled with deep breathing, prayer, or meditation

6:00 to 6:30—Dinner preparation

6:30 to 7:15—Dinner

7:15 to 10:30—Engaging in social activities, development of relationships, and enjoyment of personal interests

10:30—Bedtime

Plugging in the Health-Promoting Components

The sample routine above probably bears little resemblance to your daily routine. There are undoubtedly time obstacles in your life that will require you to modify the routine. The key point is that you absolutely must commit to engaging in a routine that supports your health if you want maximum protection against cancer. There are many variables in the construction of your own personal routine, but what is not variable is that to fully protect yourself from cancer you will need to plug in positive social and personal relationships, regular exercise, time for enough sleep, a health-promoting diet, and nutritional supplementation. Make no excuses. You must find a way to address each of these factors and incorporate them into your daily routine.

Diet: Putting It All Together

As a reminder, the key dietary goals that we want to achieve in order to reduce the risk for cancer are to

1. Eat a "rainbow" assortment of fruits and vegetables.
2. Reduce exposure to pesticides.
3. Reduce the intake of meat and other animal foods.
4. Eat the right types of fats by increasing the intake of omega-3 fatty acids.
5. Avoid high-calorie, low-nutrient foods such as junk foods, candy, and soft drinks.
6. Keep salt intake low, potassium intake high.
7. Choose foods that help your body detoxify and eliminate waste.

In an effort to encourage Americans to eat in a more healthful manner, as well as to try to address the growing epidemic of diet-related diseases like cancer and heart disease, the U.S. government developed the Food Guide Pyramid. It basically replaces the old Four Basic Food Groups model that many of us grew up with as kids. The goal of the pyramid is to increase the intake of breads, fruits, and vegetables while reducing the intake of meat, dairy, sugar, and fats.

While the USDA Food Guide Pyramid is a step in a better dietary direction, we do not feel it is ideal. Instead, we encourage you to follow the innovative food guide pyramids developed by Oldways (www.oldwayspt. org). Jointly with the Harvard School of Public Health and other institutions, Oldways has published the Healthy Eating Pyramids, a set of unique dietary guides based on worldwide dietary traditions closely associated with good health. Individual pyramids are based on Mediterranean, Asian, and Latin American food. Any of these food guides can be followed individually, or you can simply choose to take the basic principles from all of them, as they coincide with our recommendations as well. These dietary pyramids are more in line with optimal dietary recommendations to lower cancer risk. For example, the Mediterranean diet pyramid has received a great deal of attention for its association with a reduced rate of heart disease, but it also is protective against cancer.[1] The traditional Mediterranean diet is characterized by high consumption of plant foods, relatively low consumption of red meat, and high consumption of olive oil, which in several studies has been reported to offer some of its own protection against cancer.

Foods to avoid entirely
- Smoked or cured meats: bacon, hot dogs, smoked luncheon meats, sausages, ham, Spam, and so on
- Meats cooked at extremely high temperatures or cooked to well-done
- Heavily sweetened or artificially sweetened soft drinks, sweet powdered drink mixes, juice-flavored drinks, and so on
- Fried foods, including French fries, potato chips, corn chips, and doughnuts
- Processed foods packed full of empty calories (sugar and fat) or salt (e.g., canned soups, theater-style popcorn, chips)
- Refined- white-flour products: pastas, cakes, muffins, pretzels
- Refined sugar-loaded cereals, candies, and baked goods
- Margarine, butter, and vegetable shortening

Our Daily Food Prescription

Here is your daily food prescription based on a 2000-calorie-a-day diet. If you need to increase your caloric intake, try to get the extra calories by increasing the number of servings of vegetables, whole grains, and legumes. For athletes or people engaged in heavy physicial labor or exercise, drinking a soy-protein or whey-protein smoothie is a great way to provide your body with the extra 25 to 30 g of protein that you may require (see Appendix B for recipe suggestions). Otherwise, be sure to add another serving of seafood, meat, or poultry to your daily intake.

FOODS TO EAT EVERY DAY   DAILY SERVINGS (2000-CALORIE DIET)

Vegetables: 1 serving equals 1 cup raw leafy vegetables (such as lettuce or spinach) or ½ cup raw nonleafy or cooked vegetables or fresh vegetable juice.

Green leafy and cruciferous vegetables—2 to 4 servings daily:

Alfalfa sprouts	Dandelion
Beet greens	Endive
Bok choy	Escarole
Broccoli	Kale
Brussels sprouts	Lettuce (the darker, the better)
Cabbage	Mustard greens
Cauliflower	Parsley
Chard	Spinach
Chinese cabbage	Turnip greens
Collard greens	Watercress

Carotene and flavonoid-rich vegetables—2 to 3 servings daily:

Beets	Winter, acorn, or butternut squash
Bell peppers	
Carrots	Yams or sweet potatoes
Eggplant	Zucchini
Summer squash	

Other vegetables—2 to 3 servings daily:

Artichoke (1 medium)	Peas (fresh or frozen)
Asparagus	Radishes
Bean sprouts	Rhubarb

Celery   Rutabaga
Cucumber   String beans, green or yellow
Fennel   Tomatoes, tomato paste, tomato
Mushrooms   sauce, tomato juice, vegetable
Okra   juice cocktail
Onions

Whole grains—6 to 8 servings
One of the following equals one serving:

Bread	
Whole-wheat, rye, or other whole-grain	1 slice
Cereals	
Whole-grain	½ cup
Corn	
Cooked whole-kernel	½ cup
On cob	1 small
Flour and flour products	
Whole-wheat flour (uncooked)	2½ tablespoons
Whole-grain pasta (cooked)	½ cup
Puffed cereal (unsweetened)	1 cup
Whole grains (cooked)	
Rice, oats, wheat, barley, quinoa, spelt, etc.	½ cup
Beans (½ cup cooked)	2 to 3

Black-eyed peas	Lima beans
Chickpeas	Pinto beans
Garbanzo beans	Soybeans, including tofu
Kidney beans	Split peas
Lentils	

Fruit (1 serving equals approximately 1 cup raw, ½ cup cooked, or ½ cup dried fruit)	3 to 4
Nuts and seeds (1 serving equals 3 tablespoons)	2
Olive, flaxseed, or canola oil (1 serving equals 1 tablespoon)	2
Dairy (1 serving equals 1 cup milk, yogurt, or cottage cheese; or 1 ounce cheese)	1 (optional)

Foods to eat 2–3 times a week:
    Seafood (1 serving size equals 4 ounces,
        about the size of a deck of cards)   1

Foods to eat no more than twice a week:
    Poultry (1 serving size equals 4 ounces, about
        the size of a deck of cards; or two eggs)   1 (optional)

Foods to eat no more than once a week:
    Meats (1 serving size equals 4 ounces, about
        the size of a deck of cards)   1 (optional)
  Low-fat (less than 15% fat content):
    Beef: baby beef, chipped beef, chuck, steak
        (flank, plate), tenderloin plate ribs, round
        (bottom, top), all cuts rump, spareribs, tripe
    Lamb: leg, rib, sirloin, loin (roast and chops),
        shank, shoulder
    Veal: leg, loin, rib, shank, shoulder, cutlet
  Medium-fat:
    Beef: ground (15% fat), rib eye, round
        (ground commercial)
    Pork: loin (all tenderloin), Boston butt
  High-fat:
    Beef: brisket, corned beef, ground beef (more than 20% fat):
        roasts (rib), steaks (club and rib)
    Lamb: breast
    Pork: spareribs, loin, ground pork, country-style ham
    Veal: chop

Supplements

The following charts contain all the vitamin, mineral, and antioxidant dosages you will need. Read labels carefully to find multiple vitamin and mineral formulas that contain doses in these ranges. Be aware that you will not find a formula that provides all these nutrients at these levels in one single pill—it would simply be too big. Usually, you'll need to take at least three to six tablets a day to meet these levels. While many "one-a-day" supplements provide good levels of vitamins, they tend to be insufficient in the amount of some of the minerals they provide. Your body needs the minerals as much as the vitamins—remember: the two work hand in hand.

When to Take Your Supplements

- Multiple vitamin and mineral supplements are best taken with meals. Whether you take it at the beginning or end of a meal is up to you. If you are taking more than a couple of pills, you may find that taking them at the beginning of a meal is more comfortable. Taking a handful of pills on a full stomach may cause a little stomach upset.
- Flavonoid-rich herbal extracts can be taken with meals or anytime desired.
- Green drinks make great between-meal snacks (especially if you are trying to lose a little weight, as they can quell an overactive appetite).
- For maximum benefit, enteric-coated probiotics should be taken with meals. If the product is not enteric-coated, it should be taken at least 5 minutes before or 1 hour after a meal.
- Fish oil supplements are best taken at or near the beginning of a meal to avoid any fishy aftertaste. Some people experience burping up a little of the oil if they take it at the end of the meal on a full stomach.
- Always take vitamin E, vitamin C, selenium, and zinc in combination with one another, never separately. This is why we recommend a high-quality multivitamin.

The following recommendations provide an optimum intake range to guide you in selecting a high-quality multiple. (Note that vitamins and minerals are measured in different units. IU = International Units; mg = milligrams; mcg = micrograms.)

VITAMIN	DAILY DOSE FOR ADULTS
Vitamin A (retinol)[a]	5000 IU
Vitamin A (from beta-carotene)	5000–25,000 IU
Vitamin B$_1$ (thiamin)	10–100 mg
Vitamin B$_2$ (riboflavin)	10–50 mg
Vitamin B$_3$ (niacin)	10–100 mg
Vitamin B$_5$ (pantothenic acid)	25–100 mg
Vitamin B$_6$ (pyridoxine)	25–100 mg
Vitamin B$_{12}$ (cobalamin)	400 mcg
Vitamin C (ascorbic acid)[b]	250–1000 mg
Vitamin D[c]	400–800 IU
Vitamin E (d-alpha tocopherol)[d]	100–800 IU
Vitamin K (phytonadione)	60–300 mcg
Biotin	100–300 mcg
Choline	10-100 mg
Folic acid	400–800 mcg
Inositol	10–100 mg
Niacinamide	10–30 mg
MINERALS	**RANGE FOR ADULTS**
Boron	1–6 mg
Calcium[e]	250–1500 mg
Chromium[f]	200–400 mcg
Copper	1–2 mg
Iodine	50–150 mcg
Iron[g]	15–30 mg
Magnesium	250–500 mg

a. Women of childbearing age who may become pregnant should not take more than 2500 IU of retinol daily because of the possible risk of birth defects.
b. It may be easier to take vitamin C separately.
c. Elderly people in nursing homes living in northern latitudes should supplement at the high range.
d. It may be more cost-effective to take vitamin E separately rather than as a component of a multiple vitamin.
e. Women who have or who are at risk for osteoporosis may need to take a separate calcium supplement to achieve the recommended level of 1000 to 1500 mg daily.
f. For diabetes and weight loss, doses of 600 mcg of chromium can be used.
g. Most men as well as most women who have gone through menopause rarely need supplemental iron.

MINERALS	RANGES FOR ADULTS
Manganese	10–15 mg
Molybdenum	10–25 mcg
Potassium	200–500 mg
Selenium	100–200 mcg
Silica	1–5 mg
Vanadium	50–100 mcg
Zinc	15–45 mg

Selecting a Flavonoid Supplement

FLAVONOID-RICH EXTRACT	DAILY DOSE FOR ANTI-OXIDANT SUPPORT	INDICATION
Green tea extract (60–70% total polyphenols)	150–300 mg	Systemic antioxidant. May provide the best protection against cancer. Best choice if there is a family history of cancer. Also protects against damage to cholesterol.
Quercetin	200–400 mg	Allergies, symptoms of prostate enlargement or bladder irritation, eczema.
Grape seed extract (95% procyanidolic oligomers)	50–100 mg	Systemic antioxidant; best choice for most people under age 50. Also specific for the lungs, diabetes, varicose veins, and protection against heart disease.
Ginkgo biloba extract (24% ginkgo flavon-glycosides)	120–240 mg	Best choice for most people over age 50. Protects brain and vascular lining.
Milk thistle extract (70% silymarin)	100–300 mg	Best choice for additional antioxidant protection of liver or skin needs.
Bilberry extract (25% anthocyanidins)	80–160 mg	Best choice to protect the eyes.
Hawthorn extract (10% procyanidins)	150–300 mg	Best choice in heart disease or high blood pressure.

DAILY GREEN DRINKS

3 cups green tea or 1 green drink daily
   Green drinks usually contain one or more of the following:
   dehydrated barley grass
   wheat grass
   algae sources such as chorella or spirulina

Some of the more popular brands are Enriching Greens, Green Magma, Kyo-Green, Greens +, Barlean's Greens, and ProGreens. Drinks should be taken 20 minutes before or 2 hours after a meal.

PROBIOTICS

Lactobacillus acidophilus, Bifidobacterium bifidum, or *Propionibacterium freudenrichi*—5 to 10 billion viable cells daily

FISH OIL SUPPLEMENTS

Take enough capsules to provide 120 to 360 mg EPA and 80 to 240 mg DHA daily.

FOR EXTRA PROTECTION AGAINST LUNG CANCER

Curcumin—200 to 400 mg daily
   or
Quercetin—200 to 400 mg daily

FOR EXTRA PROTECTION AGAINST COLON CANCER

Curcumin—200 to 400 mg daily
Calcium—1000 to 1500 mg daily
Vitamin D—400 to 800 IU daily

FOR EXTRA PROTECTION AGAINST BREAST OR PROSTATE CANCER

Ground flaxseed or flax mix—2 tablespoons daily
Indole-3-carbinol—300 to 400 mg daily
Lycopene—5 to 15 mg daily
Calcium d-glucarate—200 to 400 mg daily

Sample Menu

To help you design your diet, we offer the following basic framework followed by a four-day sample menu (including shopping lists) and recipes.

SAMPLE MENU

BREAKFAST
Supplements: multiple vitamin (½ daily dosage); probiotic supplement
Whole-grain cereal with nuts and seeds, and soymilk or nonfat yogurt
Cup of herbal tea

MIDMORNING SNACK
Green drink
One cup raw, cut-up vegetables

LUNCH
Supplement: flavonoid-rich herbal extract
Salad
Bowl of soup (bean or vegetable soups, noncream base)

MIDAFTERNOON SNACK
Serving of fruit

DINNER
Supplements: Multiple vitamin (½ daily dosage); fish oil supplement
Salad
Vegetable side dish
Main entrée (vegetarian 3 nights a week, fish 2 to 3 nights a week, poultry or meat once a week)
Dessert (fresh berries or fresh fruit—e.g., mango, pineapple, or orange slices)

EVENING TEA
One or two cups of herbal tea (no caffeine)

Shopping List

The following shopping list represents the items needed in order to follow the four-day meal plan.

HERBAL TEA
Most of the major brands of herbal tea (e.g., Celestial Seasons, Bigelow, Republic of Tea, Traditional Medicinals) provide a sampler pack to help

you identify teas that appeal to you. In general, avoid black teas. Try to choose decaffeinated varieties, especially with your nighttime cup of tea. If you feel you need a little caffeine in the morning, go with a cup of regular green tea.

PRODUCE

Try to buy organic, if possible, and be sure to wash all produce before consumption.

Apples—2 red, 2 green
Apricots—4
Asparagus—1 bunch
Bananas—2
Bell peppers—3 green, 2 red
Blueberries—1 cup
Broccoli—1 head
Carrots—1 large bag
Celery—2 bunches
Cilantro—1 bunch
Cucumbers—2
Fennel—1 small bulb
Garlic—2 bulbs
Green onions—1 bunch
Jicama—1
Kale—1 large bunch
Lemons—8
Mango—1

Mint (fresh)—½ cup
Mixed field greens—8 cups
Onions—4
Oranges—4
Parsley—1 bunch
Pear—1 red
Pineapple—1 medium
Plums—4 medium
Radishes—1 bunch
Raspberries—1 cup
Red or green grapes—1 cup
Red pears—2
Romaine lettuce—1 head
Shiitake mushrooms—2 cups
Tomatoes—6 medium-sized
Tomatoes, cherry—6
Yam—1 or 2 small sweet
    potatoes

FISH

Salmon—8 ounces fresh salmon
Tuna—1 can (or foil pouch) of low-sodium, chunk white tuna in spring water

MISCELLANEOUS GROCERY ITEMS

Balsamic vinegar—8 to
    12 ounces
Dijon mustard—8 ounces
Honey (raw)—8 ounces
Kalamata olives—1 small jar

Rice milk, soymilk, nonfat
    milk, or nonfat yogurt—
    32 ounces
Tofu—1 container (15 ounces)
    of firm variety

NUTS, SEEDS, AND DRIED FRUIT

Almonds (raw)—1 cup

Flaxseed (raw)—1 cup

Pumpkin seeds (raw)—1 cup

Raisins—1 small box

Sunflower seeds (raw)—1 cup

Walnuts (raw)—1 cup

OILS

Flaxseed oil—12 to 16 ounces

Olive oil (extra-virgin)—12 to 16 ounces

GRAINS AND PASTA

Brown rice (quick)—1 box

Rolled oats—1 small
container

Ry-Vita or WASA whole-grain
rye crackers—1 packet

Whole-grain cereal—1 box

Whole-wheat pasta—
1 8-ounce package of fresh
pasta or dried whole-wheat
pasta

Whole-wheat tortillas—
1 pack of 8

FROZEN FOODS

Corn (frozen)—2 cups

CANNED FOODS

Black beans—2 (15-ounce) cans

Chicken or vegetable broth—
6 (11-ounce) cans

Garbanzo beans—1 (8-ounce) can

Red kidney beans—1 (11-ounce)
can

Tomatoes, diced—
1 (7.5-ounce) can

Tomato sauce—
1 (4-ounce) can low-
sodium; 1 (12-ounce)
can low-sodium

Tomato soup—1 (11-ounce)
can low-sodium

White beans—1 (15-ounce)
can

SPICES AND SEASONINGS

Capers

Chili powder

Crushed red pepper

Cumin

Curry powder

Ginger (dried)

Ground black pepper

Italian herbs (seasoning)

No Salt or Nu-Salt—
chloride)
potassium chloride salts
regular salt (sodium
to use as a substitute for

Soy sauce (low-sodium)

Four-Day Sample Menus and Recipes

We have chosen to provide a four-day sample menu to get you started in planning out your own daily menus. Since most people do not have the time to get to the grocery store every day, we wanted to show you how to shop for a four-day period. That way you can get in the habit of planning out your meals well in advance and replenishing your perishables every three to four days.

We have chosen recipes that can be prepared and cooked within 30 minutes or less. We have also chosen recipes that have a short list of ingredients or readily available ingredients with no difficult steps to fol-

DAY 1	
BREAKFAST *Supplements: multiple vitamin (½ daily dosage); probiotic supplement* Happy Apple Breakfast (see p. 295) Cup of herbal tea **MIDMORNING SNACK** Green drink 1 cup celery sticks **LUNCH** *Supplement: flavonoid-rich herbal extract* Field Greens Salad with Olive (or Flaxseed) Oil Dressing (see p. 295) Red Bean and Tomato Soup (see p. 296) Ry-Vita or WASA whole-grain rye crackers	**MIDAFTERNOON SNACK** 1 medium orange **DINNER** *Supplements: Multiple vitamin (½ daily dosage); fish oil supplement* Field Greens Salad with Bell Peppers, Carrots, and Radishes (see p. 297) Minted Carrots with Pumpkin Seeds (see p. 297) Steamed Broccoli (see p. 297) Asian Salmon (see p. 297) Whole-grain bread or roll Fresh Raspberries (see p. 298) **EVENING TEA** One or two cups of herbal tea (no caffeine)

DAY 2

BREAKFAST

Supplements: multiple vitamin (½ daily dosage); probiotic supplement
Power Smoothie (see p. 298)

MIDMORNING SNACK

Green drink
3 tablespoons almonds

LUNCH

Supplement: flavonoid-rich herbal extract
Tuna Salad Wrap
(see p. 299)

MIDAFTERNOON SNACK

2 medium plums

DINNER

Supplements: Multiple vitamin (½ daily dosage); fish oil supplement
Jicama Salad (see p. 299)
Black Bean Chili (see p. 300)
Whole-wheat tortillas
Blueberries (see p. 301)

EVENING TEA

One or two cups of herbal tea
(no caffeine)

DAY 3

BREAKFAST

Supplements: multiple vitamin (½ daily dosage); probiotic supplement
Grape and Apricot Muesli
(see p. 301)
Cup of herbal tea (no caffeine)

MIDMORNING SNACK

Green drink
1 cup celery sticks

LUNCH

Supplement: flavonoid-rich herbal extract
Orange and Fennel Salad
(see p. 302)
Italian White Bean Soup
(see p. 302)

MIDAFTERNOON SNACK

1 medium red pear

DINNER

Supplements: multiple vitamin (½ daily dosage); fish oil supplement
Asparagus Salad
(see p. 303)
Mashed Yams (see p. 303)
Curried Chicken or Tofu
over Brown Rice
(see p. 304)
Sliced Pineapple
(see p. 304)

EVENING TEA

One or two cups of herbal tea
(no caffeine)

DAY 4	
BREAKFAST Whole-grain cereal with nuts and seeds, with soymilk or nonfat yogurt (see p. 305) Sliced Pineapple (see p. 304) Cup of herbal tea **MIDMORNING SNACK** Green drink 1 cup carrot sticks **LUNCH** *Supplement: flavonoid-rich herbal extract* Black Bean Salad (see p. 305) **MIDAFTERNOON SNACK** 1 medium red apple	**DINNER** *Supplements: Multiple vitamin (½ daily dosage); fish oil supplement* Mediterranean Salad (see p. 306) Dr. Murray's Favorite Greens (see p. 306) Pasta Puttanesca with Tofu (see p. 307) Whole-grain bread or roll Fresh Mango Slices (see p. 307) **EVENING TEA** One or two cups of herbal tea (no caffeine)

low. They are easy. In our own experiences we have been frustrated by vegetarian and cookbooks designed for healthier eating that were packed full of difficult (or nearly impossible-to-get ingredients), took too long to prepare, and required too many steps to prepare.

Recipes

The recipes that we are providing also allow for substitutions and modifications based on your own tastes. For example, if a recipe contains a vegetable that you don't like, substitute one that you do like. The recipes are based on providing two servings, but you can adjust the number of servings up or down as needed (e.g., for four servings simply double the recipe).

Day 1

Happy Apple Breakfast

1½ cups rolled oats
2½ cups water
1 medium green or golden apple, chopped
¼ cup raw pumpkin or sunflower seeds
2 tablespoons organic flaxseed oil, or to taste
1 tablespoon raw honey, or to taste
Nonfat yogurt, for topping (optional)

Combine all the ingredients except the flaxseed oil and honey and simmer for 10 minutes. Turn off the heat, cover, and let steam for 5 minutes. Stir in the flaxseed oil and honey. Top with nonfat yogurt if desired.

Green drink
1 cup celery sticks

Field Greens Salad with Olive (or Flaxseed) Oil Dressing

4 cups mixed field greens

Most supermarkets and grocery stores now have mixed field greens in the produce section or in pre-packaged plastic bags. This convenience makes a simple mixed field green salad a perfect quick and easy salad. Your serving size should be 2 cups along with 1 tablespoon of olive (or flaxseed) oil salad dressing.

Olive (or Flaxseed) Oil Salad Dressing

8 ounces olive or organic flaxseed oil
2 tablespoons lemon juice
2 tablespoons balsamic vinegar
2 garlic cloves, finely minced
1 tablespoon Italian herbs
1 teaspoon salt (use No Salt or Nu-Salt)
1 teaspoon black pepper

Place all the ingredients in a blender and blend for 2 to 3 minutes. Store in your refrigerator for a quick and easy health-promoting salad dressing.

Red Bean and Tomato Soup

½ cup onion, chopped
1 garlic clove, chopped
1 stalk celery, chopped in small chunks
1 tablespoon olive oil
1 (8-ounce) can red kidney beans, drained
1 (11-ounce) can low-sodium tomato soup
2 tablespoons Italian herbs
Salt (use No Salt or Nu-Salt) and pepper to taste

Sauté the onions, garlic, and celery in olive oil over medium-low heat for about 5 minutes in a medium soup pot, stirring often. Blend the kidney beans, tomato soup, and herbs in a blender for 2 to 3 minutes, and then add to the soup pot and cook for 15 minutes. Add salt (use No Salt or Nu-Salt) and pepper to taste.

Ry-Vita or WASA whole-grain rye crackers—2 crackers

• MIDAFTERNOON SNACK •

1 medium orange

• DINNER •

Field Greens Salad with Bell Peppers, Carrots, and Radishes

3 cups mixed field greens
1 green bell pepper, chopped
½ cup carrots, chopped
½ cup radishes, chopped

Your serving size should be 2 cups. Toss with 1 tablespoon Olive (or Flaxseed) Oil Salad Dressing (see above).

Minted Carrots with Pumpkin Seeds

3 medium carrots, peeled and cut into round slices
1 tablespoon parsley, chopped
1 tablespoon mint, chopped
2 tablespoons pumpkin seeds, coarsely chopped
1 tablespoon lemon juice
1 tablespoon olive oil
Salt (use No Salt or Nu-Salt) and pepper to taste

Steam the carrots until still slightly crunchy. Chop the rest of the ingredients and toss with the carrots.

Steamed Broccoli

½ head broccoli

Slice the broccoli head lengthwise to separate out the florets of the head.

Asian Salmon

2 teaspoons low-sodium soy sauce
1 tablespoon Dijon mustard
8 ounces salmon, cut into 2 pieces
½ cup onions, sliced
1 garlic clove, chopped
¼ teaspoon dried ginger (or ½ tablespoon fresh ginger, minced)
2 cups fresh shiitake mushrooms, sliced

Preheat the oven to 375°F. Mix the soy sauce into the mustard and coat the salmon. Sauté the onion, garlic, ginger, and mushrooms in a medium sauté pan for about 5 minutes. Bake the salmon in a baking dish, depending on how thick it is (about 7 minutes if less than an inch thick). When cooked, place on a bed of the mushroom mixture.

Fresh Raspberries

1 cup fresh raspberries

Served chilled for a ½-cup serving size. A little vanilla soymilk or non-fat yogurt can be used to soak the berries as well.

• EVENING TEA •

One or two cups of herbal tea (no caffeine)

Day 2

• BREAKFAST •

Power Smoothie

1 cup rice milk, soymilk, or nonfat milk
1 orange, peeled and sliced
1 banana, sliced
4 ice cubes
1 tablespoon flaxseed oil
20 grams whey or soy protein powder (optional)

Combine the ingredients in a blender and blend at high speed until liquefied.

Green drink
3 tablespoons almonds

Tuna Salad Wrap

1 can (or foil pouch) low-sodium, chunk white tuna in spring water
¼ cup onion, minced
1 celery stalk, chopped
1 teaspoon fresh lemon juice
1 tablespoon olive oil
1 tablespoon parsley, chopped
¼ cup Dijon mustard
½ teaspoon salt (use No Salt or Nu-Salt)
½ teaspoon pepper
2 whole-wheat tortillas

Mix all the ingredients except the tortillas in a bowl, spoon on to the tortillas, and wrap. Whole-grain bread can be substituted for the tortillas to make a sandwich.

2 medium plums

Jicama Salad

1 cup jicama, julienne-cut and peeled
1 orange, peeled, sectioned, and cut into chunks (remove membrane)
1 cucumber, seeded and thinly sliced

¼ *cup green onion, chopped*
¼ *cup cilantro, chopped*
1 *tablespoon mint, chopped*
¼ *cup fresh orange juice*
¼ *cup fresh lemon or lime juice*
¼ *teaspoon salt (use No Salt or Nu-Salt)*
¼ *teaspoon pepper*
¼ *teaspoon chili powder*

Combine jicama, orange, cucumber, green onion, cilantro, and mint in a large bowl. In another bowl, mix the orange juice, lemon or lime juice, salt, pepper, and chili powder. Pour the juice mixture over the jicama mixture and toss gently. Cover and chill for at least 20 minutes.

Black Bean Chili

½ *medium onion, chopped*
2 *garlic cloves, chopped*
1 *green pepper, diced*
1 *(15-ounce) can black beans, drained*
1 *cup corn kernels, frozen*
1 *cup chicken broth or light vegetable broth*
1 *(4-ounce) can low-sodium tomato sauce*
2 *tablespoons cumin*
2 *tablespoons chili powder*
2 *tablespoons Italian herbs*
1 *tablespoon olive oil*
½ *teaspoon salt (use No Salt or Nu-Salt)*
½ *teaspoon pepper*
¼ *cup cilantro, chopped*
Whole-wheat tortillas, for serving

Sauté the onion, garlic, and bell pepper in a medium soup pot over medium-low heat for about 5 minutes, stirring frequently. Starting with the chicken broth, add the rest of ingredients (except the cilantro) and simmer for 15 minutes. Add the cilantro as garnish and season with additional salt and pepper if needed. Serve with heated whole-wheat tortillas.

Blueberries

1 cup fresh blueberries

Served chilled for a ½-cup serving size. A little vanilla soymilk or non-fat yogurt can be used as well to soak the berries.

• EVENING TEA •

One or two cups of herbal tea (no caffeine)

Day 3

• BREAKFAST •

Grape and Apricot Muesli

2 tablespoons rolled oats
4 teaspoons water
1 cup nonfat yogurt or vanilla soymilk
1 tablespoon fresh lemon or orange juice
1 cup red or green grapes
4 apricots, chopped into small chunks
1 tablespoon raisins
3 tablespoons walnuts or almonds, chopped
2 tablespoons sunflower seeds
1 tablespoon organic flaxseed oil

Soak the rolled oats overnight in 4 teaspoons water. Combine all the ingredients and mix well.

Cup of herbal tea (no caffeine)

Green drink
1 cup celery sticks

• LUNCH •

Orange and Fennel Salad

1 orange, sliced
1 small bulb fennel, sliced
1 head of romaine lettuce, cut up
¼ cup parsley, chopped
1 tablespoon Olive (or Flaxseed) Oil Salad Dressing (see p. 296)

Toss the orange and fennel with the greens and dressing in a large bowl.

Italian White Bean Soup

½ onion, cut in half and thinly sliced
4 garlic cloves, sliced
2 cups chicken stock or light vegetable stock
2 cups collard greens or kale, finely chopped (stems cut out)
1 (7.5-ounce) can diced tomatoes
2 tablespoons Italian herb mixture
1 (15-ounce) can navy beans, drained
1 tablespoon olive oil
Salt (use No Salt or Nu-Salt) and pepper to taste

Sauté the onion in a medium soup pot over medium-low heat for 5 minutes, stirring frequently. Add the garlic and continue to sauté for another minute. Add the stock, greens, tomatoes, and herb mixture. Simmer for 15 minutes over medium heat. Add the beans, salt, and pepper. Cook for another 5 minutes. Taste, and adjust salt and pepper if necessary.

1 medium red pear

Asparagus Salad

1 bunch asparagus
2 cup fresh tomato, seeds and excess pulp removed, and chopped
1 garlic clove, pressed
1 teaspoon balsamic vinegar
1 teaspoon fresh lemon juice
½ teaspoon salt (use No Salt or Nu-Salt)
½ teaspoon cracked black pepper
1 tablespoon olive oil

Discard the bottom fourth of the asparagus stalks and cut the rest into 2-inch lengths. Lightly steam the asparagus for about 2 to 3 minutes, depending on thickness. The goal is to cook the asparagus but still maintain the crispness. Immediately place in ice water after steaming.

Mix the other ingredients in a large bowl. Pat the asparagus dry with paper towels and mix it in with the other ingredients.

Mashed Yams

1 large yam or 2 small sweet potatoes, peeled and sliced
1 tablespoon honey
1 tablespoon olive oil or vegetable spread
¼ teaspoon salt (use No Salt or Nu-Salt)

Steam (or microwave) the yam or sweet potatoes. When tender, mash with a potato masher or mixer and add the rest of the ingredients. Add a little vanilla soymilk or nonfat yogurt if needed and mix well.

Curried Chicken or Tofu over Brown Rice

½ cup uncooked quick brown rice

7.5 ounces firm tofu cut into small cubes OR 1 boneless, skinless chicken breast cut into bite-sized pieces OR ½ cup chopped onion

1 garlic clove, minced

1 cup chicken stock or vegetable stock

1 medium red bell pepper, chopped

½ cup coconut milk (make sure it is mixed well before using)

½ head broccoli

2 teaspoons curry powder

1 tablespoon olive oil

Salt (use No Salt or Nu-Salt) and pepper to taste

Follow the instructions on the package of quick brown rice. While the water for the rice is coming to a boil, cut up the tofu or chicken and the other ingredients. Sauté the onion with olive oil in a medium sauté pan over medium-low heat for about 5 minutes, stirring frequently. Add the garlic and continue to sauté for another minute, then remove from heat and add the curry powder. Mix well. Return to heat and add stock, tofu or chicken, bell peppers, and coconut milk. Simmer until tofu or chicken is done, about 10 minutes. Salt (use No Salt or Nu-Salt) and pepper to taste.

Place rice on plate and top with the curry mixture.

Sliced Pineapple

Slice a whole pineapple into bite-sized pieces. Place half of the sliced pineapple in the refrigerator for breakfast the next morning and serve the other half as a dessert.

• EVENING TEA •

One or two cups of herbal tea (no caffeine)

Day 4

Whole-grain cereal with nuts and seeds, with soymilk or nonfat yogurt

For each serving:

1 cup whole-grain cereal
1 teaspoon flaxseeds
1 teaspoon sunflower seeds
1 teaspoon coarsely chopped walnuts or almonds
1 cup vanilla soymilk or nonfat yogurt

Mix all ingredients together.

Sliced Pineapple

Make good use of the sliced pineapple from the night before.

Green drink
1 cup carrot sticks

Black Bean Salad

1 (15-ounce) can black beans, drained and rinsed
1 cup frozen corn, thawed
6 cherry tomatoes, quartered
½ cup minced green onion
1 garlic clove, pressed
½ cup diced red bell pepper
½ cup chopped cilantro
2 cups mixed field greens

1 tablespoon olive or flaxseed oil
2 tablespoons fresh lemon juice
¼ cup chopped cilantro
Salt (use No Salt or Nu-Salt) and pepper to taste

Mix all the ingredients together in a large bowl and serve.

• MIDAFTERNOON SNACK •

1 medium red apple

• DINNER •

Mediterranean Salad

1 cup chopped fresh tomato (cut out excess flesh if pulpy)
1 cup peeled and chopped cucumber
½ cup finely minced green onion
1 garlic clove, finely minced
1 (8-ounce) can garbanzo beans, drained and rinsed
1 tablespoon fresh lemon juice
1 tablespoon chopped parsley
1 teaspoon Italian herbs
1 tablespoon olive oil

Mix all the ingredients together and chill. This is best if it chills for at least 15 minutes.

Dr. Murray's Favorite Greens

1 tablespoon olive oil
1 teaspoon balsamic vinegar
1 large bunch kale, washed, trimmed, and coarsely chopped
½ cup chopped green onion
1 garlic clove, thinly sliced
½ cup coarsely chopped walnuts or almonds
¼ teaspoon salt (use No Salt or Nu-Salt), or to taste
½ teaspoon black pepper, or to taste
Lemon wedges, for serving

Heat the olive oil and balsamic vinegar in large skillet or wok over medium-high heat. Add the kale, green onion, garlic, and walnuts and sauté until softened. Season with salt and pepper. Serve with lemon wedges.

Pasta Puttanesca with Tofu

PASTA:

8 ounces fresh whole-wheat pasta (or 2 ounces dried whole-wheat pasta)

SAUCE:

1 (12-ounce) can tomato sauce
7.5 ounces firm tofu, cut into small cubes
1 onion, diced
1 garlic clove, crushed or minced
1 green bell pepper, diced
1 tablespoon Italian herbs
1 tablespoon crushed red pepper
2 tablespoons capers, rinsed and drained
8 to 10 pitted Kalamata olives
1 tablespoon finely chopped parsley
¼ teaspoon salt (use No Salt or Nu-Salt)
½ teaspoon black pepper
1 tablespoon olive oil

Prepare the pasta as directed on the package. In a large saucepan, sauté the onion and garlic in the olive oil over medium heat for 3 to 4 minutes. Add the peppers and sauté for 3 to 4 more minutes. Add the rest of the ingredients and simmer for 15 minutes, stirrring occasionally. Remove from heat and allow to cool. Serve reheated or cold over pasta.

Fresh Mango Slices

1 fresh mango

Slice up 1 fresh mango for a refreshing dessert.

• EVENING TEA •

One or two cups of herbal tea (no caffeine)

Daily Plan for Beating Cancer

A daily plan for beating cancer should be based on the unique needs of each cancer patient. Given the spectrum of severity of cancer cases, there are many variables in constructing this daily plan. Some cancer patients are able to go about their normal lives, while others are severely limited in their energy levels and activities. Generally speaking, the more serious the cancer, the more aggressive your focus has to be in getting well. If you are able to continue to work, that is great. If not, you need to make getting well your number-one job.

For someone with a good energy level, appetite, and nutritional status, following the daily plan provided in Appendix A may be all that is necessary. For example, a woman with localized breast cancer undergoing only a lumpectomy will probably only need to modify the daily plan given in Appendix A for preventing any recurrence. Likewise, a woman with more advanced breast cancer or those electing to also go through radiation and chemotherapy will need more aggressive dietary and supplemental support. In any case, you should follow the supplement program in Appendix A and add the recommendations included here. People with advanced cancers and most people going through chemotherapy will usually be challenged with such things as low energy levels, loss of appetite, and nausea (and possibly even vomiting).

Here are the dietary suggestions that can help improve nutritional status in cancer patients, especially those experiencing anorexia or cachexia:

- Eat small frequent meals (every 1 to 2 hours), rather than larger meals less often.

- Stay well hydrated and drink 18 to 24 ounces of fresh vegetable juice daily. The juice can be taken with food, or better yet, take a midmorning juice break.
- Drink a high-protein smoothie once or twice daily (see page 153). Smoothies can take the place of breakfast or be a midafternoon snack.
- Try ginger—nature's nausea and vomiting remedy—as a tea or in rice (see recipes on page 158).
- Use extra seasonings, spices, and flavorings to improve food's taste appeal. A higher sensitivity to the taste of food may cause them to be unappealing.
- Avoid flavorings that are very sweet or very bitter.
- Eat soft, moist foods, such as smoothies, bananas, brown rice, and yams, and avoid hard, dry foods, such as cereals, crackers, and hard candies.
- Take small bites and chew completely.
- Take enough fish oil capsules to provide 700 to 1200 mg of EPA and 400 to 800 mg DHA each day.

Exercise and the Cancer Patient

Fatigue is one of the most common and distressing symptoms reported by cancer patients, especially during and following completion of chemotherapy or radiation therapy. One of the best measures to reduce fatigue is participation in regular exercise. Several clinical trials have proved quite convincingly that exercise goes a very long way in reducing the daily fatigue experienced by so many cancer patients.[1-4] In addition, exercise also relieves anxiety, promotes a better night's sleep, and raises self-esteem.

We do not recommend that our cancer patients train as if preparing for the Olympics, however. The studies have specifically looked at the benefits of low- to moderate-intensity exercises, such as walking, riding a stationary bike, or participation in low-impact aerobic exercises. Because of the many benefits of walking, yoga, and tai chi (see page 209), we recommend these activities as the exercise of choice to our cancer patients.

Basic Supplementation Program for the Cancer Patient

Supplements to take before a meal:

- Proteolytic enzymes (see page 313 for dosage).
- Quercetin or curcumin. Depending on the type of cancer (see page 242), dosage for either is 200 to 400 mg one to three times daily.

Supplements to take with a meal:

- High-potency multiple vitamin and mineral supplement according to the guidelines given on page 312.
- Extra vitamin C—500 to 1000 mg three times daily.
- Extra vitamin E—400 IU daily.
- Fish oil supplement—take enough capsules to provide 700 to 1200 mg of EPA and 400 to 800 mg of DHA. Take fish oils at the beginning of a meal to reduce any aftertaste.
- Probiotic supplement—5 to 10 billion live *Lactobacillus* species, *Bifidobacteria* species, and/or *Propionibacterium freudenrichi* daily.
- Whey protein (20 to 30 g twice daily) or glutamine (1.5 to 5 g twice daily). See page 154 for more information.

Supplements to take between meals or on an empty stomach:

- Green drink (described below)—2 servings daily.
- Green tea extract—300 to 400 mg of polyphenols daily.
- Maitaike D- or MD-fraction or PSP (dosage given below). Best taken between meals. Can be taken 5 to 10 minutes before taking your green drink or juice break or 30 minutes before meals.

At night before retiring (at least 1 hour after last meal):

Modified citrus pectin (6 g) or Ip6 with inositol (4800 to 7200 mg and 1200 to 1800 mg, respectively).

If you have breast or prostate cancer, add the following (can be taken with meals):

- Ground flaxseeds or flaxseed meal—2 tablespoons daily.
- Indole-3-carbinol—300 to 400 mg daily.
- Lycopene—30 mg daily.
- Calcium d-glucarate—400 mg daily.

Optional supplements:

Polyerga

People up to 140 pounds body weight should take one Polyerga tablet three times per day. For every additional 40 pounds body weight, add an additional tablet (e.g., a 220-pound person would take 5 tablets daily in divided dosages). For best results, take Polyerga on an empty stomach before meals. Also, do not take Polyerga at the same time you take digestive enzymes like pancreatin, bromelain, or papain. Polyerga can be taken at the same time as MD-fraction or PSK/PSP.

Co-enzyme Q10

Take 50 to 100 mg daily with meals to enhance absorption. Note: Higher dosages may be required in patients being treated with chemotherapy drugs, especially doxorubicin.

Additonal items:

- Herbal teas can be consumed any time throughout the day.
- Be sure to stay well hydrated and make a point to drink at least 6 glasses of bottled, filtered, or distilled water throughout the day.

Green Drinks

Green drinks contain dehydrated barley grass, wheat grass, and/or algae sources such as chorella or spirulina that are rehydrated by mixing with water or juice. Some of the more popular brands are Enriching Greens, Green Magma, Kyo-Green, Greens +, Barlean's Greens, and ProGreens. The cancer patient should drink two servings of a green drink daily.

Vitamins and Minerals

The following recommendations provide an optimum intake range to guide you in selecting a high-quality multiple. (Note that vitamins and minerals are measured in different units. IU = International Units; mg = milligrams; mcg = micrograms.)

VITAMIN	DAILY DOSE FOR ADULTS
Vitamin A (retinol)[a]	5000 IU
Vitamin A (from beta-carotene)	5000–25,000 IU
Vitamin B_1 (thiamin)	10–100 mg
Vitamin B_2 (riboflavin)	10–50 mg
Vitamin B_3 (niacin)	10–100 mg
Vitamin B_5 (pantothenic acid)	25–100 mg
Vitamin B_6 (pyridoxine)	25–100 mg
Vitamin B_{12} (cobalamin)	400 mcg
Vitamin C (ascorbic acid)[b]	250–1000 mg
Vitamin D[c]	400–800 IU
Vitamin E (d-alpha tocopherol)[d]	100–800 IU
Vitamin K (phytonadione)	60–300 mcg
Niacinamide	10–30 mg
Biotin	100–300 mcg
Folic acid	400–800 mcg
Choline	10–100 mg
Inositol	10–100 mg
MINERAL	RANGE FOR ADULTS
Boron	1–6 mg
Calcium[e]	250–1500 mg

a. Women of childbearing age who might become pregnant should not take more than 2500 IU of retinol daily, because of the possible risk of birth defects.

b. It may be easier to take vitamin C separately.

c. Elderly people in nursing homes living in northern latitudes should supplement at the high range.

d. It may be more cost-effective to take vitamin E seperately rather than as a component of a multiple vitamin.

e. Women who have or who are at risk of osteoporosis may need to take a separate calcium supplement to achieve the recommended level of 1000 to 1500 mg daily.

MINERAL	RANGE FOR ADULTS
Chromium[f]	200–400 mcg
Copper	1–2 mg
Iodine	50–150 mcg
Iron[g]	15–30 mg
Magnesium	250–500 mg
Manganese	10–15 mg
Molybdenum	10–25 mcg
Potassium	200–500 mg
Selenium	100–200 mcg
Silica	1–5 mg
Vanadium	50–100 mcg
Zinc	15–45 mg

f. For diabetes and weight loss, doses of 600 mcg of chromium can be used.
g. Most men as well as most women who have gone through menopause rarely need supplemental iron.

Proteolytic Enzymes

When used for reasons other than as a digestive aid, proteolytic enzymes should be taken on an empty stomach just before a meal. The following recommendations are dosages for patients with cancer. We recommend

Dosages for Individual Proteolytic Enzymes*

ENZYME	DOSAGE	NOTES
Pancreatin	300–900 mg 3x/day	Dosage is for full-strength product (8X USP)
Chymotrypsin	180–540 mg 3x/day	1 mg = 1000 USP units
Trypsin	3–9 mg 3x/day	1 mg = 25,000 USP units
Bromelain	250–750 mg 3x/day	1200–1800 mcu or gdu
Fungal proteases	15,000–45,000 USP 3x/day	
Papain	50–150 mg 3x/day	1 mg = 30,000 USP units
Serratia peptidase	50–150 mg 3x/day	200,000 serratia peptidase units per gram

*We recommend using combination products like Wobenzyme or Zymactive to provide a broader range of activity compared to any single proteolytic enzyme.

starting at the lower dosage level and working up to the higher dosage level in weekly increments. After remission of cancer, we recommend using the lowest dosage as a maintenance therapy. For best results, take 15 to 20 minutes before meals.

Sample Daily Routine with Basic Supplementation Program for the Cancer Patient

8:00 A.M.—Wake up.

8:00—Take before-meal supplements:

- Proteolytic enzymes
- Quercetin or curcumin

8:00 to 8:30—Gentle exercise (may range from simply performing breathing exercises in bed to light stretching, yoga, or tai chi)

8:30—Breakfast smoothie

With-meal supplements:

- High-potency multiple vitamin and mineral formula according to the guidelines given on page 312.
- Extra vitamin C—500 to 1000 mg
- Extra vitamin E—400 IU
- Fish oil supplement
- Probiotic supplement—5 to 10 billion

8:45 to 9:15—Personal time for taking a shower or bath and getting cleaned up for the day

9:15 to 10:15—Reading inspirational books or watching comedies

10:15—Take any between-meal supplement such as maitake MD-fraction or PSK/PSP

10:30—Green drink (2 servings)

Supplements to take with juice or greens:

- Green tea extract

10:35 to 11:30—Engage in enjoyable but relaxing activities

11:30—Before-meal supplements (take with glass of water):

- Proteolytic enzymes
- Quercetin or curcumin

12:00 P.M.—Fresh juice break (8 to 12 ounces)

12:30—Lunch (see menu suggestions)

With-meal supplements:

- Extra vitamin C (500 to 1000 mg)
- Fish oil supplement

12:30 to 2:30—Engage in enjoyable but relaxing activities

2:30—Green drink or additional smoothie with whey protein (if muscle wasting and weight loss are occurring, definitely go with the smoothie)

2:30 to 3:00—Low-intensity exercise—walking, yoga, or tai chi

3:00 to 4:00—Quiet time filled with deep breathing, relaxation exercises, prayer, or meditation

4:00—Take any between-meal supplement

4:00 to 5:00—Rest and relaxation

5:00—Before-meal supplements:
- Proteolytic enzymes
- Quercetin or curcumin

5:30—Fresh juice break (8 to 12 ounces)

6:00—Dinner (see menu suggestions)
With-meal supplements:
- Extra vitamin C (500 to 1000 mg)
- Fish oil supplement

6:00 to 9:00—Engage in social activities, development of relationships, and enjoyment of personal interests

9:00—Herbal tea nightcap

10:00—Get to bed early

Shopping List

The following shopping list represents the items needed in order to follow the four-day meal plans. Take a look in your cupboards, pantry, and refrigerator to see if you already have some of these items on hand. Look over all the recipes for any optional items that you may want to add. You will also need to make a list for the health food store for your supplements and whey protein.

HERBAL TEA

Most of the major brands of herbal tea (e.g., Celestial Seasons, Bigelow, Republic of Tea, Traditional Medicinals, etc.) provide a sampler pack to help you identify teas that appeal to you. In general, avoid black teas. Try to choose decaffeinated varieties, especially with your nighttime cup of tea. If you feel you need a little caffeine in the morning, go with a cup of regular green tea.

PRODUCE

Try to buy organic, if possible, and be sure to wash all produce before consumption.

Acorn squash—1

Apples—2 red, 2 green

Bananas—2

Basil—1 bunch

Bell peppers—4 green, 2 red

Blueberries—1 cup

Broccoli—1 head

Cabbage—½ head

Carrots—3 large bags

Celery—2 bunches

Cucumber—1

Garlic—2 bulbs

Green onions—1 bunch

Kale—2 bunches

Leek—1

Lemons—8

Mushrooms—2 ounces

Onions—3

Oranges—3

Parsley—1 bunch

Pears—2 Bartlett

Potato—1 small white

Raspberries—1 cup

Strawberries—2 cups

Tomatoes, roma (plum)—
2 medium

Yam—2, or 4 small sweet
potatoes

FISH

Salmon—2½ pounds salmon fillets

MISCELLANEOUS GROCERY ITEMS

Balsamic vinegar—8 ounces

Honey (raw)—8 ounces

Instant pudding packets
(sugar-free, nonfat
preferred)

Nonfat yogurt—8 ounces

Rice milk, soymilk, or nonfat
milk—64 ounces

Tofu—1 container (15 ounces)
of firm variety

Vegetable boullion—enough
for 64 ounces

NUTS, SEEDS, AND DRIED FRUIT

Flaxseed, raw or ground—1 cup

OILS

Flaxseed oil—12 to 16 ounces

Olive oil (extra-virgin)—12 to 16 ounces

GRAINS AND PASTA
Brown rice (quick)—1 box
Rolled oats—1 small container
Whole-wheat tortillas—1 pack of 8

FROZEN FOODS
Corn (frozen)—10-ounce package

CANNED FOODS
Garbanzo beans—
    1 (7.5-ounce) can
Red kidney beans—
    1 (7.5-ounce) can

Refried black beans—
    1 (15-ounce) can
White beans—
    1 (7.5-ounce) can

SPICES AND SEASONINGS
Allspice or nutmeg
Capers
Chili powder
Cinnamon
Crushed red pepper
Cumin
Curry powder
Ginger (dried)

Ground black pepper
No Salt or Nu-Salt—
    potassium chloride salts to
    use as a substitute for
    regular salt (sodium
    chloride)
Soy sauce (low-sodium)
Thyme

Sample Menus

Just as we did in Appendix A Daily Plan for Preventing Cancer, we are providing four-day sample menus to get you started in planning out your own daily menus. Since the guidelines given in Appendix A still apply for someone with less severe symptoms or dietary challenges, the sample daily menus below are for someone with a more advanced cancer or someone going through chemotherapy who is in need of maximum nutritional support. Notice that we are focusing on smoothies, fresh juices, and rather simple foods that are soft and easy to chew, including substituting fresh vegetable juice for salads. The reason we are recommending drinking the juice before lunch or dinner is that drinking during the meal may reduce the intake of solid foods. Sip water during the meal if you need some additional liquid to help get the food down.

DAY 1	
BREAKFAST Apple-Cinnamon Shake Smoothie (see p. 320) Cup of herbal tea **MIDMORNING SNACK** Green drink (2 servings) **LUNCH** Cruciferous Surprise (see p. 320) French White Bean Soup (see p. 321) **MIDAFTERNOON SNACK** Strawberry Banana Smoothie (see p. 321)	**DINNER** Popeye's Power Drink (see p. 322) Pan-Seared Salmon (see p. 322) Quick Acorn Squash (see p. 322) Whey-Enhanced Yogurt (see p. 323) **EVENING TEA** One or two cups of herbal tea (no caffeine)

DAY 2	
BREAKFAST Whey-Enhanced Oatmeal (see p. 323) **MIDMORNING SNACK** Green drink (2 servings) **LUNCH** Cleansing Cocktail Juice: (see p. 324) Warm Mediterranean Bean Salad (see p. 324)	**MIDAFTERNOON SNACK** Peach Smoothie (see p. 325) **DINNER** Pineapple Kale Juice (see p. 325) Coconut Curry with Tofu or Chicken (see p. 325) Whey-Enhanced Instant Pudding (see p. 326) **EVENING TEA** One or two cups of herbal tea (no caffeine)

DAY 3	
BREAKFAST Peanut Butter Chocolate Truffle Smoothie (see p. 326)	**MIDAFTERNOON SNACK** Orange Jubilee Smoothie (see p. 328)
MIDMORNING SNACK Green drink (2 servings)	**DINNER** Super V-7 Juice (see p. 328) Steamed Broccoli with Lemon (see p. 328) Baked Salmon (see p. 329)
LUNCH Pineapple Strawberry Juice (see p. 327) Sweet Potato and Pear Soup (see p. 327)	**EVENING TEA** One or two cups of herbal tea (no caffeine)

DAY 4	
BREAKFAST Tri-berry Boost Smoothie (see p. 330)	**DINNER** Pineapple Blueberry Juice (see p. 331) Yam and Bean Burritos (see p. 331) Whey-Enhanced Instant Pudding (see p. 332)
MIDMORNING SNACK Green drink (2 servings)	
LUNCH Ginger Hopper (see p. 330)	
MIDAFTERNOON SNACK Vanilla Ice Smoothie (see p. 331)	**EVENING TEA** One or two cups of herbal tea (no caffeine)

Recipes

These recipes are designed to be quick and easy. The smoothie and juice recipes can be tailored to your tastes as well as size of serving (simply increase or decrease the ingredients), based on need. For example, if you are a 100-pound woman, you may find that the serving size for these smoothies and juices is too large. Simply reduce the ingredients proportionally. Please be aware that the smoothies and juices are single servings while the lunch entrées and dinner dishes are 2 servings.

Day 1

Apple-Cinnamon Shake Smoothie

25 to 30 grams whey protein
8 ounces nonfat milk, rice milk, or soymilk (vanilla)
1 small red apple, chopped
¼ to ½ teaspoon cinnamon
1 tablespoon flaxseed oil or ground flaxseed (optional)

Mix in a blender and liquefy.

Green drink (2 servings)

Cruciferous Surprise

JUICE THE FOLLOWING:
3 or 4 kale leaves
½ cup broccoli florets with stems
½ head cabbage, sliced into wedges
4 carrots
2 apples, cut into wedges

French White Bean Soup

½ cup onion, chopped
1 leek, chopped
1 garlic clove, minced
1 tablespoon olive oil
1 (7.5-ounce) can white beans, drained and rinsed
1 small white potato
½ teaspoon dried thyme
2 cups vegetable broth (low-sodium)
¼ cup chopped fresh parsley
2 teaspoons fresh lemon juice
Dash of No Salt or Nu-Salt
Ground pepper to taste

In a large saucepan or Dutch oven, sauté the onions, leeks, and garlic in the olive oil for about 5 minutes over medium-high heat. Add the beans, the potato, ¼ teaspoon of thyme, and 1 cup of the vegetable broth; simmer 20 minutes. Purée in a blender or food processor. When smooth, return to the saucepan, add the remaining broth, and heat through. If necessary, add water or more broth to reach the desired thickness. Before serving, stir in the chopped parsley, lemon juice, salt and pepper, and the remaining ¼ teaspoon thyme.

• MIDAFTERNOON SNACK •

Strawberry Banana Smoothie

25 to 30 grams whey protein (any flavor, e.g., strawberry, vanilla, chocolate)
½ cup fresh strawberries
8 ounces cold water or vanilla soymilk
½ cup sliced frozen banana
1 tablespoon flaxseed oil or ground flaxseed (optional)

Mix in a blender and liquefy.

· DINNER ·

Popeye's Power Drink

JUICE THE FOLLOWING:
Handful of parsley
4 carrots
Handful of spinach

Pan-Seared Salmon

8 ounces salmon fillet, cut in half
1 tablespoon olive oil
1 tablespoon drained capers
2 lemon slices, for garnish
1 tablespoon chopped parsley
Salt (use No Salt or Nu-Salt) and pepper to taste

Preheat a large skillet over moderate heat for 3 minutes. Coat the salmon fillets with olive oil. Place the fillets in the skillet, raise the heat to high, and cook for 3 minutes. Add the capers and turn over the salmon. Cook for an additional 5 minutes or until well browned. Transfer the fillets and capers to individual plates and garnish with lemon slices and parsley.

Quick Acorn Squash

1 acorn squash, cut in half with seeds removed
1 tablespoon honey
Dash of cinnamon

Place the squash in a microwave-safe dish with cup side up. Cover and cook in the microwave for 10 to 13 minutes on high or until fork-tender. Top with the honey and cinnamon.

Whey-Enhanced Yogurt

8 ounces nonfat yogurt (any desired flavor)
10 to 15 grams whey protein
1 tablespoon flaxseed oil or ground flaxseed (optional)

Stir the ingredients into a medium-size cup. Makes 1 serving.

• EVENING TEA •

One or two cups of herbal tea (no caffeine)

Day 2

• BREAKFAST •

Whey-Enhanced Oatmeal

1 cup cooked oatmeal
25 to 30 grams whey protein (vanilla)
¼ cup water, soymilk, or nonfat yogurt
1 tablespoon flaxseed oil (optional)
Raisins, nuts, and cinnamon (optional)

Prepare 1 cup oatmeal according to the instructions on the package. While the oatmeal is cooking, stir the whey protein into the ¼ cup water. Adding additional liquid will thin the oatmeal, if desired. Top with raisins, nuts, flaxseed oil, and cinnamon if desired. Makes 1 serving.

• MIDMORNING SNACK •

Green drink (2 servings)

• LUNCH •

Cleansing Cocktail

JUICE THE FOLLOWING:
4 carrots
1 apple, cut into wedges
2 celery ribs
½ cup chopped parsley
2 beets (with top)

Warm Mediterranean Bean Salad

1 (7.5-ounce) can red kidney beans, rinsed and drained
1 (7.5-ounce) can garbanzo beans, rinsed and drained
2 cups low-sodium vegetable broth
½ medium onion, diced
¼ cup balsamic vinegar
1 garlic clove, minced
1 tablespoon lemon juice
¼ cup red bell pepper, diced
¼ cup green bell pepper, diced
¼ cup frozen corn kernels, thawed
¼ cup chopped celery
¼ cup chopped parsley
Salt (use No Salt or Nu-Salt) and pepper to taste

In a large pot combine the kidney beans, garbanzo beans, broth, and onions; bring to a boil and drain. Add the remaining ingredients and mix well, seasoning with salt (use No Salt or Nu-Salt) and pepper to taste. The salad should be served and enjoyed while still warm.

• MIDAFTERNOON SNACK •

Peach Smoothie

25 to 30 grams whey protein (vanilla)
1 ripe peach (washed and sliced)
3 or 4 ice cubes
1 tablespoon flaxseed oil or ground flaxseed (optional)

Mix in a blender and liquefy.

• DINNER •

Pineapple Kale Juice

JUICE THE FOLLOWING:
½ pineapple, sliced lengthwise in strips that fit in juicer
1 cup kale or spinach

Coconut Curry with Tofu or Chicken

1 (7-ounce) can coconut milk
2 tablespoons soy sauce (low-sodium)
½ teaspoon curry powder
1 teaspoon minced fresh ginger
1 teaspoon chili powder
1 (15-ounce) package firm tofu, cut into ¾-inch cubes (or use 1 cup
cubed, cooked chicken breast)
2 roma (plum) tomatoes, chopped
1 green bell pepper, thinly sliced
2 ounces fresh mushrooms, chopped
1 bunch green onions, chopped
¼ cup chopped fresh basil
¼ teaspoon salt (use No Salt or Nu-Salt)

In a large wok or heavy skillet over medium heat, mix the coconut milk, soy sauce, curry powder, ginger, and chili powder and bring to a boil. Mix the tofu, tomatoes, bell pepper, mushrooms, and half of the chopped green onion into the wok. Cover and cook 5 minutes, stirring occasionally. Mix in the basil. Season with salt and continue cooking 5 minutes, or until the vegetables are tender but firm. Garnish with the remaining green onion pieces.

Whey-Enhanced Instant Pudding

2 cups nonfat milk, rice milk, or soymilk (vanilla or chocolate)
1 packet instant pudding (sugar-free and fat-free preferred)
25 to 30 grams whey protein (vanilla or chocolate)

Mix the nonfat milk, pudding mix, and whey protein in blender on low speed for approximately 2 minutes. Pour into 2 medium-size bowls and refrigerate for 7 to 10 minutes.

• EVENING TEA •

One or two cups of herbal tea (no caffeine)

Day 3

• BREAKFAST •

Peanut Butter Chocolate Truffle Smoothie

25 to 30 grams chocolate-flavored whey protein powder
1 tablespoon creamy peanut butter
8 ounces nonfat milk, rice milk, or soymilk (chocolate)
4 ounces water

3 or 4 ice cubes
1 tablespoon flaxseed oil or ground flaxseed (optional)

Mix in a blender and liquefy.

• MIDMORNING SNACK •

Green drink (2 servings)

• LUNCH •

Pineapple Strawberry Juice

JUICE THE FOLLOWING:
½ pineapple, sliced lengthwise in strips that fit in juicer
1 cup fresh strawberries

Sweet Potato and Pear Soup

1 large yam or 2 small sweet potatoes, cut into small chunks
½ onion, chopped
1 tablespoon olive oil
2 cups vegetable broth (low-sodium)
2 large Bartlett pears, cut into small chunks
Dash of allspice or nutmeg

Microwave the yam until soft (usually 6 to 8 minutes) and mash with a potato masher or hand mixer. In a medium-sized soup pot, sauté the onion in the olive oil. Add the broth, pears, and allspice and heat through.

Orange Jubilee Smoothie

2 oranges, peeled and sliced
¼ cup fresh orange juice
25 to 30 grams whey protein (vanilla)
4 ounces water, nonfat milk, or soymilk
3 or 4 ice cubes or ½ cup sliced frozen banana
1 tablespoon flaxseed oil or ground flaxseed (optional)

Mix the orange slices and the orange juice in a blender and liquefy. Add the whey protein and blend, then add the water, ice cubes, and flaxseed oil and liquefy.

• DINNER •

Super V–7 Juice

JUICE THE FOLLOWING:
Handful of parsley
4 carrots
Handful of spinach
2 celery ribs
2 tomatoes, quartered
½ cup chopped cucumber
½ green or red bell pepper

Mix in a blender and liquefy.

Steamed Broccoli with Lemon

1 head broccoli, cut into large florets
2 teaspoons fresh lemon or lime juice
⅛ teaspoon salt (use No Salt or Nu-Salt)
⅛ teaspoon pepper

Place the broccoli florets in a vegetable steamer and sprinkle with the lemon juice, salt (use No Salt or Nu-Salt), and pepper. Lightly steam the broccoli until it is just warmed through.

Baked Salmon

8 ounces salmon fillet
1 cup cooked brown rice
Juice of 1 orange
½ teaspoon dried dill weed
½ teaspoon dried rosemary
½ teaspoon dried basil
½ teaspoon pepper
1 tablespoon chopped parsley

Preheat oven to 350° F. Cover the bottom of a large pan with water, just enough to cover the bottom. Lay the salmon fillet in the pan, flesh side up. Place the cooked rice around the outside of the fish. Sprinkle the orange juice over the fish and rice. In a small bowl, combine the dill weed, rosemary, basil, and pepper and sprinkle over the fish and rice. Cover with aluminum foil. Bake for 30 to 40 minutes, or until the salmon is tender and flaky. Garnish with the parsley.

• EVENING TEA •

One or two cups of herbal tea (no caffeine)

Day 4

Tri-berry Boost Smoothie

25 to 30 grams whey protein
8 ounces nonfat milk, rice milk, or soymilk (vanilla)
½ cup strawberries (fresh or frozen)
½ cup raspberries (fresh or frozen)
½ cup blueberries (fresh or frozen)
3 or 4 ice cubes (optional)
1 tablespoon flaxseed oil or ground flaxseed (optional)

Mix in a blender and liquefy.

Green drink (2 servings)

Ginger Hopper

JUICE THE FOLLOWING:
4 carrots
1 apple, cut into wedges
Handful of parsley
¼-inch slice fresh ginger

Vanilla Ice Smoothie

25 to 30 grams whey protein (vanilla)
8 ounces vanilla soymilk
½ teaspoon vanilla extract
3 or 4 ice cubes OR ½ cup frozen berries
1 tablespoon flaxseed oil or ground flaxseed (optional)

Mix in a blender and liquefy.

• DINNER •

Pineapple Blueberry Juice

JUICE THE FOLLOWING:
½ pineapple, sliced lengthwise in strips that fit in juicer
1 cup fresh blueberries

Yam and Bean Burritos

½ onion, chopped
1 garlic clove, minced
1 tablespoon olive oil
1 (15-ounce) can black refried beans (nonfat)
1 cup water
1 tablespoon chili powder
½ teaspoon ground cumin
1 tablespoon soy sauce (low-sodium)
1 cup cooked and mashed sweet potatoes
4 whole-wheat flour tortillas, warmed
4 ounces grated low-fat cheddar cheese (optional)
Salsa or picante sauce to taste (optional)

Preheat oven to 350° F. Sauté the onion and garlic in the olive oil until soft. Stir in the refried beans and mash in the garlic and onion. Gradually stir in the water and heat until warm. Remove from the heat and stir in the chili powder, cumin, and soy sauce. Fill each tortilla with some of the bean mixture and some of the mashed sweet potatoes. Top with cheese if desired. Fold up the tortillas burrito style and bake for 12 minutes, then serve.

Whey-Enhanced Instant Pudding

2 cups nonfat milk, rice milk, or soymilk (vanilla or chocolate)
1 packet instant pudding (sugar-free and fat-free preferred)
25 to 30 grams whey protein (vanilla or chocolate)

Mix the nonfat milk, pudding mix, and whey protein in a blender on low speed for approximately 2 minutes. Pour into 2 medium-size bowls and refrigerate for 7 to 10 minutes.

• EVENING TEA •

One or two cups of herbal tea (no caffeine)

Appendix C

Presurgical Supplement Recommendations

For two weeks prior to surgery, take:

- High-potency multiple vitamin and mineral formula

Note: Keep vitamin E doses below 200 IU per day

- Vitamin C: 500 mg three times a day
- Grape seed extract: 150 mg twice a day
- Gotu kola *(Centella asiatica)* extract: Dosage is based on triterpenic acid content of 30 to 60 mg twice daily. Read labels carefully to make sure that you are getting the proper dosage.
- Probiotic supplement (e.g., *Lactobacillus rhamnosus*): 5 to 10 billion live organisms daily

For one to seven days before surgery, take:

- Whey protein: 25 to 50 grams per day
- Modified citrus pectin (MCP): 6 g of MCP dissolved by blending in water or juice twice daily for one week prior to surgery.

Postsurgical Supplemental Recommendations

For at least two weeks after surgery, take:

- High-potency multiple vitamin and mineral formula

Note: Keep vitamin E level below 200 IU per day

- Vitamin C: 500 mg three times daily
- Grape seed extract: 150 mg twice daily
- Proteolytic enzymes: See page 313 for dosage information.
- Gotu kola *(Centella asiatica)* extract: Dosage is based on triterpenic acid content of 30 to 60 mg twice daily. Read labels carefully to make sure you are getting the proper dosage.
- Probiotic supplement (e.g., *Lactobacillus rhamnosus*): 10 to 20 billion live organisms daily
- Whey protein: 25 to 50 g per day
- Take modified citrus pectin (MCP) at a dosage of 6 g dissolved by blending in water or juice twice daily. To ensure the best absorption, MCP should be taken on an empty stomach.

Before Surgery Avoid:

Garlic	7 days prior
Ginkgo	36 hours prior
Ginseng	7 days prior
Kava	24 hours prior
Proteolytic enzymes	2 days prior
St. John's wort	5 days prior
Valerian	5 days prior

Before Surgery or Biopsy Add:

MCP	6 grams in water or juice twice daily

After Surgery Add:

Gotu kola	See above
Proteolytic enzymes	See page 313 for dosage information

Supplemental Support for Radiation Therapy

The following supplement recommendations are designed to support your body as you undergo radiation therapy:

- Use a high-potency multiple vitamin and mineral formula according to the guidelines given on page 312.
- Consume one to two servings of a green drink daily (see page 311 for description).
- Take extra vitamin C—a total of 500 to 1000 mg three times a day.
- Make sure that your daily vitamin E intake is in the 400-to-800 mg range.
- Take an extra 75 mg of natural beta-carotene and 10,000 IU of vitamin A daily for one week prior to radiation therapy. After this one-week usage, discontinue these supplements at this dosage.
- For head and neck cancers, take quercetin (200 to 400 mg daily). For other cancers being treated by radiation, take curcumin (200 to 400 mg daily). Continue for at least one month after your last radiation treatment. After this period, choose either quercetin or curcumin, depending on the type of cancer (see page 242).
- Take either maitake D-fraction, maitake MD-fraction, or PSK/PSP at either 1 mg per 2.2 pounds per day for the maitake products or 3000 mg for the PSK/PSP products. Continue at this dosage until the cancer is in remission, then cut the dosage in half.

- Take melatonin at a dosage of 20 mg a day one week prior to radiation. Continue at this dosage until the cancer is in remission.
- Take alkylglycerols at a dosage of 1200 mg a day for at least one week before and after treatment. A dosage of 600 mg a day should be continued until normal white blood cell counts are achieved.

Before radiation (begin 1 week prior)

Use a high-potency multiple vitamin and mineral formula according to the guidelines given on page 312.

In addition, take:

Beta-carotene (natural)	75 mg daily
Vitamin A	10,000 IU, daily

During radiation

Use a high-potency multiple vitamin and mineral formula according to the guidelines given on page 312.

In addition,

take:

Vitamin C	500 to 1000 mg three times daily
Vitamin E	400 to 800 IU daily
Quercetin	200 to 400 mg daily
or	
Curcumin	200 to 400 mg daily
Maitake MD-fraction	1mg daily per 2.2 pounds of body weight
or	
PSK	3000 mg a day
or	
PSP	3000 mg a day (take until cancer is in remission)

| Melatonin | 20 mg a day (begin one week prior to radiation and continue until cancer is in remission) |
| Alkylglyercols | 1200 mg a day at least one week before and after treatment and 600 mg a day until normal white blood cell count is achieved |

Basic Chemotherapy
Supplementation Program

- Before meals:
  a. Take proteolytic enzymes according to the dosage recommendations on page 313. Best taken 15 to 20 minutes before meals.
  b. Take either quercetin (200 to 400 mg daily) or curcumin based on the type of cancer and the chemotherapy agent used (see page 242). Can be taken before meals along with the proteolytic enzymes.

- With meals:
  a. Use a high-potency multiple vitamin and mineral according to the guidelines given on page 312. Best taken with food.
  b. Take extra vitamin C—a total of 500 to 1000 mg three times a day.
  c. Make sure that your daily vitamin E intake is in the 400-to-800 mg range.
  d. Use fish oil supplements at a daily dosage to provide at least 700 to 1200 mg of EPA and 400 to 800 mg of DHA. Take fish oils at the beginning of a meal to reduce any aftertaste.
  e. Take probiotics according to the guidelines on page 221.

- With fresh vegetable juice or green drink breaks:
  a. Take green tea extract—enough to provide 300 to 400 mg of polyphenols. Best taken when you drink your vegetable juice or green drink.
  b. Consume one to two servings of a green drink daily (see page 311 for description). Can be used as a between-meal snack.

- Between meals:
  a. Take either maitake MD-fraction or PSK/PSP (discussed below). Best taken between meals. Can be taken 5 to 10 minutes before taking your green drink or juice break or 30 minutes before meals.

- At bedtime:
  a. Take 20 to 40 mg daily of melatonin. Best taken 30 to 45 minutes before bedtime.

If taking alkylating agents and platinum compounds, add:

- Polyerga to prevent the reduction of white blood cell counts. For people of up to 140 pounds body weight, take 1 Polyerga tablet three times a day. For every additional 40 pounds body weight, add an additional tablet (e.g., a 220-pound person would take 5 tablets daily in divided dosages). For best results, take Polyerga on an empty stomach before meals. Also, do not take Polyerga at the same time you take digestive enzymes like pancreatin, bromelain, or papain. Polyerga can be taken the same time as MD-fraction or PSK/PSP.

If taking platinum compounds:

- Do not take N-acetylcysteine (NAC), a derivative of the naturally occurring amino acid cysteine.
- Do not take dosages of vitamin B_6 greater than 200 mg a day.

If taking antitumor antibiotics, add:

- Co-enzyme Q10 (CoQ10) at a dosage of 100 mg twice daily. Take CoQ10 with meals to enhance absorption.

If taking antimetabolites:

- Do not take dosages of folic acid greater than 800 mcg a day.

If taking biological response modifiers:

- Follow the basic chemotherapy supplementation program above.

If taking hormones or hormone inhibitors:

- Do not use supplements containing soy phytoestrogens if taking tamoxifen.

For breast and prostate cancers, add the following (best with meals):

- Lycopene: 30 mg daily
- Calcium D-glucarate: 400 mg daily
- Indole-3-carbinol: 400 mg daily
- Ground flaxseed or flaxseed meal: 2 tablespoons daily

If taking microtubule and chromatin inhibitors, add:

- Polyerga (see on p. 339 under alkylating agents).

If taking new-breed chemotherapy agents:

- Follow the basic chemotherapy supplementation program above.

For bone marrow suppression, add:

- Polyerga (see on p. 339 under alkylating agents).

For mouth ulcers, add:

- A special licorice extract, DGL: Take 400 mg three times daily 15 to 20 minutes before meals.

For hand-foot syndrome, add:

- Vitamin B_6: 50 mg twice daily with meals.

Optional supplements:

- Modified citrus pectin or IP6 with inositol: Best taken between meals or at night before going to bed (can be taken along with the melatonin), according to the dosage recommendations given on page 184 and 185, respectively.

During chemotherapy

Maitake MD-fraction	1 mg per 2.2 pounds of body weight
or	
PSK	3000 mg a day
or	
PSP	3000 mg a day
Curcumin	200 to 400 mg one to daily
or	
Quercetin (see chart on page 242)	200 to 400 mg one to daily
Melatonin	20 mg once daily at bedtime

For hand-foot syndrome

Vitamin B$_6$	50 mg twice daily
Aloe vera gel	Topically

If you take a platinum-based chemotherapy agent, avoid (see on page 253 for more information):

N-acetylcysteine (NAC)	
Vitamin B$_6$	over 200 g a day

For mouth ulcers

DGL (deglycyrrhizinated licorice)	400 mg a day (chew tablets 20 minutes before meals)

If you take antitumor antibiotics:

AVOID:

Quercetin if being treated for colon cancer

TAKE:

CoQ10	100 mg twice daily
Melatonin	20 mg once daily at bedtime

Open Letter to Physicians

Consider taking a copy of this letter to your physicians when you discuss the use of alternative and complementary strategies for cancer treatment.

Dear Doctor,

We have written the book *How to Prevent and Treat Cancer with Natural Medicine* as a guide that includes valuable and sensible information for cancer patients on how to incorporate diet, nutritional supplements, herbal medicine, and other strategies, such as acupuncture, into their conventional treatment program. Our goals are simple but important:

- Reduce the toxicity of conventional treatment strategies while enhancing their effectiveness, thus dramatically lowering the risk of side effects, including mouth sores, fatigue, vomiting, hair loss, and organ toxicity
- Eliminate or dramatically reduce malnutrition and tissue wasting as a result of treatment
- Bolster the immune system
- Significantly increase the chances for remission and cure while simultaneously lowering the risk of recurrence

Having painstakingly reviewed the medical literature, we base our recommendations on current scientific evidence and reasoning as well as our own clinical experience. Should you wish to review the research that helped us form our opinions, please consult the references listed in the back of this book.

We urge you to work cooperatively with your patient to achieve the goal we all seek: the best possible outcome of care.

Sincerely,

Michael T. Murray, N.D.
Joseph E. Pizzorno, N.D.
Tim Birdsall, N.D.
Paul Reilly, N.D.

Dietary Fiber Content
of Selected Foods

FOOD	SERVING	CALORIES	GRAMS OF FIBER
Fruits			
Apple (with skin)	1 medium	81	3.5
Banana	1 medium	105	2.4
Cantaloupe	¼ melon	30	1.0
Cherries, sweet	10	49	1.2
Grapefruit	½ medium	38	1.6
Orange	1 medium	62	2.6
Peach (with skin)	1	37	1.9
Pear (with skin)	½ large	61	3.1
Prunes	3	60	3.0
Raisins	¼ cup	106	3.1
Raspberries	½ cup	35	3.1
Strawberries	1 cup	45	3.0
Vegetables, raw			
Bean sprouts	½ cup	13	1.5
Celery, diced	½ cup	10	1.1
Cucumber	½ cup	8	0.4
Lettuce	1 cup	10	0.9
Mushrooms	½ cup	10	1.5
Pepper, green	½ cup	9	0.5
Spinach	1 cup	8	1.2
Tomato	1 medium	20	1.5
Vegetables, cooked			
Asparagus, cut	1 cup	30	2.0
Beans, green	1 cup	32	3.2
Broccoli	1 cup	40	4.4
Brussels sprouts	1 cup	56	4.6
Cabbage, red	1 cup	30	2.8
Carrots	1 cup	48	4.6
Cauliflower	1 cup	28	2.2
Corn	½ cup	87	2.9

FOOD	SERVING	CALORIES	GRAMS OF FIBER
Vegetables, cooked *(continued)*			
Kale	1 cup	44	2.8
Parsnip	1 cup	102	5.4
Potato (with skin)	1 medium	106	2.5
Potato (without skin)	1 medium	97	1.4
Spinach	1 cup	42	4.2
Sweet potatoes	1 medium	160	3.4
Zucchini	1 cup	22	3.6
Legumes			
Baked beans	½ cup	155	8.8
Dried peas, cooked	½ cup	115	4.7
Kidney beans, cooked	½ cup	110	7.3
Lentils, cooked	½ cup	97	3.7
Lima beans, cooked	½ cup	64	4.5
Navy beans, cooked	½ cup	112	6.0
Rice, breads, pastas, and flour			
Bran muffins	1 muffin	104	2.5
Bread, white	1 slice	78	0.4
Bread, whole-wheat	1 slice	61	1.4
Crisp bread, rye	2 crackers	50	2.0
Rice, brown, cooked	½ cup	97	1.0
Rice, white, cooked	½ cup	82	0.2
Spaghetti, regular, cooked	½ cup	155	1.1
Spaghetti, whole-wheat, cooked	½ cup	155	3.9
Breakfast cereals			
All-Bran	⅓ cup	71	8.5
Bran Chex	⅔ cup	91	4.6
Corn Bran	⅔ cup	98	5.4
Corn flakes	1¼ cups	110	0.3
Grape-Nuts	¼ cup	101	1.4
Oatmeal	¾ cup	108	1.6
Raisin bran	⅔ cup	115	4.0
Shredded wheat	⅔ cup	102	2.6
Nuts			
Almonds	10 nuts	79	1.1
Filberts	10 nuts	54	0.8
Peanuts	10 nuts	105	1.4

Are You an Optimist?

What distinguishes an optimist from a pessimist is the way in which they explain both good and bad events. Martin Seligman has developed a simple test to determine your level of optimism (from *Learned Optimism,* Knopf, 1981). Take as much time as you need. There are no right or wrong answers. It is important that you take the test before you read the interpretation. Read the description of each situation and vividly imagine it happening to you. Choose the response that most applies to you by circling either A or B. Ignore the letter and number codes for now; they will be explained later.

1. The project you are in charge of is a great success.   PsG
   A. *I kept a close watch over everyone's work.*   1
   B. *Everyone devoted a lot of time and energy to it.*   0

2. You and your spouse (boyfriend/girlfriend) make up
   after a fight.   PmG
   A. *I forgave him/her.*   0
   B. *I'm usually forgiving.*   1

3. You get lost driving to a friend's house.   PsB
   A. *I missed a turn.*   1
   B. *My friend gave me bad directions.*   0

4. Your spouse (boyfriend/girlfriend) surprises you
   with a gift.   PsG
   A. *He/she just got a raise at work.*   0
   B. *I took him/her out to a special dinner the night before.* 1

5. You forget your spouse's (boyfriend's/girlfriend's) birthday.   PmB
   A. *I'm not good at remembering birthdays.*   1
   B. *I was preoccupied with other things.*   0

6. You get a flower from a secret admirer.   PvG
   A. *I am attractive to him/her.*   0
   B. *I am a popular person.*   1

7. You run for a community office position and you win.   PvG
   A. *I devote a lot of time and energy to campaigning.*   0
   B. *I work very hard at everything I do.*   1

8. You miss an important engagement.   PvB
   A. *Sometimes my memory fails me.*   1
   B. *I sometimes forget to check my appointment book.*   0

9. You run for a community office position and you lose.   PsB
   A. *I didn't campaign hard enough.*   1
   B. *The person who won knew more people.*   0

10. You host a successful dinner.   PmG
    A. *I was particularly charming that night.*   0
    B. *I am a good host.*   1

11. You stop a crime by calling the police.   PsG
    A. *A strange noise caught my attention.*   0
    B. *I was alert that day.*   1

12. You were extremely healthy all year.   PsG
    A. *Few people around me were sick, so I wasn't exposed.*   0
    B. *I made sure I ate well and got enough rest.*   1

13. You owe the library $10 for an overdue book.   PmB
    A. *When I am really involved in what I am reading,*
       I often forget when the book is due.   1
    B. *I was so involved in writing the report that I forgot to*
       return the book.   0

14. Your stocks make you a lot of money.   PmG
    A. *My broker decided to take on something new.*   0
    B. *My broker is a top-notch investor.*   1

15. You win an athletic contest.   PmG
    A. *I was feeling unbeatable.*   0
    B. *I trained hard.*   1

16. You fail an important examination.   PsB
    A. *I wasn't as smart as the other people taking the exam.* 1
    B. *I didn't prepare for it well.*   0

17. You prepared a special meal for a friend and he/she
    barely touched the food.   PvB
    A. *I wasn't a good cook.*   1
    B. *I made the meal in a rush.*   0

18. You lose a sporting event for which you have been
    training for a long time.   PvB
    A. *I'm not very athletic.*   1
    B. *I'm not good at that sport.*   0

19. Your car runs out of gas on a dark street late at night.   PsB
    A. *I didn't check to see how much gas was in the tank.*   1
    B. *The gas gauge was broken.*   0

20. You lose your temper with a friend.   PmB
    A. *He/she is always nagging me.*   1
    B. *He/she was in a hostile mood.*   0

21. You are penalized for not returning your
    income-tax forms on time.   PmB
    A. *I always put off doing my taxes.*   1
    B. *I was lazy about getting my taxes done this year.*   0

22. You ask a person out on a date and he/she says no.   PvB
    A. *I was a wreck that day.*   1
    B. *I got tongue-tied when I asked him/her on the date.*   0

23. A game-show host picks you out of the audience to
participate in the show. PsG
    A. *I was sitting in the right seat.* 0
    B. *I looked the most enthusiastic.* 1

24. You are frequently asked to dance at a party. PmG
    A. *I am outgoing at parties.* 1
    B. *I was in perfect form that night.* 0

25. You buy your spouse (boyfriend/girlfriend) a gift
he/she doesn't like. PsB
    A. *I don't put enough thought into things like that.* 1
    B. *He/she has very picky tastes.* 0

26. You do exceptionally well in a job interview. PmG
    A. *I felt extremely confident during the interview.* 0
    B. *I interview well.* 1

27. You tell a joke and everyone laughs. PsG
    A. *The joke was funny.* 0
    B. *My timing was perfect.* 1

28. Your boss gives you too little time in which to finish
a project, but you get it finished anyway. PvG
    A. *I am good at my job.* 0
    B. *I am an efficient person.* 1

29. You've been feeling run-down lately. PmB
    A. *I never get a chance to relax.* 1
    B. *I was exceptionally busy this week.* 0

30. You ask someone to dance and he/she says no. PsB
    A. *I am not a good enough dancer.* 1
    B. *He/she doesn't like to dance.* 0

31. You save a person from choking to death. PvG
    A. *I know a technique to stop someone from choking.* 0
    B. *I know what to do in crisis situations.* 1

32. Your romantic partner wants to cool things off for a while.   PvB
    A. *I'm too self-centered.*   1
    B. *I don't spend enough time with him/her.*   0

33. A friend says something that hurts your feelings.   PmB
    A. *She always blurts things out without thinking of others.*   1
    B. *My friend was in a bad mood and took it out on me.*   0

34. Your employer comes to you for advice.   PvG
    A. *I am an expert in the area about which I was asked.*   0
    B. *I'm good at giving useful advice.*   1

35. A friend thanks you for helping him/her get through
    a bad time.   PvG
    A. *I enjoy helping him/her through tough times.*   0
    B. *I care about people.*   1

36. You have a wonderful time at a party.   PsG
    A. *Everyone was friendly.*   0
    B. *I was friendly.*   1

37. Your doctor tells you that you are in good physical shape.   PvG
    A. *I make sure I exercise frequently.*   0
    B. *I am very health-conscious.*   1

38. Your spouse (boyfriend/girlfriend) takes you away for
    a romantic weekend.   PmG
    A. *He/she needed to get away for a few days.*   0
    B. *He/she likes to explore new areas.*   1

39. Your doctor tells you that you eat too much sugar.   PsB
    A. *I don't pay much attention to my diet.*   1
    B. *You can't avoid sugar, it's in everything.*   0

40. You are asked to head an important project.   PmG
    A. *I just successfully completed a similar project.*   0
    B. *I am a good supervisor.*   1

41. You and your spouse (boyfriend/girlfriend) have been
    fighting a great deal.   PsB
    A. *I have been feeling cranky and pressured lately.*   1
    B. *He/she has been hostile lately.*   0

42. You fall down a great deal while skiing.   PmB
    A. *Skiing is difficult.*   1
    B. *The trails were icy.*   0

43. You win a prestigious award.   PvG
    A. *I solved an important problem.*   0
    B. *I was the best employee.*   1

44. Your stocks are at an all-time low.   PvB
    A. *I didn't know much about the business climate at
       the time.*   1
    B. *I made a poor choice of stocks.*   0

45. You win the lottery.   PsG
    A. *It was pure chance.*   0
    B. *I picked the right numbers.*   1

46. You gain weight over the holidays and you can't lose it.   PmB
    A. *Diets don't work in the long run.*   1
    B. *The diet I tried didn't work.*   0

47. You are in the hospital and few people come to visit.   PsB
    A. *I'm irritable when I am sick.*   1
    B. *My friends are negligent about things like that.*   0

48. They won't honor your credit card at a store.   PvB
    A. *I sometimes overestimate how much money I have.*   1
    B. *I sometimes forget to pay my credit card bill.*   0

SCORING KEY

PmB	_____	PmG	_____
PvB	_____	PvG	_____
PsB	_____	PsG	_____

Total B _____   Total G _____

G – B _____

Interpreting Your Test Results

The test results will give you a clue as to your explanatory style. In other words, the results will tell you about the way in which you explain things to yourself. It tells you your habit of thought. Again, remember that there are no right or wrong answers.

There are three crucial dimensions to your explanatory style: permanence, pervasiveness, and personalization. Each dimension, plus a couple of others, will be scored from your test.

Permanence. When pessimists are faced with challenges or bad events, they view these events as being permanent. In contrast, people who are optimists tend to view the challenges or bad events as temporary. Here are some statements that reflect the subtle differences:

PERMANENT (PESSIMISTIC)	TEMPORARY (OPTIMISTIC)
"My boss is always a jerk."	"My boss is in a bad mood today."
"You never listen."	"You are not listening."
"This bad luck will never stop."	"My luck has got to turn."

To determine how you view bad events, look at the eight items coded PmB (for Permanent Bad): 5, 13, 20, 21, 29, 33, 42, and 46. Each one with a "0" after it is optimistic; each one followed by a "1" is pessimistic. Total the numbers at the right-hand margin of the questions coded PmB, and write the total on the PmB line on the scoring key.

If you totaled 0 or 1, you are very optimistic on this dimension; 2 or 3 is a moderately optimistic score; 4 is average; 5 or 6 is quite pessimistic; and 7 or 8 is extremely pessimistic.

Now let's take a look at the difference in explanatory style between pessimists and optimists when there is a positive event in their lives. It's just the opposite of what happened with a bad event. Pessimists view positive events as temporary, while optimists view them as permanent. Here again are some subtle differences in how pessimists and optimists might communicate their good fortune:

TEMPORARY (PESSIMISTIC)	PERMANENT (OPTIMISTIC)
"It's my lucky day."	"I am always lucky."
"My opponent was off today."	"I am getting better every day."
"I tried hard today."	"I always give my best."

Now total all the questions coded PmG (for Permanent Good): 2, 10, 14, 15, 24, 26, 38, and 40. Write the total on the line in the scoring key marked PmG.

If you totaled 7 or 8, you are very optimistic on this dimension; 6 is a moderately optimistic score; 4 or 5 is average; 3 is pessimistic; and 0, 1, or 2 is extremely pessimistic.

Are you starting to see a pattern? If you are scoring as a pessimist, you may want to learn how to be more optimistic. Your anxiety may be due to your belief that bad things are always going to happen, while good things are only a fluke.

Pervasiveness. Pervasiveness refers to the tendency to describe things either in universals (everyone, always, never, etc.) versus specifics (a specific individual, a specific time, etc.). Pessimists tend to describe things in universals, while optimists describe things in specifics:

UNIVERSAL (PESSIMISTIC)	SPECIFIC (OPTIMISTIC)
"All lawyers are jerks."	"My attorney was a jerk."
"Instruction manuals are worthless."	"This instruction manual is worthless."
"He is repulsive."	"He is repulsive to me."

Total your score for the questions coded PvB (for Pervasive Bad): 8, 17, 18, 22, 32, 44, and 48. Write the total on the PvB line.

If you totaled 0 or 1, you are very optimistic on this dimension; 2 or 3 is a moderately optimistic score; 4 is average; 5 or 6 is quite pessimistic; and 7 or 8 is extremely pessimistic.

Now let's look at the level of pervasiveness of good events. Optimists tend to view good events as universal, while pessimists view them as specific. Again, it's just the opposite of how each views a bad event.

Total your score for the questions coded PvG (for Pervasive Good): 6, 7, 28, 31, 34, 35, 37, and 43. Write the total on the line labeled PvG.

If you totaled 7 or 8, you are very optimistic on this dimension; 6 is a moderately optimistic score; 4 or 5 is average; 3 is pessimistic; and 0, 1, or 2 is extremely pessimistic.

Hope. Our level of hope or hopelessness is determined by our combined level of permanence and pervasiveness. Your level of hope may be the most significant score for this test. Take your PvB and add it to your PmB score. This is your hope score.

If it is 0, 1, or 2, you are extraordinarily hopeful; 3, 4, 5, or 6 is a moderately hopeful score; 7 or 8 is average; 9, 10, or 11 is moderately hopeless; and 12, 13, 14, 15, or 16 is severely hopeless.

People who make permanent and universal explanations for their troubles tend to suffer from stress, anxiety, and depression; they tend to collapse when things go wrong. According to Dr. Seligman, no other score is as important as your hope score.

Personalization. The final aspect of explanatory style is personalization. When bad things happen, we can either blame ourselves (internalize) and lower our self-esteem as a consequence, or we can blame things beyond our control (externalize). Although it may not be right to deny personal responsibility, people who tend to externalize blame in relation to bad events have higher self-esteem and are more optimistic.

Total your score for those questions coded PsB (for Personalization Bad): 3, 9, 16, 19, 25, 30, 39, 41, and 47. Write the total on the PsB line.

A score of 0 or 1 indicates very high self-esteem and optimism; 2 or 3 indicates moderate self-esteem; 4 is average; 5 or 6 indicates moderately low self-esteem; and 7 or 8 indicates very low self-esteem.

Now let's take a look at personalization and good events. Again, just the exact opposite occurs compared with bad events. When good things happen, the person with high self-esteem internalizes, while the person with low self-esteem externalizes.

Total your score for those questions coded PsG (for Personalization Good): 1, 4, 11, 12, 23, 27, 36, and 45. Write your score on the line marked PsG on your scoring key.

If you totaled 7 or 8, you are very optimistic on this dimension; 6 is a moderately optimistic score; 4 or 5 is average; 3 is pessimistic; and 0, 1, or 2 is extremely pessimistic.

Your Overall Scores. To compute your overall scores, first add the three B's (PmB + PvB + PsB). This is your B (bad event) score. Do the same for all of the G's (PmG + PvG + PsG). This is your G score. Subtract B from G; this is your overall score.

If your B score is from 3 to 6, you are marvelously optimistic when bad events occur; 10 or 11 is average; 12 to 14 is pessimistic; anything above 14 is extremely pessimistic.

If your G score is 19 or above, you think about good events extremely optimistically; 14 to 16 is average; 11 to 13 indicates pessimism; and a score of 10 or less indicates great pessimism.

If your overall score (G minus B) is above 8, you are very optimistic across the board; if it's from 6 to 8, you are moderately optimistic; 3 to 5 is average; 1 or 2 is pessimistic; and a score of 0 or below is very pessimistic.

Seven Steps to Creating an Effective Exercise Routine

Step 1. Recognize the Importance of Physical Exercise

The first step is realizing just how important it is to get regular exercise. We cannot stress enough just how vital regular exercise is to your health. But as much as we stress this fact, it means nothing unless it really sinks in and you accept it, too. You must make regular exercise a top priority in your life.

Step 2. Consult Your Physician

If you are not currently on a regular exercise program, get medical clearance if you have health problems or if you are over forty years of age. The main concern is the functioning of your heart. Exercise can be quite harmful (and even fatal) if your heart is not able to meet the increased demands placed on it.

It is especially important to see a physician if any of the following applies to you:

- Heart disease
- Smoking
- High blood pressure
- Extreme breathlessness with physical exertion
- Pain or pressure in chest, arm, teeth, jaw, or neck with exercise
- Dizziness or fainting
- Abnormal heart action (palpitations or irregular beat)

Step 3. Select an Activity You Enjoy

If you are fit enough to begin, the next thing to do is select an activity that you will enjoy. Using the list below, choose from one to five of the activities that you think you may enjoy—or fill in a choice or two of your own. Make a commitment to do one activity a day for at least 20 minutes, and preferably an hour. Make your goal be to enjoy the activity. The important thing is to move your body enough to raise your pulse a bit above its resting rate.

Bicycling	Jogging
Bowling	Stair climbing
Cross-country skiing	Stationary bicycling
Dancing	Swimming
Gardening	Tennis
Golfing	Treadmill
Heavy housecleaning	Walking
Jazzercise	Weight lifting

In general, the best exercises are the ones that get your heart moving. Aerobic activities such as walking briskly, jogging, bicycling, cross-country skiing, swimming, aerobic dance, and racquet sports are good examples. Brisk walking (4 to 5 miles per hour) for approximately 30 minutes may be the very best form of exercise for most people. Walking can be done anywhere, and the risk of injury is extremely low. It doesn't require any expensive equipment—just comfortable clothing and well-fitting shoes. If you are going to walk on a regular basis, we strongly urge you to first purchase a pair of high-quality walking or jogging shoes. They will not only make walking more enjoyable and comfortable but also reduce the risk of injury.

Step 4. Monitor Exercise Intensity

Exercise intensity is determined by measuring your heart rate (the number of times your heart beats per minute). This determination can quickly be made by placing the index and middle fingers of one hand on your opposite wrist, or on the side of your neck just below the angle of your jaw. Beginning with zero, count the number of heartbeats for six seconds. Simply add a zero to this number, and you have your pulse rate. For example, if you counted fourteen beats, your heart rate would be 140.

Would this be a good number? It depends on your "training zone." A quick and easy way to determine your maximum training heart rate is to simply subtract your age from 185. For example, if you are 40 years old, your maximum heart rate would be 145. To determine the bottom of the training zone, simply subtract 20 from this number. In the case of a 40-year-old, this would be 125. So the training range for a 40-year-old would be between 125 and 145 beats per minute. For maximum health benefits, you must stay within your training zone or range and never exceed it.

Step 5. Do It Often

You don't get in good physical condition by exercising once; it must be done on a regular basis. A minimum of 15 to 20 minutes of exercising at your training heart rate at least three times a week is necessary to gain any significant cardiovascular benefits. It is better to exercise at the lower end of your training zone for longer periods of time than it is to exercise at a higher intensity for a shorter period of time. It is also better if you can make exercise a part of your daily routine.

Step 6. Make It Fun

The key to getting the maximum benefit from exercise is to make it enjoyable. Choose an activity that you enjoy and have fun with. If you can find enjoyment in exercise, you are much more likely to exercise regularly. One way to make it fun is to get a workout partner. For example, if you choose walking as your activity, here is a great way to make it fun:

Find one or two people in your neighborhood whom you would enjoy walking with. If you are meeting others, you will certainly be more regular than if you depend solely on your own intentions. Commit to walking three to five mornings or afternoons each week, and increase the exercise duration from an initial 10 minutes to at least 30 minutes.

Step 7. Stay Motivated

No matter how committed you are to regular exercise, at some point in time you are going to be faced with a loss of enthusiasm for working out. Here is a suggestion: take a break. Not a long break; just skip one or two workouts. It gives your enthusiasm and motivation a chance to recoup, so that you can come back with an even stronger commitment. Here are some other things to help you to stay motivated:

- Read or thumb through fitness magazines like *Shape, Runner's World, Men's Fitness, Muscle & Fitness,* and *Muscular Development.* Looking at pictures of people in fantastic shape is really inspiring. In addition, these magazines typically feature articles on interesting new exercise routines.
- Set exercise goals. Goals really help keep you motivated. Success breeds success, so set a lot of small goals that can easily be achieved. Write down your daily exercise goal, and check it off when you have it completed. Vary your routine. Variety is important to help you stay interested in exercise. Doing the same thing every day becomes monotonous and drains motivation. Continually find new ways to enjoy working out.
- Keep a record of your activities and progress. Sometimes it is hard to see the progress you are making, but if you write in a journal, you'll have a permanent record of your progress. Keeping track of your progress will motivate you to continued improvement.

Insurance issues

Without insurance, most people would be unable to pay for cancer therapies, which—no surprise here—can be extremely expensive. (Some of the newer biological therapies can cost $3,000 to $10,000 per week.) Getting and using insurance coverage is complicated because so many entities are involved. The federal government, state governments, employers, unions, and insurance companies themselves all have a say in insurance policies, and the levels of bureaucracy can be intimidating. We are naturopathic physicians, not insurance brokers, so we don't have all the answers. But we can suggest a few things to consider concerning your policy.

First of all, confirm that you do have insurance coverage. Become familiar with the terms of your policy. Pay attention to details—time limits for filing claims, deadlines for dispute resolution, and so on. If you need to speak with someone about your insurance policy, make note of names and dates, and keep a record of what you spoke about. Some people find it convenient to use a spiral or loose-leaf notebook or to keep track of their files on a computer or personal digital assistant such as a PalmPilot.

Keep a record of all your contacts, as well as copies of all bills and other documents to confirm their accuracy. Be sure to address any overcharges or duplicate billings. Knowing how much you spend is important, because many policies set lifetime limits for certain treatments. You don't want to reach that limit too soon because of accounting errors (which, alas, are all too common).

If you are unfortunate enough to receive a diagnosis of cancer while uninsured, it can be very difficult to get a policy. In such cases, consider applying for coverage under one or more government assistance programs such as Medicaid. Also explore getting coverage under a group policy through work or an organization you belong to, such as a union or professional society. It's also possible to be covered under a spouse's workplace insurance policy.

Many policies will have a pre-existing condition clause that limits coverage for a condition present at the time the policy was put into place. This limitation may be for a brief period of several months or may be indefinite. Consider this when looking into changes of coverage. Sometimes even switching policies within the same company can trigger this clause, so consult carefully with your agent.

Workplace insurance will usually cover you only for the time you are actually employed. If illness forces you to stop work, try to get a temporary leave of absence rather than quitting your job, as it may be easier to keep your insurance in effect. There is also a federal law (called COBRA) that allows you to continue your workplace insurance for up to 18 months if you pay the fees out of pocket. Most larger companies or unions have human resource (HR) departments with people who specialize in helping employees with these types of problems. Take advantage of their expertise, because these individuals will know the most about the details of your particular insurance policy terms and state laws.

If you feel that your insurance company is not delivering the coverage it's supposed to provide, contact the ombudsman for the company. Activate the dispute-resolution process for the insurance company. Your company's HR department can act as your advocate. Since that department has a voice in selecting companies for future contracts, it can often get favorable rulings in cases where an individual policyholder would be powerless.

In some cases it may be necessary to seek legal advice. An attorney can often move dispute resolution along faster. If you need to go this route, look for a lawyer who specializes in health care and insurance law. As a last resort, contact your state insurance commissioner; these officials have the authority to enforce insurance laws and regulations.

Complementary Care Costs

Although the situation is different in each state, many insurance companies will not cover services of complementary medicine providers such as naturopathic doctors, acupuncturists, and mental health counselors. In Washington State, where three of the authors of this book practice, state-regulated insurance companies do have to cover the services of naturopathic physicians, but federally regulated policies such as Medicare do not. Even when a naturopath's services are covered, most policies will not pay for natural medicines. Our patients must pay for these out of pocket.

Not surprisingly, we feel this policy is shortsighted, because the use of the natural therapies can reduce the risk of expensive complications and hospitalizations during treatments, potentially saving insurance companies large sums of money. As an example, at the outpatient treatment center in Seattle where one of the authors practice, we rarely have to hospitalize patients for complications, because our approach to integrated therapy seems to protect patients from most of the serious problems that can occur during cancer therapy.

We generally advise our patients that whether insurance pays or not, the benefits of natural medicines are great enough to justify using them, to maximize your chances of full recovery.

Experimental Natural Therapies

Many cancer patients facing a poor prognosis often look to alternative treatments hoping for a "miracle." Sometimes they travel outside the country (usually to Mexico or Europe) to undergo questionable therapies at the hands of practitioners who have little or no medical expertise. If you elect to go outside the country for treatment, make sure the clinic is run by well-trained and reputable physicians.

In our experience, and in our reading of the scientific literature, there is encouraging evidence that three experimental treatments may ultimately prove to be worthwhile. These therapies are antineoplastons, mistletoe preparations, and Ukrain.

Antineoplastons

Antineoplastons are a group of synthetic compounds that were originally isolated from human blood and urine by Stanislaw Burzynski, M.D., Ph.D., in Houston. Dr. Burzynski has used antineoplastons to treat patients with a variety of cancers. In 1991, the National Cancer Institute (NCI) conducted a review to evaluate the clinical responses in a group of patients treated with antineoplastons at the Burzynski Research Institute in Houston.

The investigators studied the medical records of seven patients with brain tumors who appeared to benefit from antineoplaston therapy. Because they found some evidence of antitumor activity, the NCI recommended conducting formal clinical trials. These NCI-sponsored studies began in 1993 at the Memorial Sloan-Kettering Cancer Center, the

Mayo Clinic, and the Warren Grant Magnuson Clinical Center at the National Institutes of Health. But two years later, only nine patients had been recruited. The researchers and Dr. Burzynski could not agree on a strategy for improving recruitment, so the studies were shut down. As a result, no definitive conclusions can be drawn at this time about the effectiveness of treatment with antineoplastons. The most promising preliminary evidence is in the use of antineoplastons for brain tumors. At this time we cannot recommend their use for other types of cancers.

The Burzynski Research Institute is currently conducting trials using antineoplastons for a variety of cancers. Unfortunately, treatment requires going to Houston and can be extremely expensive. Information about these trials is available from the Cancer Information Service or on the Internet at http://cancertrials.nci.nih.gov. You can also contact the Burzynski Clinic directly:

The Burzynski Clinic
9432 Old Katy Road, Suite 200
Houston, TX 77055
Phone: 713-335-5697
Fax: 713-335-5699
E-mail: info@burzynskiclinic.com

Mistletoe Preparations

Mistletoe is a parasitic plant that has been used since ancient times to treat a variety of human ailments. Extracts of mistletoe have been shown to kill cancer cells in the laboratory and to stimulate the immune system in both animals and humans. Three components of mistletoe (lectins, alkaloids, and viscotoxins) may be responsible for its biologic effects.

In Europe, commercially available products have been used clinically for the treatment of cancer since 1926 when Iscador, a fermented product made from the crude pressed juice of mistletoe, was introduced. Currently, there are several mistletoe preparations being used in addition to Iscador, including the nonfermented preparations Eurixor, Helixor, Isorel, Vysorel, and ABNOBAviscum. These new-generation unfermented mistletoe preparations contain standardized concentrations of an active ingredient, mistletoe lectin-1 (ML1), to ensure consistent potency and activity. None of these preparations is sold commercially in the United States.

We must stress that mistletoe plants and berries are toxic to humans and should never be used (see Warning box). Furthermore, in the clinical studies, mistletoe preparations have been administered by intramuscular injection, subcutaneous injection (sometimes in the vicinity of a tumor), or intravenous infusion. The mistletoe compounds apparently responsible for the anticancer effects do not seem to be absorbed orally.

Warning

Oral preparations of mistletoe can be very toxic. Adverse effects at lower dosages include low blood pressure and a slowing of the heart rate. At higher levels, adverse effects can include hallucinations, delirium, hypertension, gastroenteritis, nausea, vomiting, and diarrhea. At toxic levels, adverse effects include bursting of red blood cells (hemolysis), hemorrhage, convulsions, and even death.

Cases of fatal poisoning have resulted from eating the leaves or berries of mistletoe plants. This is a special problem with children, who may be drawn to the bright red berries and who are more susceptible to the toxins. Never use real mistletoe for holiday decorations, especially if children or pets are present.

We believe that eventually one or more of these newer mistletoe preparations will be approved for use in the United States. There's a growing body of scientific evidence showing that mistletoe may be effective in a variety of cancers, including breast cancer. In these studies, mistletoe increased the levels of several white blood cell types, raised the level of immune system activators in the blood, and induced apoptosis (cell death) in tumors. Although mistletoe can be toxic, there appears to be a lower risk of side effects than with some conventional therapies, and treatment has been associated with a higher quality of life (as determined by use of a standardized questionnaire). Common side effects found with mistletoe injection include soreness and inflammation at the injection site, headache, fever, and chills.

Ukrain

Ukrain is a derivative of alkaloids from the plant called greater celandine *(Chelidonium majus)*. Numerous scientific tests have demonstrated that the preparation destroys cancer cells through apoptosis without attacking healthy cells. Like mistletoe preparations, Ukrain is given via injection.

More than 120 scientific papers from 16 countries have found evidence that Ukrain offers benefits as a cancer therapy. In laboratory studies, researchers from the NCI demonstrated that Ukrain exhibits significant anticancer activity against all sixty human cancer cell lines tested from eight main cancer types (brain, ovary, colon, and kidney carcinomas; small-cell and non-small-cell lung carcinomas; melanoma; leukemia; and lymphoma). Clinical studies in several types of cancer, most notably breast cancer, have shown that Ukrain may cause tumor regression, prevent metastases, and prolong and improve the quality of life. For a current list of scientific articles on Ukrain, see www.ukrin. com. *[sic]*

Ukrain is not available for use in the United States, although approval currently is being sought here and in several European countries and in Australia.

Resources

Acupuncture

Accreditation Commission for Acupuncture
and Oriental Medicine (ACAOM)
7501 Greenway Center Drive, Suite 820
Greenbelt, MD 20770
301-313-0855, fax: 301-313-0912
www.ACAOM.org

American Association of Oriental Medicine (AAOM)
433 Front Street
Catasauqua, PA 18032
610-266-1433
www.aaom.org

Council of Colleges of Acupuncture and Oriental Medicine
(CCAOM)
7501 Greenway Center Drive, Suite 820
Greenbelt, MD 20770
301-313-0868
www.CCAOM.org

Cancer Centers

Cancer Treatment Centers of America (CTCA)
Web site: www.cancercenter.com. Two of the authors, Drs. Birdsall and Reilly, are key physicians at Cancer Treatment Centers of America. Currently, there are five centers coast to coast (Zion, IL; Tulsa, OK; Hampton Roads, VA; Seattle, WA; and Goshen, IN) that accommodate over 60,000 patient visits annually. For over ten years, CTCA has combined complementary and alternative medicine (CAM)—including naturopathic medicine, therapeutic nutrition, herbal medicine, mind-body approaches, massage, exercise and physical therapies, and spiritual care—with leading-edge conventional oncology care. For more information, visit their Web site or call 800-342-3810.

The National Comprehensive Cancer Network (NCCN)

Web site: www.nccn.org. The NCCN is an alliance of the world's leading cancer centers. The members include:

City of Hope National Medical Center
Los Angeles, California
800-359-8111
www.cityofhope.org

Dana-Farber/Partners CancerCare
Boston, Massachusetts
800-320-0022
www.dana-farber.org

Duke Comprehensive Cancer Center
Durham, North Carolina
888-275-3853 (888-ASK-DUKE)
www.cancer.duke.edu

Fred Hutchinson Cancer Research Center
Seattle, Washington
800-804-8824
www.fhcrc.org

MD Anderson Cancer Center
The University of Texas
Houston, Texas
800-392-1611
www.mdanderson.org

Memorial Sloan-Kettering Cancer Center
New York, New York
800-525-2225
www.mskcc.org

St. Jude Children's Research Hospital
Memphis, Tennessee
901-495-3306
www.stjude.org

The Sidney Kimmel Comprehensive Cancer Center at Johns
  Hopkins
600 North Wolfe Street
Baltimore, Maryland 21287-8943
410-955-8964
www.hopkinscancercenter.org

Stanford Hospital and Clinics
Stanford, California
877-668-7535
www.cancer.stanfordhospital.com

UCSF Comprehensive Cancer Center
Clinical Cancer Program
San Francisco, California
800-888-8664
http://cc.ucsf.edu

University of Michigan Comprehensive Cancer Center
Ann Arbor, Michigan
800-865-1125
www.cancer.med.umich.edu

NCI Cancer Centers Program

Web site: www3.cancer.gov/cancercenters. The Cancer Centers Program of the NCI supports major academic and research institutions throughout the United States to sustain broad-based, coordinated, interdisciplinary programs in cancer research. Currently, there are thirty-seven centers nationwide designated as Comprehensive Cancer Research Centers. To find the nearest major center, go to the Web site.

Cancer Organizations

American Cancer Society (ACS)

Web site: www.cancer.org. The American Cancer Society (ACS) is a nationwide, community-based voluntary health organization. Headquartered in Atlanta, the ACS has state divisions and more than 3400 local offices. The ACS Web site provides a plethora of information for patients, family members, and professionals.

National Cancer Institute (NCI)

This is the federal government's principal agency for cancer research. Web site: cancernet.nci.nih.gov. You will find information on types of cancer, treatment, clinical trials, genetics, causes, risk factors, prevention, testing, coping, and more. If you can't locate the cancer information you need, you can also call the NCI's Cancer Information Service, toll-free, to speak with a trained information specialist (Monday through Friday, 9:00 A.M. to 4:30 P.M., EST) at 800-4-CANCER (800-422-6237) or (TTY: 800-332-8615).

Web site: www.clinicaltrials.gov. Provides the latest information on current studies on virtually all types of cancer.

The National Coalition for Cancer Survivorship

Web site: www.cansearch.org. The National Coalition for Cancer Survivorship is a patient-led advocacy organization working on behalf of people with all types of cancer and their families.

Diet and Nutrition Web Sites

National Cancer Institute
Web site: www.5aday.gov

Oldways
Web site: www.olwayspt.org

Faith, Prayer, and Spirituality in Medicine

Bastyr University
Department of Spirituality in Health and Medicine
14500 Juanita Drive
Kenmore, WA 98028
425-602-3000
Web site: www.bastyr.edu

International Center for the Integration of Health and Spirituality
(ICIHS)
6110 Executive Boulevard, Suite 680
Rockville, MD 20852
Web site: www.nihr.com

Spindrift
2407 La Jolla Drive NW
Salem, OR 97304
Web site: www.home.xnet.com/~spindrif/index.htm

Guided Imagery

The Academy for Guided Imagery
P.O. Box 2070
Mill Valley, CA 94942
800-726-2070
Web site: www.interactiveimagery.com.

Innervisions Studio
Web site: www.innervisionstudioinc.com

Health Food Store Locator

The National Nutritional Foods Association (NNFA)

Web site: www.nnfa.org. The NNFA, founded in 1936, represents the manufacturers and retailers of the natural foods industry. To find a health food store retailer in your area, go to the NNFA Web site.

Naturopathic Medical Schools

Bastyr University
14500 Juanita Drive
Kenmore, WA 98028
425-602-3000
Web site: www.bastyr.edu

Canadian College of Naturopathic Medicine
1255 Sheppard Avenue East
North York, Ontario M2K 1E2
Canada
416-498-1255
Web site: www.ccnm.edu

National College of Naturopathic Medicine
049 S.W. Porter
Portland, OR 97201
503-499-4343
Web site: www.ncnm.edu

Southwest College of Naturopathic Medicine & Health Sciences
2140 E. Broadway Road
Tempe, AZ 85282
480-858-9100
Web site: www.scnm.edu

Naturopathic Physician Associations and Referrals

The American Association of Naturopathic Physicians
8201 Greensboro Drive, Suite 300
McLean, VA 22102
877-969-2267
Web site: www.naturopathic.org

Canadian Naturopathic Association
1255 Sheppard Avenue East
North York, Ontario M2K 1E2
Canada
416-496-8633
Web site: www.naturopathicassoc.ca

Psychoneuroimmunology

The PsychoNeuroImmunology Research Society
Web site: www.pnirs.org

Qi Gong

Qi Gong Association of America
Web site: www.qi.org

Reiki

International Association of Reiki Professionals
P.O. Box 481
Winchester, MA 01890
781-729-3530
Web site: www.iarp.org

Tai Chi

EasyTai Chi
Web site: www.easytaichi.com

Work-Related Issues

Equal Employment Opportunity Commission
800-669-3362
Web site: www.eeoc.gov

References and Notes

The references provided are by no means designed to represent a complete reference list for all of the studies reviewed or mentioned in *How to Prevent and Treat Cancer with Natural Medicine*. We have chosen to focus on key studies and comprehensive review articles. In general, these sorts of scientific references are usually of value only to health care professionals.

In addition to finding the articles listed here useful, we encourage interested parties to access the Internet site for the National Library of Medicine (NLM): gateway.nlm.nih.gov for additional studies.

The NLM Gateway is a Web-based system that lets users search simultaneously in multiple retrieval systems at the NLM. From this site, you can access all of the NLM databases, including the PubMed database. This database was developed in conjunction with publishers of biomedical literature as a search tool for accessing literature citations and linking to full-text journal articles at Web sites of participating publishers. Publishers participating in PubMed electronically supply the NLM with their citations prior to or at the time of publication. If the publisher has a Web site that offers full text of its journals, PubMed provides links to that site as well as sites to other biological data, sequence centers, and the like. User registration, a subscription fee, or some other type of fee may be required to access the full text of articles in some journals.

PubMed provides access to bibliographic information, which includes MEDLINE—the NLM's premier bibliographic database covering the fields of medicine, nursing, dentistry, veterinary medicine, the health care system, and the preclinical sciences. MEDLINE contains bibliographic citations and author abstracts from more than 4,000 medical journals published in the United States and in seventy other countries. The file contains over 11 million citations, dating back to the mid-1960s. Coverage is worldwide, but most records are from English-language sources or have English abstracts (summaries). Conducting a search is quite easy, and the site has a link to a tutorial that fully explains the process.

Another valuable resource for professionals as well as the public is the Web site of the National Cancer Institute (NCI), the federal government's principal agency for cancer research: http://cancernet.nci.nih.gov. You will find on this site information on types of cancer, treatment, clinical trials, genetics, causes, risk factors, prevention, testing, coping, and more. If you can't locate the cancer information you need, you can also call the NCI's Cancer Information Service, toll-free, to speak with a trained information Specialist (Monday through Friday, 9:00 A.M. to 4:30 P.M., EST) at 800-4-CANCER (800-422-6237) or TTY: 800-332-8615.

Finally, in regard to the discussion of conventional aspects of cancer—such as basic features, statistics, epidemiology, risk factors, and conventional treatments—we utilized mainstream oncology texts.

Chapter 1. An Ounce of Prevention
1. Lash TL, Aschengrau A. Active and passive cigarette smoking and the occurrence of breast cancer. Am J Epidemiol 1999;149:5–12.
2. Caplan LS, Schoenfeld ER, O'Leary ES, Leske MC. Breast cancer and electromagnetic fields—a review. Ann Epidemiol 2000;10(1):31–44.
3. Terry P, Lichtenstein P, Feychting M, Ahlbom A, Wolk A. Fatty fish consumption and risk of prostate cancer. Lancet 2001;357(9270):1764–66.
4. Singh PN, Fraser GE. Dietary risk factors for colon cancer in a low-risk population. Am J Epidemiol 1998;148:761–74.
5. Zheng W, Gustafson DR, Sinha R, et al. Well-done meat intake and the risk of breast cancer. J Natl Cancer Inst 1998;90:1724–29.
6. Terry P, Giovannucci E, Michels KB, et al. Fruit, vegetables, dietary fiber, and risk of colorectal cancer. J Natl Cancer Inst 2001;93:525–33.
7. Silverman DT, Swanson CA, Gridley G, et al. Dietary and nutritional factors and pancreatic cancer: a case-control study based on direct interviews. J Natl Cancer Inst 1998;90:1710–19.
8. Zhang S, Folsom AR, Sellers TA, Kushi LH, Potter JD. Breast cancer survival for postmenopausal women who are less overweight and eat less fat. Cancer 1995;76:275–83.

9. Slattery ML, Benson J, Berry TD, et al. Dietary sugar and colon cancer. Cancer Epidemiol Biomarkers Prev 1997;6(9):677–85.

10. Levi F, Pasche C, La Vecchia C, Lucchini F, Franceschi S. Food groups and colorectal cancer risk. Br J Cancer 1999;79:1283–87.

11. Franceschi S, Dal Maso L, Augustin L, et al. Dietary glycemic load and colorectal cancer risk. Ann Oncol 2001;12:173–78.

12. Penninx BW, Guralnik JM, Pahor M, et al. Chronically depressed mood and cancer risk in older persons. J Natl Cancer Inst 1998;90:1888–93.

13. Bruske-Hohlfeld I, Mohner M, Ahrens W, et al. Lung cancer risk in male workers occupationally exposed to diesel motor emissions in Germany. Am J Ind Med 1999;36:405–14.

14. Johnson K. Dairy products linked to ovarian cancer risk. Family Practice News, June 15, 2000:8.

15. Chan JM, Giovannucci EL. Dairy products, calcium, phosphorus, vitamin D, and risk of prostate cancer. Cancer Causes and Control 1998;9:559–66.

16. Levi F, Pasche C, La Vecchia C, Lucchini F, Franceschi S. Food groups and colorectal cancer risk. Br J Cancer 1999;79:1283–87.

17. La Vecchia C, Favero A, Franceschi S. Monounsaturated and other types of fat, and the risk of breast cancer. Eur J Cancer Prev 1998;7:461–64.

18. Zhong L, Goldberg MS, Gao YT, Jin F. Lung cancer and indoor air pollution arising from Chinese-style cooking among nonsmoking women living in Shanghai, China. Epidemiology 1999;10:488–94.

19. Prescott E, Gronbaek M, Becker U, Sorensen TI. Alcohol intake and the risk of lung cancer: influence of type of alcoholic beverage. Am J Epidemiol 1999;149:463–70.

20. Garland M, Hunter DJ, Colditz GA, et al. Alcohol consumption in relation to breast cancer risk in a cohort of United States women 25–42 years of age. Cancer Epidemiol Biomarkers Prev 1999;8:1017–21.

21. Mannisto S, Virtanen M, Kataja V, Uusitupa M, Pietinen P. Lifetime alcohol consumption and breast cancer: a case-control study in Finland. Public Health Nutr 2000;3:11–18.

22. Giovannucci EL, Stampfer MJ, Colditz GA, et al. Multivitamin use, folate, and colon cancer in women in the Nurses' Health Study. Ann Intern Med 1998;129(7):517–24.

23. Michaud DS, Spiegelman D, Clinton SK, et al. Fluid intake and the risk of bladder cancer in men. New Engl J Med 1999;340:1390–97.

24. Combs GF Jr, Clark LC, Turnbull BW. Reduction of cancer risk with an oral supplement of selenium. Biomed Environ Sci 1997;10:227–34.

25. Bougnoux P. N-3 polyunsaturated fatty acids and cancer. Curr Opin Clin Nutr Metab Care 1999;2:121–26.

26. van Poppel G, Verhoeven DT, Verhagen H, Goldbohm RA. Brassica vegetables and cancer prevention. Epidemiology and mechanisms. Adv Exp Med Biol 1999;472:159–68.

27. Michaud DS, Spiegelman D, Clinton SK, et al. Fruit and vegetable intake and incidence of bladder cancer in a male prospective cohort. J Natl Cancer Inst 1999;91:605–13.

28. Jacobsen BK, Knutsen SF, Fraser GE. Does high soymilk intake reduce prostate cancer incidence? The Adventist Health Study (United States). Cancer Causes and Control 1998;9:553–57.

29. Messina MJ. Legumes and soybeans: overview of their nutritional profiles and health effects. Am J Clin Nutr 1999;70(Suppl. 3):439S–50S.

30. Kristal AR, Stanford JL, Cohen JH, Wicklund K, Patterson RE. Vitamin and mineral supplement use is associated with reduced risk of prostate cancer. Cancer Epidemiol Biomarkers Prev 1999;8:887–92.

31. Hardman AE. Physical activity and cancer risk. Proc Nutr Soc 2001;60(1):107–13.

32. Cohen JH, Kristal AR, Stanford JL. Fruit and vegetable intakes and prostate cancer risk. J Natl Cancer Inst 2000;92(1):61–68.

33. Clinton SK. The dietary antioxidant network and prostate carcinoma. Cancer 1999;86:1629–31.

34. Michaud DS, Spiegelman D, Clinton SK, et al. Prospective study of dietary supplements, macronutrients, micronutrients, and risk of bladder cancer in US men. Am J Epidemiol 2000;152:1145–53.

35. Inoue M, Tajima K, Mizutani M, et al. Regular consumption of green tea and the risk of breast cancer recurrence: follow-up study from the Hospital-based Epidemiologic Research Program at Aichi Cancer Center (HERPACC), Japan. Cancer Lett 2001;167:175–82.

36. Setiawan VW, Zhang ZF, Yu GP, et al. Protective effect of green tea on the risks of chronic gastritis and stomach cancer. Int J Cancer 2001;92:600–4.

37. Nakachi K, Matsuyama S, Miyake S, Suganuma M, Imai K. Preventive effects of drinking green tea on cancer and cardiovascular disease: epidemiological evidence for multiple targeting prevention. Biofactors 2000;13:49–54.

38. Fleischauer AT, Poole C, Arab L. Garlic consumption and cancer prevention: meta-analyses of colorectal and stomach cancers. Am J Clin Nutr 2000;72:1047–52.

39. German JB, Walzem RL. The health benefits of wine. Annu Rev Nutr 2000;20:561–93.

40. Greenlee RT, Murray T, Bolden S, Wingo PA. Cancer Statistics 2000. CA Cancer J Clin 2000;50:7–33.

41. Hackshaw AK, Law MR, Wald NJ. The accumulated evidence on lung cancer and environmental tobacco smoke. BMJ 1997;315:980–88.

42. Thune I, Furberg AS. Physical activity and cancer risk: dose-response and cancer, all sites and site-specific. Med Sci Sports Exerc 2001;33(Suppl. 6): 530S–50S.

43. Hardman AE. Physical activity and cancer risk. Proc Nutr Soc 2001; 60(1):107–13.

44. Segerstrom SC. Personality and the immune system: models, methods, and mechanisms. Ann Behav Med 2000;22:180–90.

45. Imai K, Nakachi K. Personality types, lifestyle, and sensitivity to mental stress in association with NK activity. Int J Hyg Environ Health 2001; 204:67–73.

46. Sturm R, Wells KB. Does obesity contribute as much to morbidity as poverty or smoking? Public Health 2001;115:229–35.

Chapter 2. Seven Tips for Creating an Environment
That Is Hostile to Cancer

1. Steinmetz KA, Potter JD. Vegetables, fruit, and cancer prevention: a review. J Am Diet Assoc 1996;96:1027–39.

2. La Vecchia C, Tavani A. Fruit and vegetables, and human cancer. Eur J Cancer Prev 1998;7:3–8.

3. Van Duyn MA, Pivonka E. Overview of the health benefits of fruit and vegetable consumption for the dietetics professional: selected literature. J Am Diet Assoc 2000;100(12):1511–21.

4. Eaton SB, Konner M. Paleolithic nutrition. A consideration of its nature and current implications. New Engl J Med 1985;312:283–89.

5. Ryde D. What should humans eat? Practitioner 1985;232:415–18.

6. Steinmetz KA, Potter JD: Vegetables, fruit, and cancer. II. Mechanisms. Cancer Causes and Control 1991;2:427–42.

7. Krinsky NI. The antioxidant and biological properties of the carotenoids. Ann NY Acad Sci 1998;854:443–47.

8. Rao AV, Agarwal S. Role of antioxidant lycopene in cancer and heart disease. J Am Coll Nutr 2000;19(5):563–69.

9. Johnston CS, Taylor CA, Hampl JS. More Americans are eating "5 a day" but intakes of dark green and cruciferous vegetables remain low. J Nutr 2000;130(12):3063.

10. Xue H, Aziz RM, Sun N, et al. Inhibition of cellular transformation by berry extracts. Carcinogenesis 2001;22(2):351–56.

11. Lin SS, Hung CF, Ho CC, et al. Effects of ellagic acid by oral administration on N-acetylation and metabolism of 2-aminofluorene in rat brain tissues. Neurochem Res 2000;25(11):1503–8.

12. Barch DH, Rundhaugen LM, Stoner GD, et al. Structure-function rela-

tionships of the dietary anticarcinogen ellagic acid. Carcinogenesis 1996; 17(2):265–69.

13. de Ancos B, Gonzalez EM, Cano MP. Ellagic acid, vitamin C, and total phenolic contents and radical scavenging capacity affected by freezing and frozen storage in raspberry fruit. J Agric Food Chem 2000;48(10): 4565–70.

14. Sen CK. Nutritional biochemistry of cellular glutathione. Nutr Biochem 1997;8:660–72.

15. Jones DP, Coates RJ, Flagg EW, et al. Glutathione in foods listed in the National Cancer Institutes Health Habits and History Food Frequency Questionnaire. Nutr Cancer 1995;17:57–75.

16. Witschi A, Reddy S, Stofer B, Lauterburg BH. The systemic availability of oral glutathione. Eur J Clin Pharmacol 1992;43(6):667–69.

17. Johnston CJ, Meyer CG, Srilakshmi JC. Vitamin C elevates red blood cell glutatione in healthy adults. Am J Clin Nutr 1993;58:103–5.

18. Jaga K, Brosius D. Pesticide exposure: human cancers on the horizon. Rev Environ Health 1999;14(1):39–50.

19. Blair A, Zahm SH. Agricultural exposures and cancer. Environ Health Perspect 1995;103(Suppl. 8):205–8.

20. Mao Y, Hu J, Ugnat AM, White K. Non-Hodgkin's lymphoma and occupational exposure to chemicals in Canada. Canadian Cancer Registries Epidemiology Research Group. Ann Oncol 2000;11(Suppl. 1):69–73.

21. Baris D, Zahm SH. Epidemiology of lymphomas. Curr Opin Oncol 2000; 12(5):383–94.

22. Zhang SM, Hunter DJ, Rosner BA, et al. Intakes of fruits, vegetables, and related nutrients and the risk of non-Hodgkin's lymphoma among women. Cancer Epidemiol Biomarkers Prev 2000;9(5):477–85.

23. Zhang S, Hunter DJ, Rosner BA, et al. Dietary fat and protein in relation to risk of non-Hodgkin's lymphoma among women. J Natl Cancer Inst 1999;91(20):1751–58.

24. Tavani A, Pregnolato A, Negri E, et al. Diet and risk of lymphoid neoplasms and soft tissue sarcomas. Nutr Cancer 1997;27(3):256–60.

25. Chiu BC, Cerhan JR, Folsom AR, et al. Diet and risk of non-Hodgkin's lymphoma in older women. JAMA 1996;275(17):1315–21.

26. Falck F, Ricci A, Wolff MS. Pesticides and polychlorinated biphenyl residues in human breast lipids and their relation to breast cancer. Archives of Environmental Health 1992; 47:143–46.

27. Aronson KJ, Miller AB, Woolcott CG, et al. Breast adipose tissue concentrations of polychlorinated biphenyls and other organochlorines and breast cancer risk. Cancer Epidemiol Biomarkers Prev 2000;9:55–63.

28. Fan AM, Jackson RJ. Pesticides and food safety. Regulatory Toxicol Pharmacol 1989;9:158–74.

29. Bingham SA. High-meat diets and cancer risk. Proc Nutr Soc 1999;58(2):243–48.

30. Whigham LD, Cook ME, Atkinson RL. Conjugated linoleic acid: implications for human health. Pharmacol Res 2000;42:503–10.

31. Blot WJ, Henderson BE, Boice JD Jr. Childhood cancer in relation to cured meat intake: review of the epidemiological evidence. Nutr Cancer 1999;34:111–18.

32. Preston-Martin S, Pogoda JM, Mueller BA, et al. Maternal consumption of cured meats and vitamins in relation to pediatric brain tumors. Cancer Epidemiol Biomarkers Prev 1996;5:599–605.

33. Bougnoux P. N-3 polyunsaturated fatty acids and cancer. Curr Opin Clin Nutr Metab Care 1999;2:121–26.

34. Fernandez E, Chatenoud L, La Vecchia C, Negri E, Franceschi S. Fish consumption and cancer risk. Am J Clin Nutr 1999;70:85–90.

35. Rose DP, Connolly JM. Omega-3 fatty acids as cancer chemopreventive agents. Pharmacol Therapeutics 1999;83:217–44.

36. Argiles JM, Lopez-Soriano FJ. Insulin and cancer (review). Int J Oncol 2001;18:683–87.

37. Jansson B. Potassium, sodium, and cancer: a review. J Env Pathol Toxicol Oncol 1996;15:65–73.

38. Medina MA, Quesada AR, Nunez de Castro I, Sanchez-Jimenez F. Histamine, polyamines, and cancer. Biochem Pharmacol 1999;57:1341–44.

39. Wallace HM, Caslake R. Polyamines and colon cancer. Eur J Gastroenterol Hepatol 2001;13(9):1033–39.

40. Canizares F, Salinas J, de las Heras M, et al. Prognostic value of ornithine decarboxylase and polyamines in human breast cancer: correlation with clinicopathologic parameters. Clin Cancer Res 1999;5:2035–41.

41. Singh J, Rivenson A, Tomita M, et al. Bifidobacterium longum, a lactic acid-producing intestinal bacterium inhibits colon cancer and modulates the intermediate biomarkers of colon carcinogenesis. Carcinogenesis 1997 18(4):833–41.

42. Haddox M, Frassir K, Russel D. Retinol inhibition of ornithine decarboxylase induction and G1 progression in CHD cells. Cancer Res 1979;39:4930–38.

43. McGarrity TJ, Peiffer LP, Hartle RJ. Effect of selenium on growth, S-adenosylmethionine and polyamine biosynthesis in human colon cancer cells. Anticancer Res 1993;13:811–15.

44. Carnesecchi S, Schneider Y, Ceraline J, et al. Geraniol, a component of

plant essential oils, inhibits growth and polyamine biosynthesis in human colon cancer cells. J Pharmacol Exp Ther 2001;298:197–200.

45. Kuwano S, Yamauchi K. Effect of berberine on tyrosine decarboxylase activity of Streptococcus faecalis. Chem Pharm Bull 1960;8:491–96.

46. Clapper ML. Genetic polymorphism and cancer risk. Curr Oncol Rep 2000;2:251–56.

47. Surh Y. Molecular mechanisms of chemopreventive effects of selected dietary and medicinal phenolic substances. Mutat Res 1999;428:305–27.

48. Polasa K, Raghuram TC, Krishna TP, Krishnaswamy K. Effect of turmeric on urinary mutagens in smokers. Mutagenesis 1992;7:107–9.

49. Kleiner SM. Water: an essential but overlooked nutrient. J Am Diet Assoc 1999;99:200–6.

Chapter 3. Taking the Right Natural Products to Prevent Cancer

1. Lamson DW, Brignall MS. Natural agents in the prevention of cancer. Part 1: human chemoprevention trials. Altern Med Rev. 2001;6:7–19.

2. Lee IM. Antioxidant vitamins in the prevention of cancer. Proc Assoc Am Physicians 1999;111:10–15.

3. Albanes D, Heinonen OP, Huttunen JK, et al. Effects of alpha-tocopherol and beta-carotene supplements on cancer incidence in the Alpha-Tocopherol, Beta-Carotene Cancer Prevention Study. Am J Clin Nutr 1996; 62:1427S–30S.

4. Omenn GS, Goodman GE, Thornquist MD, et al. Effects of a combination of beta-carotene and vitamin A on lung cancer and cardiovascular disease. N Engl J Med 1996;334:1150–55.

5. Lamm DL, Riggs DR, Shriver JS, et al. Megadose vitamins in bladder cancer: a double-blind clinical trial. J Urol 1994;151:21–26.

6. Cameron E, Pauling L. Supplemental ascorbate in the supportive treatment of cancer: prolongation of survival times in terminal human cancer. Proc Natl Acad Sci 1976;73:3685–89.

7. Cameron E, Pauling L. Supplemental ascorbate in the supportive treatment of cancer: reevaluation of prolongation of survival times in terminal human cancer. Proc Natl Acad Sci 1978;75:4538–42.

8. Cameron E, Campbell A. The orthomolecular treatment of cancer. II. Clinical trial of high-dose ascorbic acid supplements in advanced human cancer. Chem-Biol Interactions 1974;9:285–315.

9. Morishige F, Murata A. Prolongation of survival times in terminal human cancer by administration of supplemental ascorbate. J Interntl Acad Prev Med 1979;5:47–52.

10. Murata A, Morishige F, Yamaguchi H. Prolongation of survival times of

terminal cancer patients by administration of large doses of ascorbate. Int J Vitam Nutr Res Suppl 1982;23:103–13.

11. Creagan ET, Moertel CG, O'Fallon JR, et al. Failure of high-dose vitamin C (ascorbic acid) therapy to benefit patients with advanced cancer. N Engl J Med 1979;301:687–90.

12. Moertel CG, Fleming TR, Creagan ET, et al. High-dose vitamin C versus placebo in the treatment of patients with advanced cancer who have had no prior chemotherapy. N Engl J Med 1985;312:137–41.

13. Patterson RE, White E, Kristal AR, Neuhouser ML, Potter JD. Vitamin supplements and cancer risk: the epidemiologic evidence. Cancer Causes and Control 1997;8:786–802.

14. Greenwald P, Clifford CK, Milner JA. Diet and cancer prevention. Eur J Cancer 2001;37:948–65.

15. Shklar G, Oh SK. Experimental basis for cancer prevention by vitamin E. Cancer Invest 2000;18:214–22.

16. Bechoua S, Dubois M, Nemoz G, et al. Very low dietary intake of n-3 fatty acids affects the immune function of healthy elderly people. Lipids 1999;34(Suppl.):143S.

17. De Waart FG, Portengen L, Doekes G, Verwaal CJ, Kok FJ. Effect of 3 months vitamin E supplementation on indices of the cellular and humoral immune response in elderly subjects. Br J Nutr 1997;78:761–74.

18. Meydani SN, Meydani M, Blumberg JB, et al. Vitamin E supplementation and in vivo immune response in healthy elderly subjects. A randomized controlled trial. JAMA 1997;277(17):1380–86.

19. Moyad MA, Brumfield SK, Pienta KJ. Vitamin E, alpha- and gamma-tocopherol, and prostate cancer. Semin Urol Oncol 1999;17:85–90.

20. Neuzil J, Weber T, Terman A, Weber C, Brunk UT. Vitamin E analogues as inducers of apoptosis: implications for their potential antineoplastic role. Redox Rep 2001;6:143–51.

21. Combs GF, Gray WP. Chemopreventive agents: selenium. Pharmacol Ther 1998;79:179–92.

22. Combs GF Jr, Clark LC, Turnbull BW. Reduction of cancer risk with an oral supplement of selenium. Biomed Environ Sci 1997;10:227–34.

23. Kiremidjian-Schumacher L, Roy M, Wishe HI, Cohen MW, Stotzky G. Supplementation with selenium and human immune cell functions. II. Effect on cytotoxic lymphocytes and natural killer cells. Biol Trace Elem Res 1994;41(1–2):115–27.

24. Krinsky NI. The antioxidant and biological properties of the carotenoids. Ann NY Acad Sci 1998;854:443–47.

25. Rock CL. Carotenoids: biology and treatment. Pharmacol Ther 1997; 75(3):185–97.

26. Duthie SJ. Folic acid deficiency and cancer: mechanisms of DNA instability. Br Med Bull 1999;55(3):578–92.

27. Duthie SJ. Folic-acid-mediated inhibition of human colon-cancer cell growth. Nutrition 2001;17:736–37.

28. Thomson SW, Heimburger DC, Cornwell PE, et al. Effect of total plasma homocysteine on cervical dysplasia risk. Nutr Cancer 2000;37:128–33.

29. Kato I, Dnistrian AM, Schwartz M, et al. Serum folate, homocysteine and colorectal cancer risk in women: a nested case-control study. Br J Cancer 1999;79:1917–22.

30. Giovannucci E, Stampfer MJ, Colditz GA, et al. Multivitamin use, folate, and colon cancer in women in the Nurses' Health Study. Ann Intern Med 1998;129(7):517–24.

31. Garland CF, Garland FC, Gorham ED. Calcium and vitamin D. Their potential roles in colon and breast cancer prevention. Ann NY Acad Sci 1999;889:107–19.

32. Narvaez CJ, Zinser G, Welsh J. Functions of 1alpha,25-dihydroxyvitamin D(3) in mammary gland: from normal development to breast cancer. Steroids 2001;66:301–8.

33. Zhao XY, Feldman D. The role of vitamin D in prostate cancer. Steroids 2001;66:293–300.

34. Pietta PG. Flavonoids as antioxidants. J Nat Prod 2000;63:1035–42.

35. Nijveldt RJ, van Nood E, van Hoorn DE, et al. Flavonoids: a review of probable mechanisms of action and potential applications. Am J Clin Nutr 2001;74:418–25.

36. Di Carlo G, Mascolo N, Izzo AA, Capasso F. Flavonoids: old and new aspects of a class of natural therapeutic drugs. Life Sci 1999;65:337–53.

37. Middleton E Jr, Kandaswami C, Theoharides TC. The effects of plant flavonoids on mammalian cells: implications for inflammation, heart disease, and cancer. Pharmacol Rev 2000;52:673–751.

38. Emerit I, Oganesian N, Sarkisian T, et al. Clastogenic factors in the plasma of Chernobyl accident recovery workers: anticlastogenic effect of Ginkgo biloba extract. Radiat Res 1995;144:198–205.

39. Nihal A, Hasan M. Green tea polyphenols and cancer: biological mechanisms and practical implications. Nutr Rev 1999;57:78–83.

40. Imai K, Suga K, Nakachi K. Cancer-preventive effects of drinking tea among a Japanese population. Prev Med 1997;26:769–75.

41. Nakachi K, Suemasu K, Suga K, et al. Influence of drinking green tea on breast cancer malignancy among Japanese patients. Jpn J Cancer Res 1998;89:254–61.

42. Gupta S, Ahmad N, Mukhtar H. Prostate cancer chemoprevention by green tea. Semin Urol Oncol 1999;17:70–76.

43. Paschka AG, Butler R, Young CY. Induction of apoptosis in prostate cancer cell lines by the green tea component, (-)-epigallocatechin-3-gallate. Cancer Lett 1998;130:1–7.

44. Wollowski I, Rechkemmer G, Pool-Zobel BL. Protective role of probiotics and prebiotics in colon cancer. Am J Clin Nutr 2001;73(Suppl. 2):451S–55S.

45. Horie H, Kanazawa K, Kobayashi E, et al. Effects of intestinal bacteria on the development of colonic neoplasm II. Changes in the immunological environment. Eur J Cancer Prev 1999;8:533–37.

46. Aso Y, Akaza H, Kotake T, et al. Preventive effect of a Lactobacillus casei preparation on the recurrence of superficial bladder cancer in a double-blind trial. The BLP Study Group. Eur Urol 1995;27:104–9.

47. Bouglé D, Roland D, Lebeurrier N, Arhan F. Effect of propionibacteria supplementation on fecal bifidobacteria and segmental colonic transic time in healthy human subjects. Scand J Gastroenterol 1999;34:144–48.

48. Chaia AP, Zarate G, Oliver G. The probiotic properties of propionibacter. Lait 1999;79:175–85.

49. Uauy R, Valenzuela A. Marine oils: the health benefits of n-3 fatty acids. Nutrition 2000;16(7–8):680–84.

Chapter 4. Special Steps for Preventing Lung, Breast, Prostate, and Colon Cancer

1. Marcus PM. Lung cancer screening: an update. J Clin Oncol 2001;19 (Suppl.18):83S–86S.

2. Takezaki T, Hirose K, Inoue M, et al. Dietary factors and lung cancer risk in Japanese: with special reference to fish consumption and adenocarcinomas. Br J Cancer 2001;84:1199–1206.

3. Matsumura Y, Yoshiike N, Yokoyama T, Tanaka H. Dietary intake and cancer mortality in Japan. Biofactors 2000;12:95–99.

4. Le Marchand L, Murphy SP, Hankin JH, Wilkens LR, Kolonel LN. Intake of flavonoids and lung cancer. J Natl Cancer Inst 2000;92:154–60.

5. Zhang J, Temme EH, Kesteloot H. Fish consumption is inversely associated with male lung cancer mortality in countries with high levels of cigarette smoking or animal fat consumption. Int J Epidemiol 2000 Aug; 29(4):615–21.

6. Combs GF Jr, Clark LC, Turnbull BW. Reduction of cancer risk with an oral supplement of selenium. Biomed Environ Sci 1997;10:227–34.

7. Miller AB. Controversies in breast cancer screening. Cancer Prev Control 1997;1:73–79.

8. Miller AB, To T, Baines CJ, Wall C. Canadian National Breast Screening

Study-2: 13–year results of a randomized trial in women aged 50–59 years. J Natl Cancer Inst 2000;92:1490–99.

9. Hartmann LC, Schaid DJ, Woods JE, et al. Efficacy of bilateral prophylactic mastectomy in women with a family history of breast cancer. N Engl J Med 1999;340:77–84.

10. Schernhammer ES, Laden F, Speizer FE, et al. Rotating night shifts and risk of breast cancer in women participating in the Nurses' Health Study. J Natl Cancer Inst 2001;93:1563–68.

11. Davis S, Mirick DK, Stevens RG. Night shift work, light at night, and risk of breast cancer. J Natl Cancer Inst 2001;93:1557–62.

12. Haller CA, Simpser E. Breastfeeding: 1999 perspective. Curr Opin Pediatr 1999;11:379–83.

13. Hebert J, Rosen A. Nutritional, socioeconomic, and reproductive factors in relation to female breast cancer mortality: findings from a cross-national study. Cancer Detection Prevention 1996;20:234–44.

14. Zheng W, Gustafson DR, Sinha R, et al. Well-done meat intake and the risk of breast cancer. J Natl Canc Inst 1998;90:1724–29.

15. Bartsch H, Nair J, Owen RW. Dietary polyunsaturated fatty acids and cancers of the breast and colorectum: emerging evidence for their role as risk modifiers. Carcinogenesis 1999;20:2209–18.

16. De Deckere EA. Possible beneficial effect of fish and fish n-3 polyunsaturated fatty acids in breast and colorectal cancer. Eur J Cancer Prev 1999; 8:213–21.

17. Rose DP. Dietary fatty acids and breast cancer. Am J Clin Nutr 1998; 66(Suppl.):998S–1003S.

18. Klein V, Chajes V, Germain E, et al. Low alpha-linolenic acid content of adipose breast tissue is associated with an increased risk of breast cancer. Eur J Cancer 2000;36:335–40.

19. Bougnoux P, Koscielny S, Chajes V, et al. Alpha-linolenic acid content of adipose breast tissue: a host determinant of the risk of early metastasis in breast cancer. Br J Cancer 1994;70:330–34.

20. Ward WE, Jiang FO, Thompson LU. Exposure to flaxseed or purified lignan during lactation influences rat mammary gland structures. Nutr Cancer 2000;37:187–92.

21. Thompson LU, Rickard SE, Orcheson LJ, Seidl MM. Flaxseed and its lignan and oil components reduce mammary tumor growth at a late stage of carcinogenesis. Carcinogenesis 1996;17:1373–76.

22. Thompson LU, Seidl MM, Rickard SE, Orcheson LJ, Fong HH. Antitumorigenic effect of a mammalian lignan precursor from flaxseed. Nutr Cancer 1996;26:159–65.

23. Haggans CJ, Hutchins AM, Olson BA, et al. Effect of flaxseed consumption on urinary estrogen metabolites in postmenopausal women. Nutr Cancer 1999;33:188–95.

24. Sirtori CR. Risks and benefits of soy phytoestrogens in cardiovascular diseases, cancer, climacteric symptoms and osteoporosis. Drug Safety 2001; 24:665–82.

25. Messina M. Soy, soy phytoestrogens (isoflavones), and breast cancer. Am J Clin Nutr 1999;70:574–75.

26. Allred CD, Allred KF, Ju YH, Virant SM, Helferich WG. Soy diets containing varying amounts of genistein stimulate growth of estrogen-dependent (MCF-7) tumors in a dose-dependent manner. Cancer Res 2001;61:5045–50.

27. Cohen LA, Zhao Z, Pittman B, Scimeca JA. Effect of intact and isoflavone-depleted soy protein on NMU-induced rat mammary tumorigenesis. Carcinogenesis 2000;21:929–35.

28. Shu XO, Jin F, Dai Q, et al. Soyfood intake during adolescence and subsequent risk of breast cancer among Chinese women. Cancer Epidemiol Biomarkers Prev 2001;10:483–88.

29. Martini MC, Dancisak BB, Haggans CJ, Thomas W, Slavin JL. Effects of soy intake on sex hormone metabolism in premenopausal women. Nutr Cancer 1999;34:133–39.

30. Wong GY, Bradlow L, Sepkovic D, Mehl S, Mailman J, Osborne MP. Dose-ranging study of indole-3-carbinol for breast cancer prevention. J Cell Biochem Suppl 1997 (28–29):111–16.

31. Shertzer HG, Senft AP. The micronutrient indole-3-carbinol: implications for disease and chemoprevention. Drug Metabol Drug Interact 2000; 17:159–88.

32. Michnovicz JJ. Increased estrogen 2-hydroxylation in obese women using oral indole-3-carbinol. Int J Obes Relat Metab Disord 1998;22(3):227–29.

33. Walaszek Z, Szemraj J, Narog M, et al. Metabolism, uptake, and excretion of a D-glucaric acid salt and its potential use in cancer prevention. Cancer Detection Prevention 1997;21:178–90.

34. Walaszek Z. Potential use of D-glucaric acid derivatives in cancer prevention. Cancer Lett 1990;54:1–8.

35. Hawk E, Breslow RA, Graubard BI. Male pattern baldness and clinical prostate cancer in the epidemiologic follow-up of the first National Health and Nutrition Examination Survey. Cancer Epidemiol Biomarkers Prev 2000;9:523–27.

36. Fair WR, Fleshner NE, Heston W. Cancer of the prostate: a nutritional disease? Urology 1997;50:840–48.

37. Gann PH, Ma J, Giovannucci E, Willett W, et al. Lower prostate cancer risk in men with elevated plasma lycopene levels: results of a prospective analysis. Cancer Res 1999;59:1225–30.

38. Kucuk O, Sarkar FH, Sakr W, et al. Phase II randomized clinical trial of lycopene supplementation before radical prostatectomy. Cancer Epidemiol Biomarkers Prev 2001;10:861–68.

39. Norrish AE, Jackson RT, Sharpe SJ, Skeaff CM. Prostate cancer and dietary carotenoids. Am J Epidemiol 2000;151:119–23.

40. Rao AV, Fleshner N, Agarwal S. Serum and tissue lycopene and biomarkers of oxidation in prostate cancer patients: a case-control study. Nutr Cancer 1999;33:159–64.

41. Pastori M, Pfander H, Boscoboinik D, Azzi A. Lycopene in association with alpha-tocopherol inhibits at physiological concentrations proliferation of prostate carcinoma cells. Biochem Biophys Res Commun 1998; 250:582–85.

42. Hayes RB, Ziegler RG, Gridley G, et al. Dietary factors and risks for prostate cancer among blacks and whites in the United States. Cancer Epidemiol Biomarkers Prev 1999;8:25–34.

43. Moyad MA. Soy, disease prevention, and prostate cancer. Semin Urol Oncol 1999;17:97–102.

44. Jacobsen BK, Knutsen SF, Fraser GE. Does high soy milk intake reduce prostate cancer incidence? The Adventist Health Study (United States). Cancer Causes and Control 1998;9:553–57.

45. Norrish AE, Skeaff CM, Arribas GL, Sharpe SJ, Jackson RT. Prostate cancer risk and consumption of fish oils: a dietary biomarker-based case-control study. Br J Cancer 1999;81:1238–42.

46. Newcomer LM, King IB, Wicklund KG, Stanford JL. The association of fatty acids with prostate cancer risk. Prostate 2001;47:262–68.

47. Gann PH, Hennekens CH, Sacks FM, Grodstein F, Giovannucci EL. Prospective study of plasma fatty acids and risk of prostate cancer. J Natl Cancer Inst 1994;86:281–86.

48. Giovannucci E, Rimm EB, Colditz GA, et al. A prospective study of dietary fat and risk of prostate cancer. J Natl Cancer Inst 1993;85:1571–79.

49. Demark-Wahnefried W, Price DT, Polascik TJ, et al. Pilot study of dietary fat restriction and flaxseed supplementation in men with prostate cancer before surgery: exploring the effects on hormonal levels, prostate-specific antigen, and histopathologic features. Urology 2001;58:47–52.

50. Heinonen OP, Albanes D, Virtamo J, et al. Prostate cancer and supplementation with α-tocopherol and ß-carotene: incidence and mortality in a controlled trial. J Natl Cancer Inst 1998;90:440–46.

51. Helzlsouer KJ, Huang HY, Alberg AJ, et al. Association between alpha-

tocopherol, gamma-tocopherol, selenium, and subsequent prostate cancer. J Natl Cancer Inst 2000;92:2018–23.

52. Clark LC, Dalkin B, Krongrad A, et al. Decreased incidence of prostate cancer with selenium supplementation: results of a double-blind cancer prevention trial. Br J Urol 1998;81:730–34.

53. Thune I, Furberg AS. Physical activity and cancer risk: dose-response and cancer, all sites and site-specific. Med Sci Sports Exerc 2001;33(Suppl.S6): 530S–50.

54. Giovannucci E, Ascherio A, Rimm EB, et al. Physical activity, obesity, and risk for colon cancer and adenoma in men. Ann Intern Med 1995;122: 327–34.

55. Slattery ML. Diet, lifestyle, and colon cancer. Semin Gastrointest Dis 2000;11:142–46.

56. Velazquez OC, Rombeau JL. Butyrate. Potential role in colon cancer prevention and treatment. Adv Exp Med Biol 1997;427:169–81.

57. Terry P, Giovannucci E, Michels KB, et al. Fruit, vegetables, dietary fiber, and risk of colorectal cancer. J Natl Cancer Inst 2001;93:525–33.

58. O'Keefe SJ, Kidd M, Espitalier-Noel G, Owira P. Rarity of colon cancer in Africans is associated with low animal product consumption, not fiber. Am J Gastroenterol 1999;94:1373–80.

59. Willett WC, Stampfer MJ, Colditz GA, Rosner BA, Speizer FE. Relation of meat, fat, and fiber intake to the risk of colon cancer in a prospective study among women. N Engl J Med 1990;323:1664–72.

60. Giovannucci E, Rimm EB, Stampfer MJ, et al. Intake of fat, meat, and fiber in relation to risk of colon cancer in men. Cancer Res 1994;54:2390–97.

61. Sinha R, Kulldorff M, Chow WH, Denobile J, Rothman N. Dietary intake of heterocyclic amines, meat-derived mutagenic activity, and risk of colorectal adenomas. Cancer Epidemiol Biomarkers Prev 2001;10:559–62.

62. Hill MJ, Caygill CP. Sugar intake and the risk of colorectal cancer. Eur J Cancer Prev 1999;8:465–68.

63. Huang YC, Jessup JM, Forse RA, et al. Omega-3 fatty acids decrease colonic epithelial cell proliferation in high-risk bowel mucosa. Lipids 1996; 31(Suppl.):313S–17S.

64. Dempke W, Rie C, Grothey A, Schmoll HJ. Cyclooxygenase-2: a novel target for cancer chemotherapy? J Cancer Res Clin Oncol 2001;127:411–17.

65. Moragoda L, Jaszewski R, Majumdar AP. Curcumin-induced modulation of cell cycle and apoptosis in gastric and colon cancer cells. Anticancer Res 2001;21:873–78.

66. Chen H, Zhang ZS, Zhang YL, Zhou DY. Curcumin inhibits cell proliferation by interfering with the cell cycle and inducing apoptosis in colon carcinoma cells. Anticancer Res 1999;19:3675–80.

67. Giovannucci E, Stampfer MJ, Colditz GA, et al. Multivitamin use, folate, and colon cancer in women in the Nurses' Health Study. Ann Intern Med 1998;129(7):517–24.

68. Baron JA, Beach M, Mande JS, et al. Calcium supplements for the prevention of colorectal adenomas. Calcium polyp prevention study group. N Engl J Med 1999;340:101–7.

69. White E, Shannon JS, Patterson RE. Relationship between vitamin and calcium supplement use and colon cancer. Cancer Epidemiol Biomarkers Prev 1997;6(10):769–74.

70. Garland CF, Garland FC, Gorham ED. Calcium and vitamin D. Their potential roles in colon and breast cancer prevention. Ann NY Acad Sci 1999;889:107–19.

71. Hofstad B, Almendingen K, Vatn M, et al. Growth and recurrence of colorectal polyps: a double-blind 3-year intervention with calcium and antioxidants. Digestion 1998;59:148–56.

72. Whelan RL, Horvath KD, Gleason NR, et al. Vitamin and calcium supplement use is associated with decreased adenoma recurrence in patients with a previous history of neoplasia. Dis Colon Rectum 1999;42:212–17.

Chapter 5. Attitude, Emotions, and Lifestyle in Cancer Prevention

1. Imai K, Nakachi K. Personality types, lifestyle, and sensitivity to mental stress in association with NK activity. Int J Hyg Environ Health 2001; 204:67–73.

2. Segerstrom SC. Personality and the immune system: models, methods, and mechanisms. Ann Behav Med 2000;22:180–90.

3. Jung W, Irwin M. Reduction of natural killer cytotoxic activity in major depression: Interaction between depression and cigarette smoking. Psychosom Med 1999;61:263–70.

4. Kiecolt-Glaser JK, McGuire L, Robles TF, Glaser R. Emotions, morbidity, and mortality: new perspectives from psychoneuroimmunology. Ann Rev Psychol 2002;53:83–107.

5. Maddock C, Pariante CM. How does stress affect you? An overview of stress, immunity, depression and disease. Epidemiol Psychiatr Soc 2001;10:153–62.

6. Cooper CL, Faragher EB. Psychosocial stress and breast cancer: the interrelationship between stress events, coping strategies and personality. Psychol Med 1993;23:653–62.

7. Kiecolt-Glaser JK, Stephens R, Lipitz P, Speicher CE, Glaser R. Distress and DNA repair in human lymphocytes. J Behav Med 1985;8:311–20.

8. Glaser R, Thorn BE, Tarr KL, Kiecolt-Glaser JK, D'Ambrosio SM. Effects of stress on methyltransferase synthesis an important DNA repair enzyme. Health Psychol 1985;4:403–12.

9. Kiecolt-Glaser JK, Glaser R. Psychoneuroimmunology and cancer: fact or fiction? Eur J Cancer 1999;35:1603–7.

10. Maruta T, Colligan RC, Malichoc M, Offord KP. Optimists vs. pessimists: survival rate among medical patients over a 30-year period. Mayo Clin Proc 2000;75:140–43.

11. Thune I, Furberg AS. Physical activity and cancer risk: dose-response and cancer, all sites and site-specific. Med Sci Sports Exerc 2001;33(Suppl. 6): 530S–50S.

12. Hardman AE. Physical activity and cancer risk. Proc Nutr Soc 2001; 60(1):107–13.

13. Shephard RJ, Shek PN. Effects of exercise and training on natural killer cell counts and cytolytic activity: a meta-analysis. Sports Med 1999;28:177–95.

14. MacKinnon LT. Special feature for the Olympics: effects of exercise on the immune system: overtraining effects on immunity and performance in athletes. Immunol Cell Biol 2000;78:502–9.

15. Li JX, Hong Y, Chan KM. Tai chi: physiological characteristics and beneficial effects on health. Br J Sports Med 2001;35:148–56.

16. Ji LL. Oxidative stress during exercise: implication of antioxidant nutrients. Free Radic Biol Med 1995;18(6):1079–86.

17. Konig D, Wagner KH, Elmadfa I, Berg A. Exercise and oxidative stress: significance of antioxidants with reference to inflammatory, muscular, and systemic stress. Exerc Immunol Rev 2001;7:108–33.

18. Savard J, Miller SM, Mills M. Association between subjective sleep quality and depression on immunocompetence in low-income women at risk for cervical cancer. Psychosom Med 1999;61:496–507.

19. Irwin M, Mascovich A, Gillin JC, et al. Partial sleep deprivation reduces natural killer cell activity in humans. Psychosom Med 1994;56:493–98.

20. Costa G. The problem: shiftwork. Chronobiol Int 1997;14:89–98.

21. Mayer G, Kroger M, Meier-Ewert K. Effects of vitamin B_{12} on performance and circadian rhythm in normal subjects. Neuropsychopharmacology 1996;15:456–64.

Chapter 6. You've Been Diagnosed: Now What?

1. Karr JP. Prostate cancer in the United States and Japan. Adv Exp Med Biol 1992;324:17–28.

2. Argiles JM, Lopez-Soriano FJ. Insulin and cancer (review). Int J Oncol 2001; 18:683–87.

3. Spiegel D, Bloom JR, Kraemer HC, Gottheil E. Effect of psychosocial treatment on survival of patients with metastatic breast cancer. Lancet 1989;2:888–91.

4. Blake-Mortimer J, Gore-Felton C, Kimerling R, Turner-Cobb JM, Spiegel

D. Improving the quality and quantity of life among patients with cancer: a review of the effectiveness of group psychotherapy. Eur J Cancer 1999; 35:1581–86.

Chapter 7. Battling Cancer Through Diet

1. Grogan M, Tabar L, Chua B, Chen HH, Boyages J. Estimating the benefits of adjuvant systemic therapy for women with early breast cancer. Br J Surg 2001;88:1513–18.

2. Kimmick GG, Muss HB. Systemic therapy for older women with breast cancer. Oncology 2001;15:280–91.

3. Sacks GS. Glutamine supplementation in catabolic patients. Ann Pharmacother 1999;33:348–54.

4. Wilmore DW. The effect of glutamine supplementation in patients following elective surgery and accidental injury. J Nutr 2001;131(Suppl. 9): 2543S–49S.

5. Miller AL. Therapeutic considerations of L-glutamine: a review of the literature. Altern Med Rev 1999;4:239–48.

6. Medina MA. Glutamine and cancer. J Nutr 2001;131(Suppl. 9):2539S–42S.

7. Calder PC, Yaqoob P. Glutamine and the immune system. Amino Acids 1999;17:227–41.

8. Bounous G. Whey protein concentrate (WPC) and glutathione modulation in cancer treatment. Anticancer Res 2000;20:4785–92.

9. Kennedy RS, Konok GP, Bounous G, Baruchel S, Lee TD. The use of a whey protein concentrate in the treatment of patients with metastatic carcinoma: a phase I-II clinical study. Anticancer Res 1995;15:2643–49.

10. Baruchel S, Viau G. In vitro selective modulation of cellular glutathione by a humanized native milk protein isolate in normal cells and rat mammary carcinoma model. Anticancer Res 1996;16:1095–99.

11. Bone ME, Wilkinson DJ, Young JR, et al. Ginger root—a new antiemetic: the effect of ginger root on postoperative nausea and vomiting after major gynaecological surgery. Anaesthesia 1990;45:669–71.

12. Phillips S, Ruggier R, Hutchingson SE. Zingiber officinale (ginger)—an antiemetic for day case surgery. Anaesthesia 1993;48:715–17.

13. Meyer K, Schwartz J, Craer D, Keyes B. Zingiber officinale (ginger) used to prevent 8-Mop associated nausea. Dermatol Nursing 1995;7:242–44.

14. Sirtori CR. Risks and benefits of soy phytoestrogens in cardiovascular diseases, cancer, climacteric symptoms and osteoporosis. Drug Safety 2001; 24:665–82.

15. Nihal A, Hasan M. Green tea polyphenols and cancer: biological mechanisms and practical implications. Nutr Rev 1999;57:78–83.

16. Paschka AG, Butler R, Young CY. Induction of apoptosis in prostate can-

cer cell lines by the green tea component, (-)-epigallocatechin-3-gallate. Cancer Lett 1998;130:1–7.

17. Bertolini F, Fusetti L, Rabascio C, et al. Inhibition of angiogenesis and induction of endothelial and tumor cell apoptosis by green tea in animal models of human high-grade non-Hodgkin's lymphoma. Leukemia 2000; 14:1477–82.

18. Sadzuka Y, Sugiyama T, Hirota S. Modulation of cancer chemotherapy by green tea. Clin Cancer Res 1998;4:153–56.

19. Sugiyama T, Sadzuka Y. Enhancing effects of green tea components on the antitumor activity of adriamycin against M5076 ovarian sarcoma. Cancer Lett 1998;133:19–26.

20. Bell MC, Crowley-Nowick P, Bradlow HL, et al. Placebo-controlled trial of indole-3-carbinol in the treatment of CIN. Gynecol Oncol 2000;78:123–29.

21. Rosen CA, Woodson GE, Thompson JW, Hengesteg AP, Bradlow HL. Preliminary results of the use of indole-3-carbinol for recurrent respiratory papillomatosis. Otolaryngol Head Neck Surg 1998;118:810–15.

22. Prasad KN, Cole WC, Kumar B, Prasad KC. Scientific rationale for using high-dose multiple micronutrients as an adjunct to standard and experimental cancer therapies. J Am Coll Nutr 2001 Oct;20(Suppl. 5):450S–63S.

23. Weijl NI, Cleton FJ, Osanto S. Free radicals and antioxidants in chemotherapy induced toxicity. Cancer Treat Rev 1997;23:209–40.

24. Conklin KA. Dietary antioxidants during cancer chemotherapy: impact on chemotherapeutic effectiveness and development of side effects. Nutr Cancer 2000;37:1–18.

25. Lamson DW, Brignall MS. Antioxidants in cancer therapy: their actions and interactions with oncologic therapies. Altern Med Rev 1999;4(5):304–29.

26. Sakamoto K, Sakka M. Reduced effect of irradiation on normal and malignant cells irradiated in vivo in mice pretreated with vitamin E. Br J Radiol 1973;46:538–40.

27. Jaakkola K, Lahteenmaki P, Laakso J, et al. Treatment with antioxidant and other nutrients in combination with chemotherapy and irradiation in patients with small-cell lung cancer. Anticancer Res 1992;12:599–606.

28. Head KA. Ascorbic acid in the prevention and treatment of cancer. Altern Med Rev 1998;3:174–86.

29. Cameron E, Pauling L. Supplemental ascorbate in the supportive treatment of cancer: prolongation of survival times in terminal human cancer. Proc Natl Acad Sci 1976;73:3685–89.

30. Cameron E, Pauling L. Supplemental ascorbate in the supportive treatment of cancer: reevaluation of prolongation of survival times in terminal human cancer. Proc Natl Acad Sci 1978;75:4538–42.

31. Morishige F, Murata A. Prolongation of survival times in terminal human

cancer by administration of supplemental ascorbate. J Interntl Acad Prev Med 1979;5:47–52.

32. Murata A, Morishige F, Yamaguchi H. Prolongation of survival times of terminal cancer patients by administration of large doses of ascorbate. Int J Vitam Nutr Res Suppl 1982;23:103–13.

33. Creagan ET, Moertel CG, O'Fallon JR, et al. Failure of high-dose vitamin C (ascorbic acid) therapy to benefit patients with advanced cancer. N Engl J Med 1979;301:687–90.

34. Moertel CG, Fleming TR, Creagan ET, et al. High-dose vitamin C versus placebo in the treatment of patients with advanced cancer who have had no prior chemotherapy. N Engl J Med 1985;312:137–41.

35. Wigmore SJ, Barber MD, Ross JA, Tisdale MJ, Fearon KC. Effect of oral eicosapentaenoic acid on weight loss in patients with pancreatic cancer. Nutr Cancer 2000;36:177–84.

36. Barber MD, McMillan DC, Preston T, et al. Metabolic response to feeding in weight-losing pancreatic cancer patients and its modulation by a fish-oil-enriched nutritional supplement. Clin Sci 2000;98:389–99.

37. Barber MD, Ross JA, Voss AC, Tisdale MJ, Fearon KC. The effect of an oral nutritional supplement enriched with fish oil on weight-loss in patients with pancreatic cancer. Br J Cancer 1999;81:80–86.

38. Burns CP, Halabi S, Clamon GH, et al. Phase I clinical study of fish oil fatty acid capsules for patients with cancer cachexia: cancer and leukemia group B study 9473. Clin Cancer Res 1999;5:3942–47.

39. Zuijdgeest-Van Leeuwen SD, Dagnelie PC, Wattimena JL, et al. Eicosapentaenoic acid ethyl ester supplementation in cachectic cancer patients and healthy subjects: effects on lipolysis and lipid oxidation. Clin Nutr 2000;19(6):417–23.

40. Gogos CA, Ginopoulos P, Salsa B, et al. Dietary omega-3 polyunsaturated fatty acids plus vitamin E restore immunodeficiency and prolong survival for severely ill patients with generalized malignancy: a randomized control trial. Cancer 1998;82:395–402.

41. Ogilvie GK, Fettman MJ, Mallinckrodt CH, et al. Effect of fish oil, arginine, and doxorubicin chemotherapy on remission and survival time for dogs with lymphoma: a double-blind, randomized placebo-controlled study. Cancer 2000;88:1916–28.

42. Rudra PK, Krokan HE. Cell-specific enhancement of doxorubicin toxicity in human tumour cells by docosahexaenoic acid. Anticancer Res 2001;21:29–38.

43. Liu QY, Tan BK. Effects of cis-unsaturated fatty acids on doxorubicin sensitivity in P388/DOX resistant and P388 parental cell lines. Life Sci 2000;67:1207–18.

Chapter 8. The Super Eight: Fighting Cancer Through Key Natural Products

1. Leipner J, Saller R. Systemic enzyme therapy in oncology: effect and mode of action. Drugs 2000;59:769–80.
2. Gonzalez NJ, Isaacs LL. Evaluation of pancreatic proteolytic enzyme treatment of adenocarcinoma of the pancreas, with nutrition and detoxification support. Nutr Cancer 1999;33:117–24.
3. Adamek J, Prausova J, Wald M. Enzyme therapy in the treatment of lymphedema in the arm after breast carcinoma surgery. Rozhl Chir 1997; 76:203–4.
4. Billigmann P. Enzyme therapy—an alternative in treatment of herpes zoster. A controlled study of 192 patients. Fortschr Med 1995;113:43–48.
5. Maurer HR. Bromelain: biochemistry, pharmacology and medical use. Cell Mol Life Sci 2001;58:1234–45.
6. Eckert K, Grabowska E, Stange R, Schneider U, Eschmann K, Maurer HR. Effects of oral bromelain administration on the impaired immunocytotoxicity of mononuclear cells from mammary tumor patients. Oncol Rep 1999;6:1191–99.
7. Li JK, Lin-Shia SY. Mechanisms of cancer chemoprevention by curcumin. Proc Natl Sci Counc Repub China B 2001;25:59–66.
8. Chen H, Zhang ZS, Zhang YL, Zhou DY. Curcumin inhibits cell proliferation by interfering with the cell cycle and inducing apoptosis in colon carcinoma cells. Anticancer Res 1999;19:3675–80.
9. Menon LG, Kuttan R, Kuttan G. Anti-metastatic activity of curcumin and catechin. Cancer Lett 1999;141:159–65.
10. Han SS, Chung ST, Robertson DA, Ranjan D, Bondada S. Curcumin causes the growth arrest and apoptosis of B cell lymphoma by downregulation of egr-1, c-myc, bcl-XL, NF-kappa B, and p53. Clin Immunol 1999;93:152–61.
11. Arbiser JL, Klauber N, Rohan R, et al. Curcumin is an in vivo inhibitor of angiogenesis. Mol Med 1998;4:376–83.
12. Inano H, Onoda M, Inafuku N, et al. Potent preventive action of curcumin on radiation-induced initiation of mammary tumorigenesis in rats. Carcinogenesis 2000;21:1835–41.
13. Sharma RA, McLelland HR, Hill KA. Pharmacodynamic and pharmacokinetic study of oral curcuma extract in patients with colorectal cancer. Clin Cancer Res 2001;7:1894–900.
14. Moragoda L, Jaszewski R, Majumdar AP. Curcumin induced modulation of cell cycle and apoptosis in gastric and colon cancer cells. Anticancer Res 2001;21:873–78.
15. Dorai T, Gehani N, Katz A. Therapeutic potential of curcumin in human

prostate cancer. II. Curcumin inhibits tyrosine kinase activity of epidermal growth factor receptor and depletes the protein. Mol Urol 2000;4:1–6.

16. Dorai T, Cao YC, Dorai B, Buttyan R, Katz AE. Therapeutic potential of curcumin in human prostate cancer. III. Curcumin inhibits proliferation, induces apoptosis, and inhibits angiogenesis of LNCaP prostate cancer cells in vivo. Prostate 2001;47:293–303.

17. Jee SH, Shen SC, Tseng CR, Chiu HC, Kuo ML. Curcumin induces a p53-dependent apoptosis in human basal cell carcinoma cells. J Invest Dermatol 1998;111:656–61.

18. Kuttan R, Sudheeran PC, Joseph CD. Turmeric and curcumin as topical agents in cancer therapy. Tumori 1987;73:29–31.

19. Navis I, Sriganth P, Premalatha B. Dietary curcumin with cisplatin administration modulates tumour marker indices in experimental fibrosarcoma. Pharmacol Res 1999;39:175–79.

20. Shankar TNB, Shantha NV, Ramesh HP, et al. Toxicity studies on turmeric (Curcuma longa): acute toxicity studies in rats, guinea pigs & monkeys. Indian J Exp Biol 1980;18:73–75.

21. Lamson DW, Brignall MS. Antioxidants and cancer, part 3: quercetin. Altern Med Rev 2000;5:196–208.

22. Yang CS, Landau JM, Huang MT, Newmark HL. Inhibition of carcinogenesis by dietary polyphenolic compounds. Annu Rev Nutr 2001;21: 381–406.

23. Choi JA, Kim JY, Lee JY, et al. Induction of cell cycle arrest and apoptosis in human breast cancer cells by quercetin. Int J Oncol 2001;19:837–44.

24. Ferry DR, Smith A, Malkhandi J, et al. Phase I clinical trial of the flavonoid quercetin: pharmacokinetics and evidence for in vivo tyrosine kinase inhibition. Clin Cancer Res 1996;2:659–68.

25. Piantelli M, Maggiano N, Ricci R, et al. Tamoxifen and quercetin interact with type II estrogen binding sites and inhibit the growth of human melanoma cells. J Invest Dermatol 1995;105:248–53.

26. Pawlikowska-Pawlega, B, Jakubowicz-Gil J, Rzymowski J, Gawron A. The effect of quercitin on apoptosis and necrosis induction in human colon adenocarcinoma cell line LS180. Folia Histochem Cytobiol 2001;39:217–18.

27. Knowles LM, Zigrossi DA, Tauber RA, Hightower C, Milner JA. Flavonoids suppress androgen-independent human prostate tumor proliferation. Nutr Cancer 2000;38:116–22.

28. Xing N, Chen Y, Mitchell SH, Young CY. Quercetin inhibits the expression and function of the androgen receptor in LNCaP prostate cancer cells. Carcinogenesis 2001;22:409–14.

29. Siess MH, Le Bon AM, Canivenc-Lavier MC, Suschetet M. Mechanisms involved in the chemoprevention of flavonoids. Biofactors 2000;12:193–99.

30. Ranelletti FO, Maggiano N, Serra FG, et al. Quercetin inhibits p21-ras expression in human colon cancer cell lines and in primary colorectal tumors. Int J Cancer 1999;85:438–45.

31. Caltagirone S, Rossi C, Poggi A, et al. Flavonoids apigenin and quercetin inhibit melanoma growth and metastatic potential. Int J Cancer 2000;87:595–600.

32. Castillo MH, Perkins E, Campbell JH, et al. The effects of the bioflavonoid quercetin on squamous cell carcinoma of head and neck origin. Am J Surg 1989;158:351–55.

33. Van Rijn J, Van den Berg J. Flavonoids as enhancers of X-ray-induced cell damage in hepatoma cells. Clin Cancer Res 1997;3:1775–79.

34. Hofmann J, Fiebig HH, Winterhalter BR, et al. Enhancement of the antiproliferative activity of cis-diamminedichloroplatinum(II) by quercetin. Int J Cancer 1990;45:536–39.

35. Scambia G, Ranelletti FO, Panici PB, et al. Inhibitory effect of quercetin on primary ovarian and endometrial cancers and synergistic activity with cis-diamminedichloroplatinum (II). Gyn Oncol 1992;45:13–19.

36. Kuhlman MK, Horsch E, Burkhardt G, et al. Reduction of cisplatin toxicity in cultured renal tubular cells by the bioflavonoid quercetin. Arch Toxicol 1998;72:536–40.

37. Scambia G, Ranelletti FO, Panici PB. Quercetin potentiates the effect of adriamycin in a multidrug-resistant MCF-7 human breast-cancer cell line: P-glycoprotein as a possible target. Cancer Chemother Pharmacol 1994;34:459–64.

38. Hofmann J, Doppler W, Jakob A, et al. Enhancement of the antiproliferative effect of cis-diamminedichloroplatinum(II) and nitrogen mustard by inhibitors of protein kinase C. Int J Cancer 1988;42:382–88.

39. Sliutz G, Karlseder J, Tempfer C, et al. Drug resistance against gemcitabine and topotecan mediated by constitutive hsp70 overexpression in vitro: implication of quercetin as sensitiser in chemotherapy. Br J Cancer 1996;74:172.

40. Shoskes DA, Zeitlin SI, Shahed A, Rajfer J. Quercetin in men with category III chronic prostatitis: a preliminary prospective, double-blind, placebo-controlled trial. Urology 1999;54:960–63.

41. Katske F, Shoskes DA, Sender M, et al. Treatment of interstitial cystitis with a quercetin supplement. Tech Urol 2001;7:44–46.

42. Hishida I, Nanba H, Kuroda H. Antitumor activity exhibited by oral administered extract from fruit body of Grifola frondosa (maitake). Chem Pharm Bull 1988;36:1819–27.

43. Nanba H, Kubo K. Antitumor substance extracted from Grifola. U.S. Patent 5,854,404, issued December 29, 1998.

44. Nanba H. Maitake D-fraction: healing and preventive potential for cancer. J Orthomol Med 1997;12:43–49.

45. Mayell M. Maitake extracts and their therapeutic potential. Altern Med Rev 2001;6:48–60.

46. Jones K. Maitake: a potent medicinal food. Alt Comp Ther 1998;4: 420–29.

47. Borchers AT, Stern JS, Hackman RM, et al. Mushrooms, tumors, and immunity. Proc Soc Exp Biol Med 1999;221:281–93.

48. Nanba H. Results of non-controlled clinical study for various cancer patients using maitake D-fraction. Explore 1995;6:19–21.

49. Ng TB. A review of research on the protein-bound polysaccharide (polysaccharopeptide, PSP) from the mushroom Coriolus versicolor (Basidiomycetes: Polyporaceae). Gen Pharmacol 1998;30:1–4.

50. Ooi VE, Liu F. Immunomodulation and anti-cancer activity of polysaccharide-protein complexes. Curr Med Chem 2000;7:715–29.

51. Torisu M, Hayashi Y, Ishimitsu T, et al. Significant prolongation of disease-free period gained by oral polysaccharide K (PSK) administration after curative surgical operation of colon cancer. Cancer Immunology Immunotherapy 1990; 31:261–68.

52. Nakazato H, Koike A, Saji S, et al. Efficacy of immunochemotherapy as adjuvant treatment after curative resection of gastric cancer. Lancet 1994; 343:122–26.

53. Mitomi T, Tsuchiya S, Iijima N, et al. Randomized, controlled study on adjuvant immunochemotherapy with PSK in curatively resected colorectal cancer. Dis Colon Rectum 1992;35:123–30.

54. Go P, Chung CH. Adjuvant PSK immunotherapy in patients with carcinoma of the nasopharynx. J Int Med Res 1989;17(2):141–49.

55. Hayakawa K, Mitsuhashi N, Saito Y, et al. Effect of Krestin (PSK) as adjuvant treatment on the prognosis after radical radiotherapy in patients with non-small cell lung cancer. Anticancer Res 1993;13:1815–20.

56. Ilino Y, Yokoe T, Maemura M, et al. Immunochemotherapies versus chemotherapy as adjuvant treatment after curative resection of operable breast cancer. Anticancer Res 1995;15:2907–12.

57. HorFerVit Pharma GMBH. Polyerga®: Supportive in Tumor Therapy. HorFerVit Pharma GMBH, Heinrich-Brockmann-Str.81, D-26131 Oldenburg, Germany, 2001. See also www.horfervit.de.

58. Berressem P, Frech S, Hartleb M. Additional therapy with Polyerga® improve immune reactivity and quality of life in breast cancer patients during rehabilitation. Tumor Diagnos Ther 1995;16:45–480.

59. Borghardt J, Rosien B, Gortelmeyer R, et al. Effects of a spleen peptide

preparation as supportive therapy in inoperable head and neck cancer patients. Arzneimittelforschung 2000;50:178–84.

60. Maar K. Improvement of the general condition of tumor patients. Erfahrungsheilkunde 1998;47:60–64.

61. Klose G, Mertens J. Long-term results of post-operative treatment of carcinoma of the stomach with Polyerga®. Therapie Woche 1977;27:5359–61.

62. de Ojeda G, Diez-Orejas R, Portoles P, et al. Polyerga, a biological response modifier enhancing T-lymphocyte-dependent responses. Res Exp Med 1994;194:261–67.

63. Klingmüller M. Spleen peptides activate natural killer cells. Erfahrungsheilkunde 1999;12:756–59.

64. Rastogi A, Singh VK, Biswas S, et al. Augmentation of human natural killer cells by splenopentin analogs. FEBS Lett 1993;317:93–95.

65. Baier JE, Neumann HA, Taufighi-Chirazi T, Gallati H, Ricken D. Thymopentin, Factor AF2, and Polyerga improve impaired mitogen-induced interferon-g release of peripheral blood mononuclear cells derived from tumor patients. Tumor Diagnos Ther 1994;15:21–26.

66. Zarkovic N, Hartleb M, Zarkovic K, et al. Spleen peptides (Polyerga) inhibit development of artificial lung metastases of murine mammary carcinoma and increase efficiency of chemotherapy in mice. Cancer Biother Radiopharm 1998;13:25–32.

67. Hartleb M, Leuschner J. Toxicological profile of a low molecular weight spleen peptide formulation used in supportive cancer therapy. Arzneimittelforschung 1997;47:1047–51.

68. Pienta KJ, Naik H, Akhtah A, et al. Inhibition of spontaneous metastasis in a rat prostate cancer model by oral administration of modified citrus pectin. J Natl Cancer Inst 1995;87:348–53.

69. Platt D, Raz A. Modulation of the lung cell colonization of B16-F1 melanoma cells by citrus pectin. J Natl Cancer Inst 1992;18:438–42.

70. Naik H, Pilat MJ, Donat T, et al. Inhibition of in vitro tumor cell-endothelial adhesion by modified citrus pectin: a pH modified natural complex carbohydrate. Proc Am Assoc Cancer Res 1995;36:Abstract 377.

71. Strum S, Scholz M, McDermed J, et al. Modified citrus pectin slows PSA doubling time: a pilot clinical trial. Presentation: International Conference on Diet and Prevention of Cancer, Tampere, Finland. May 28, 1999–June 2, 1999.

72. Shamsuddin AM. Metabolism and cellular functions of IP6: a review. Anticancer Res 1999;19:3733–36.

73. Jariwalla RJ. Inositol hexaphosphate (IP6) as an anti-neoplastic and lipid-lowering agent. Anticancer Res 1999;19:3699–702.

74. Shamsuddin AM, Vucenik I. Mammary tumor inhibition by IP6: a review. Anticancer Res 1999;19:3671–74.

Chapter 9. The Mind-Body Connection

1. Bartrop RW, Luckhurst E, Lazarus L, Kiloh LG, Penny R. Depressed lymphocyte function after bereavement. Lancet 1977;1:834–36.
2. Zisook S, Shuchter SR, Irwin M, Darko DF, Sledge P, Resovsky K. Bereavement, depression, and immune function. Psych Res 1994;52:1–10.
3. Maddock C, Pariante CM. How does stress affect you? An overview of stress, immunity, depression and disease. Epidemiol Psychiatr Soc 2001; 10:153–62.
4. Benson H. The relaxation response: therapeutic effect. Science 1997;278: 1694–51.
5. Morrow GR, Morrell C. Behavioral treatment for the anticipatory nausea and vomiting induced by cancer chemotherapy. N Engl J Med 1982;307: 1476–80.
6. Pan CX, Morrison RS, Ness J, Fugh-Berman A, Leipzig RM. Complementary and alternative medicine in the management of pain, dyspnea, and nausea and vomiting near the end of life. A systematic review. J Pain Symptom Manage 2000;20:374–87.
7. Harmon RL, Myers MA. Prayer and meditation as medical therapies. Phys Med Rehabil Clin N Am 1999;10:651–62.
8. Mock V, Dow KH, Meares CJ, et al. Effects of exercise on fatigue, physical functioning, and emotional distress during radiation therapy for breast cancer. Oncol Nurs Forum 1997;24:991–1000.
9. Schwartz AL, Mori M, Gao R, Nail LM, King ME. Exercise reduces daily fatigue in women with breast cancer receiving chemotherapy. Med Sci Sports Exerc 2001;33:718–23.
10. Demark-Wahnefried W, Rimer BK, Winer EP. Weight gain in women diagnosed with breast cancer. J Am Diet Assoc 1997;97:519–26.

Chapter 10. Other Alternative Medical Therapies

1. Ernst E, Pecho E, Wirz P, Saradeth T. Regular sauna bathing and the incidence of common colds. Ann Med 1990;22:225–27.
2. Blazickova S, Rovensky J, Koska J, Vigas M. Effect of hyperthermic water bath on parameters of cellular immunity. Int J Clin Pharmacol Res 2000;20:41–46.
3. Mayer DJ. Acupuncture: an evidence-based review of the clinical literature. Annu Rev Med 2000;51:49–63.
4. Pomeranz B. Scientific research into acupuncture for the relief of pain. J Altern Compl Med 1996;2:53–60.

5. NIH Consensus Conference. Acupuncture. JAMA 1998;280:1518–24.

6. Wong R, Sagar CM, Sagar SM. Integration of Chinese medicine into supportive cancer care: a modern role for an ancient tradition. Cancer Treat Rev 2001;27:235–46.

7. Shen J, Wenger N, Glaspy J, et al. Electroacupuncture for control of myeloablative chemotherapy-induced emesis: randomized controlled trial. JAMA 2000;284(21):2755–61.

8. Cummings M. Electroacupuncture is effective for control of myeloablative chemotherapy-induced emesis (n=104). Acupunct Med 2001;19:54–55.

9. Vickers AJ. Can acupuncture have specific effects on health? A systematic review of acupuncture antiemesis trials. JR Soc Med 1996;89:303–11.

10. Chen GB, Zhao YD, Xiao HR, et al. A study of acupuncture anesthesia in surgery on the anterior cranial fossa. J Trad Chin Med 1984;4: 189–96.

11. Kotani N, Hashimoto H, Sato Y. Preoperative intradermal acupuncture reduces postoperative pain, nausea and vomiting, analgesic requirement, and sympathoadrenal responses. Anesthesiology 2001;95(2):349–56.

12. al-Sadi M, Newman B, Julious SA. Acupuncture in the prevention of postoperative nausea and vomiting. Anaesthesia 1997;52:658–61.

13. Johnstone PA, Peng YP, May BC, Inouye WS, Niemtzow RC. Acupuncture for pilocarpine-resistant xerostomia following radiotherapy for head and neck malignancies. Int J Radiat Oncol Biol Phys 2001;50:353–57.

14. Moyad MA, Hathaway S, Ni HS. Traditional Chinese medicine, acupuncture, and other alternative medicines for prostate cancer: an introduction and the need for more research. Semin Urol Oncol 1999;17:103–10.

15. Li JX, Hong Y, Chan KM. Tai chi: physiological characteristics and beneficial effects on health. Br J Sports Med 2001;35:148–56.

Chapter 11. Natural Strategies for Support Before and After Surgery

1. Evans D. The effectiveness of music as an intervention for hospital patients: a systematic review. J Adv Nurs 2002;37(1):8–18.

2. Nilsson U, Rawal N, Unestahl LE, Zetterberg C, Unosson M. Improved recovery after music and therapeutic suggestions during general anaesthesia: a double-blind randomised controlled trial. Acta Anaesthesiol Scand 2001;45(7):812–17.

3. Pochapin M. The effect of probiotics on Clostridium difficile diarrhea. Am J Gastroenterol 2000;95(Suppl. 1):11S–13S.

4. Bergogne-Berezin E. Treatment and prevention of antibiotic associated diarrhea. Int J Antimicrob Agents 2000;16(4):521–26.

5. Kartnig T. Clinical applications of Centella asiatica (L.) Urb. Herbs Spices Med Plants 1988;3:146–73.

6. Adamek J, Prausova J, Wald M. Enzyme therapy in the treatment of lymphedema in the arm after breast carcinoma surgery. Rozhl Chir 1997; 76:203–4.

Chapter 12. Natural Strategies for Support Before, During, and After Radiation

1. Collins CE, Collins C. Roentgen dermatitis treated with fresh whole leaf Aloe vera. Am J Roentenol 1935; 33:396–97.

2. Lamson DW, Brignall MS. Antioxidants in cancer therapy; their actions and interactions with oncologic therapies. Altern Med Rev 1999;4:304–29.

3. Duchesne GM, Hutchinson LK. Reversible changes in radiation response induced by all-trans retinoic acid. Int J Radiat Oncol Biol Phys 1995;33: 875–80.

4. Mills EED. The modifying effect of beta-carotene on radiation and chemotherapy induced oral mucositis. Br J Cancer 1988;57:416–17.

5. Tannock IF, Suit HD, Marshall N. Vitamin A and the radiation response of experimental tumors: an immune mediated effect. J Natl Cancer Inst 1972;48:731–41.

6. Kennedy AR, Krinsky NI. Effects of retinoids, beta-carotene, and canthaxanthin on UV- and X-ray induced transformation of C3H10T1/2 cells in vitro. Nutr Cancer 1994;22:219–32.

7. Tewfik FA, Tewfik HH, Riley EF. The influence of ascorbic acid on the growth of solid tumors in mice and on tumor control by X-irradiation. Int J Vitam Nutr Res Suppl 1982;23:257–63.

8. Hanck AB. Vitamin C and cancer. Prog Clin Biol Res 1988;259:307–20.

9. Kennedy M, Bruninga K, Mutlu EA, et al. Successful and sustained treatment of chronic radiation proctitis with antioxidant vitamins E and C. Am J Gastroenterol 2001;96:1080–84.

10. Sakamoto K, Sakka M. Reduced effect of irradiation on normal and malignant cells irradiated in vivo in mice pretreated with vitamin E. Br J Radiology 1973;46:538–40.

11. Fonck K, Konings AWT. The effect of vitamin E on cellular survival after X irradiation of lymphoma cells. Br J Radiology 1978;51:832–33.

12. Kagreud A, Peterson HI. Tocopherol in irradiation of experimental neoplasms. Acta Radiol Oncol 1981;20:97–100.

13. Lund EL, Quistorff B, Spang-Thomsen M, Kristjansen PEG. Effect of radiation therapy on small-cell lung cancer is reduced by ubiquinone intake. Folia Microbiol 1998;43:505–6.

14. Castillo MH, Perkins E, Campbell JH, et al. The effects of the bioflavonoid quercetin on squamous cell carcinoma of head and neck origin. Am J Surg 1989;158:351–55.

15. Hayakawa K, Mitsuhashi N, Saito Y, et al. Effect of Krestin (PSK) as adju-

vant treatment on the prognosis after radical radiotherapy in patients with non-small cell lung cancer. Anticancer Res 1993;13:1815–20.

16. Neri B, DeLeonardis V, Gemelli MT, et al. Melatonin as biological response modifier in cancer patients. Anticancer Res 1998;18:1329–32.

17. Brohult A, Brohult J, Brohult S, Joesson I. Effect of alkyoxyglycerols on the frequency of injuries following radiation therapy for carcinoma of the uterine cervix. Acta Obstet Gynecol Scand 1979;58:203–7.

18. Brohult A, Brohult J, Brohult S, Joesson I. Reduced mortality in cancer patients after administration of alkoxyglycerols. Acta Obstet Gynecol Scand 1986;65:779–85.

Chapter 13. Natural Strategies for Support Before, During, and After Chemotherapy

1. Prasad KN, Cole WC, Kumar B, Prasad KC. Scientific rationale for using high-dose multiple micronutrients as an adjunct to standard and experimental cancer therapies. J Am Coll Nutr 2001 Oct;20(Suppl. 5):450S–63S.

2. Wigmore SJ, Barber MD, Ross JA, Tisdale MJ, Fearon KC. Effect of oral eicosapentaenoic acid on weight loss in patients with pancreatic cancer. Nutr Cancer 2000;36:177–84.

3. Zuijdgeest-Van Leeuwen SD, Dagnelie PC, Wattimena JL, et al. Eicosapentaenoic acid ethyl ester supplementation in cachectic cancer patients and healthy subjects: effects on lipolysis and lipid oxidation. Clin Nutr 2000;19(6):417–23.

4. Gogos CA, Ginopoulos P, Salsa B, et al. Dietary omega-3 polyunsaturated fatty acids plus vitamin E restore immunodeficiency and prolong survival for severely ill patients with generalized malignancy: a randomized control trial. Cancer 1998;82:395–402.

5. Ogilvie GK, Fettman MJ, Mallinckrodt CH, et al. Effect of fish oil, arginine, and doxorubicin chemotherapy on remission and survival time for dogs with lymphoma: a double-blind, randomized placebo-controlled study. Cancer 2000;88:1916–28.

6. Rudra PK, Krokan HE. Cell-specific enhancement of doxorubicin toxicity in human tumour cells by docosahexaenoic acid. Anticancer Res 2001; 21:29–38.

7. Liu QY, Tan BK. Effects of cis-unsaturated fatty acids on doxorubicin sensitivity in P388/DOX resistant and P388 parental cell lines. Life Sci 2000; 67:1207–18.

8. Nakazato H, Koike A, Saji S, et al. Efficacy of immunochemotherapy as adjuvant treatment after curative resection of gastric cancer. Lancet 1994; 343:1122–26.

9. Mitomi T, Tsuchiya S, Iijima N, et al. Randomized, controlled study on

adjuvant immunochemotherapy with PSK in curatively resected colorectal cancer. Dis Colon Rectum 1992;35:123–30.

10. Go P, Chung CH. Adjuvant PSK immunotherapy in patients with carcinoma of the nasopharynx. J Int Med Res 1989;17(2):141–49.

11. Hayakawa K, Mitsuhashi N, Saito Y, et al. Effect of Krestin (PSK) as adjuvant treatment on the prognosis after radical radiotherapy in patients with non-small cell lung cancer. Anticancer Res 1993;13:1815–20.

12. Ilino Y, Yokoe T, Maemura M, et al. Immunochemotherapies versus chemotherapy as adjuvant treatment after curative resection of operable breast cancer. Anticancer Res 1995;15:2907–12.

13. Navis I, Sriganth P, Premalatha B. Dietary curcumin with cisplatin administration modulates tumour marker indices in experimental fibrosarcoma. Pharmacol Res 1999;39:175–79.

14. Van Rijn J, van den Berg J. Flavonoids as enhancers of X-ray-induced cell damage in hepatoma cells. Clin Cancer Res 1997;3:1775–79.

15. Hofmann J, Fiebig HH, Winterhalter BR, et al. Enhancement of the antiproliferative activity of cis-diamminedichloroplatinum(II) by quercetin. Int J Cancer 1990;45:536–39.

16. Scambia G, Ranelletti FO, Panici PB, et al. Inhibitory effect of quercetin on primary ovarian and endometrial cancers and synergistic activity with cis-diamminedichloroplatinum (II). Gyn Oncol 1992;45:13–19.

17. Kuhlman MK, Horsch E, Burkhardt G, et al. Reduction of cisplatin toxicity in cultured renal tubular cells by the bioflavonoid quercetin. Arch Toxicol 1998;72:536–40.

18. Scambia G, Ranelletti FO, Panici PB. Quercetin potentiates the effect of adriamycin in a multidrug-resistant MCF-7 human breast-cancer cell line: P-glycoprotein as a possible target. Cancer Chemother Pharmacol 1994; 34:459–64.

19. Hofmann J, Doppler W, Jakob A, et al. Enhancement of the antiproliferative effect of cis-diamminedichloroplatinum(II) and nitrogen mustard by inhibitors of protein kinase C. Int J Cancer 1988;42:382–88.

20. Sliutz G, Karlseder J, Tempfer C, et al. Drug resistance against gemcitabine and topotecan mediated by constitutive hsp70 overexpression in vitro: implication of quercetin as sensitiser in chemotherapy. Br J Cancer 1996;74:172.

21. Neri B, DeLeonardis V, Gemelli MT, et al. Melatonin as biological response modifier in cancer patients. Anticancer Res 1998;18:1329–32.

22. Lissoni P, Paolorossi F, Ardizzoia A. A randomized study of chemotherapy with cisplatin plus etoposide versus chemoendocrine therapy with cisplatin, etoposide and the pineal hormone melatonin as a first-line treatment of advanced non-small cell lung cancer patients in a poor clinical state. J Pineal Res 1997;23:15–19.

23. Lissoni P, Barni S, Ardizzoia A, et al. Randomized study with the pineal hormone melatonin versus supportive care alone in advanced non-small cell lung cancer resistant to a first-line chemotherapy containing cisplatin. Oncology 1992;49:336–39.

24. Lissoni P, Meregalli S, Fossati V, et al. A randomized study of immunotherapy with low-dose subcutaneous interleukin-2 plus melatonin vs. chemotherapy with cisplatin and etoposide as first-line therapy for advanced non-small cell lung cancer. Tumori 1994;80:464–67.

25. Lissoni P, Barni S, Ardizzoia A, et al. A randomized study with the pineal hormone melatonin versus supportive care alone in patients with brain metastases due to solid neoplasms. Cancer 1994;73:699–701.

26. Lissoni P, Brivio O, Brivio F, et al. Adjuvant therapy with the pineal hormone melatonin in patients with lymph node relapse due to malignant melanoma. J Pineal Res 1996;21:239–42.

27. Lissoni P, Barni S, Tancini G. A randomized study with subcutaneous low-dose interleukin 2 alone vs. interleukin 2 plus the pineal neurohormone melatonin in advanced solid neoplasms other than renal cancer and melanoma. Br J Cancer 1994;69:196–99.

28. Lissoni P, Meregalli S, Nosetto L, et al. Increased survival time in brain glioblastomas by a radioneuroendocrine strategy with radiotherapy plus melatonin compared to radiotherapy alone. Oncology 1996;53:43–46.

29. Lissoni P, Paoorossi F, Tancini G, et al. Is there a role for melatonin in the treatment of neoplastic cachexia. Eur J Cancer 1996;32A:1340–43.

30. Hu YJ, Chen Y, Zhang YQ, et al. The protective role of selenium on the toxicity of cisplatin-contained chemotherapy regimen in cancer patients. Biol Trace Elem Res 1997;56:331–41.

31. Ohkawa K, Tsukada Y, Dohzono H, et al. The effects of co-administration of selenium and cis-platin (CDDP) on CDDP-induced toxicity and anti-tumor activity. Br J Cancer 1988;58:38–41.

32. Roller A, Weller M. Antioxidants specifically inhibit cisplatin cytotoxicity of human malignant glioma cells. Anticancer Res 1998;18:4493–97.

33. Marverti G, Andrews PA. Stimulation of cis-diamminedichloroplatinum(II) accumulation by modulation of passive permeability with genistein: an altered response in accumulation-defective resistant cells. Clin Cancer Res 1996;2:991–99.

34. Schwartz JA, Liu G, Brooks SC. Genistein-mediated attenuation of tamoxifen-induced antagonism from estrogen receptor-regulated genes. Bioch Biophys Res Comm 1998;253:38–43.

35. Miyajima A, Nakashima J, Tachibana M, et al. N-acetylcysteine modifies cis-dichlorodiammineplatinum induced effects in bladder cancer cells. Jpn J Cancer Res 1999;90:565–70.

36. Roller A, Weller M. Antioxidants specifically inhibit cisplatin cytotoxicity of human malignant glioma cells. Anticancer Res 1998;18:4493–97.

37. Wiernik PH, Yeap B, Vogl SE, et al. Hexamethylmelamine and low or moderate dose cisplatin with or without pyridoxine for treatment of advanced ovarian carcinoma: a study of the Eastern Cooperative Oncology Group. Cancer Invest 1992;10:1–9.

38. Das SK, Gulati AK, Singh VP. Deglycyrrhizinated liquorice in aphthous ulcers. J Assoc Physicians India 1989; 37:647.

39. Morgan AG, Pacsoo C, McAdam WA. Maintenance therapy. A two year comparison between Caved-S and cimetidine treatment in the prevention of symptomatic gastric ulcer. Gut 1985; 26:599–602.

40. Kassir ZA. Endoscopic controlled trial of four drug regimens in the treatment of chronic duodenal ulceration. Irish Med J 1985;78:153–56.

41. Tsubaki K, Horiuchi A, Kitani T, et al. Investigation of the preventive effect of CoQ10 against the side-effects of anthracycline antineoplastic agents. Gan To Kagaku Ryoho 1984;11:1420–27.

42. Iarussi D, Auricchio U, Agretto A, et al. Protective effect of coenzyme Q10 on anthracyclines cardiotoxicity: control study in children with acute lymphoblastic leukemia and non-hodgkin lymphoma. Molec Aspects Med 1994;15:207S–12S.

43. Shaeffer J, El-Mahdi AM, Nichols RK. Coenzyme Q10 and adriamycin toxicity in mice. Res Commun Chem Pathol Pharmacol 1980;29:309–15.

44. Folkers K, Brown R, Judy W, Morita M. Survival of cancer patients on therapy with coenzyme Q10. Biochem Biophys Res Comm 1993;192:241–45.

45. Lockwood K, Moesgaard S, Yamamoto T, Folkers K. Progress on therapy of breast cancer with vitamin Q10 and the regression of metastases. Biochem Biophys Res Comm 1995;212:172–77.

46. Lissoni P, Tancini G, Paolorossi F; et al. Chemoneuroendocrine therapy of metastatic breast cancer with persistent thromboaytopenia with weekly low-dose epirubicin plus melatonin: a phase II study. J Pineal Res 1999;26: 169–173.

47. Sonneveld P. Effect of alpha-tocopherol on the cardiotoxicity of adriamycin in the rat. Cancer Treat Rep 1978;62:1033–36.

48. Shimpo K, Nagatsu T, Yamada K, et al. Ascorbic acid and adriamycin toxicity. Am J Clin Nutr 1991 Dec;54(Suppl. 6):1298S–1301S.

49. Scambia G, Ranelletti FO, Panici PB, et al. Quercetin potentiates the effect of adriamycin in a multidrug-resistant MCF-7 human breast cancer cell line: P-glycoprotein as a possible target. Cancer Chemother Pharmacol 1994;34:459–64.

50. Critchfield JW, Welsh CJ, Phang JM, Yeh GC. Modulation of adriamycin

accumulation and efflux by flavonoids in HCT-15 colon cells. Biochem Pharm 1994;48:1437–45.

51. Moragoda L, Jaszewski R, Majumdar AP. Curcumin-induced modulation of cell cycle and apoptosis in gastric and colon cancer cells. Anticancer Res 2001;21:873–78.

52. Venkatesan N, Punithavathi D, Arumugam V. Curcumin prevents adriamycin nephrotoxicity in rats. Br J Pharmacol 2000;129:231–34.

53. Venkatesan N. Curcumin attenuation of acute adriamycin myocardial toxicity in rats. Br J Pharmacol 1998;124:425–27.

54. Sadzuka Y, Sugiyama T, Hirota S. Modulation of cancer chemotherapy by green tea. Clin Cancer Res 1998;4:153–56.

55. Sugiyama T, Sadzuka Y. Enhancing effects of green tea components on the antitumor activity of adriamycin against M5076 ovarian sarcoma. Cancer Lett 1998;133:19–26.

56. Sugiyama T, Sadzuka Y, Tanaka K, Sonobe T. Inhibition of glutamate transporter by theanine enhances the therapeutic efficacy of doxorubicin. Toxicol Lett 2001;121:89–96.

57. Sadzuka Y, Sugiyama T, Sonobe T. Efficacies of tea components on doxorubicin-induced antitumor activity and reversal of multidrug resistance. Toxicol Lett 2000;114:155–62.

58. Rubio IT, Cao Y, Hutchins LF, Westbrook KC, Klimberg VS. Effect of glutamine on methotrexate efficacy and toxicity. Ann Surg 1998;227:772–78.

59. Buzdar A, Howell A. Advances in aromatase inhibition: clinical efficacy and tolerability in the treatment of breast cancer. Clin Cancer Res 2001;7:2620–35.

60. Leibowitz RL, Tucker SJ. Treatment of localized prostate cancer with intermittent triple androgen blockade: preliminary results in 110 consecutive patients. Oncologist 2001;6:177–82.

61. Lissoni P, Barni S, Meregalli S, et al. Modulation of cancer endocrine therapy by melatonin: a phase II study of tamoxifen plus melatonin in metastatic breast cancer patients progressing under tamoxifen alone. Br J Cancer 1995;71:854–56.

62. Jacobson JS, Troxel AB, Evans J, et al. Randomized trial of black cohosh for the treatment of hot flashes among women with a history of breast cancer. J Clin Oncol 2001;19(10):2739–45.

63. Babu JR, Sundravel S, Arumugam G, et al. Salubrious effect of vitamin C and vitamin E on tamoxifen-treated women in breast cancer with reference to plasma lipid and lipoprotein levels. Cancer Lett 2000;151:1–5.

64. Koch E. Extracts from fruits of saw palmetto (*Sabal serrulata*) and roots of stinging nettle (*Urtica dioica*): Viable alternatives in the medical treatment

of benign prostatic hyperplasia and associated lower urinary tract symptoms. Planta Med 2001;67:489–500.

65. DiPaola RS, Zhang H, Lambert GH, et al. Clinical and biologic activity of an estrogenic herbal combination (PC-SPES) in prostate cancer. N Engl J Med 1998;339:785–91.

66. Darzynkiewicz Z, Traganos F, Wu JM, Chen S. Chinese herbal mixture PC-SPES in treatment of prostate cancer (review). Int J Oncol 2000;17:729–36.

67. Small EJ, Frohlich MW, Bok R, et al. Prospective trial of the herbal supplement PC-SPES in patients with progressive prostate cancer. J Clin Oncol 2000;18:3595–603.

68. Oh WK, George DJ, Hackmann K, Manola J, Kantoff PW. Activity of the herbal combination, PC-SPES, in the treatment of patients with androgen-independent prostate cancer. Urology 2001;57:122–26.

69. Druker BJ, Sawyers CL, Kantarjian H, et al. Activity of a specific inhibitor of the BCR-ABL tyrosine kinase in the blast crisis of chronic myeloid leukemia and acute lymphoblastic leukemia with the Philadelphia chromosome. N Engl J Med 2001;344:1038–42.

70. Druker BJ, Talpaz M, Resta DJ, et al. Efficacy and safety of a specific inhibitor of the BCR-ABL tyrosine kinase in chronic myeloid leukemia. N Engl J Med 2001;344:1031–37.

71. Van Neste DJJ, Rushton H. Hair problems in women. Clin Dermatol 1998;15:113–25.

Appendix A. Daily Plan for Preventing Cancer

1. Trichopoulou A, Lagiou P, Kuper H, Trichopoulos D. Cancer and Mediterranean dietary traditions. Cancer Epidemiol Biomarkers Prev 2000;9:869–73.

Appendix B. Daily Plan for Beating Cancer

1. Segal R, Evans W, Johnson D, et al. Structured exercise improves physical functioning in women with stages I and II breast cancer: results of a randomized controlled trial. J Clin Oncol 2001;19:657–65.

2. Schwartz AL, Mori M, Gao R, Nail LM, King ME. Exercise reduces daily fatigue in women with breast cancer receiving chemotherapy. Med Sci Sports Exerc 2001;33:718–23.

3. Dimeo FC, Stieglitz RD, Novelli-Fischer U, Fetscher S, Keul J. Effects of physical activity on the fatigue and psychologic status of cancer patients during chemotherapy. Cancer 1999;85:2273–77.

4. Mock V, Dow KH, Meares CJ, et al. Effects of exercise on fatigue, physical functioning, and emotional distress during radiation therapy for breast cancer. Oncol Nurs Forum 1997;24:991–1000.

Index